Neuroendocrine Tumors in Real Life

Annamaria Colao
Antongiulio Faggiano
Wouter de Herder
Editors

Neuroendocrine Tumors in Real Life

From Practice to Knowledge

Springer

Editors
Annamaria Colao
ENETs Center of Excellence for
Neuroendocrine Tumours
Department of Clinical
Medicine and Surgery
University of Naples Federico II
Naples, Italy

Antongiulio Faggiano
ENETs Center of Excellence for
Neuroendocrine Tumours
Department of Clinical
Medicine and Surgery
University of Naples Federico II
Naples, Italy

Wouter de Herder
Endocrine Oncology
Internal Medicine Department
Erasmus University
Rotterdam, Zuid-Holland
The Netherlands

ISBN 978-3-319-59022-6 ISBN 978-3-319-59024-0 (eBook)
https://doi.org/10.1007/978-3-319-59024-0

Library of Congress Control Number: 2018930340

Printed on acid-free paper

This Springer imprint is published by Springer Nature
The registered company is Springer International Publishing AG
The registered company address is: Gewerbestrasse 11, 6330 Cham, Switzerland

Preface

The large family of *neuroendocrine tumors* is diverse and nonhomogeneous since it includes tumors located in different organs with different functions and different degrees of differentiation. This confers a very variable diagnostic workup, treatment, and follow-up that should be appropriate to individual patients in order to ensure survival as long as possible with minimal adverse effects of the many therapeutic approaches available today. Therefore, in order to produce a comprehensive text on these heterogeneous neoplasms, a combination of basic knowledge on biology and genetics as well as an excellent familiarity with their clinical aspects is required.

This editorial initiative *Neuroendocrine Tumors in Real Life: From Practice to Knowledge* wants to overturn the classical presentation, which is only based on report and discussion of data from literature, and to take on deeply inside the real world of neuroendocrine tumors. With this impressive objective, we designed this book starting with four introductory chapters on epidemiology, pathology, biology, and staging, dedicated to clearly define and classify these tumors, and then proceeding with 20 other chapters, dedicated to prognostic factors, staging, diagnostic workup, and therapy: the common central idea is that every chapter starts from a real clinical case relative to the individual topic. Then some crucial points are answered in a dedicated section of open questions and tentative answers. In conclusion, updated evidence of literature is discussed. In this way, readers can find a large spectrum of clinical conditions which parallel with the heterogeneity of neuroendocrine tumors according to primary site, biology, and staging.

We trust that this innovative project, involving many worldwide experts of neuroendocrine tumors, can meet the learning objectives of specialists in different areas of medicine and research who are interested in being closer to the field of neuroendocrine tumors also providing some useful tools for the clinical management of patients affected with these tumors who are still diagnosed and treated in a too variable way in different parts of the world.

Antongiulio Faggiano
Annamaria Colao
Naples, Italy

Wouter de Herder
Rotterdam, The Netherlands

Contents

Contributors

Tahir Akbar
Department of Gastroenterology
Hampshire Hospitals NHS Trust
Aldermaston Rd Basingstoke, Hants, UK

Manuela Albertelli
Endocrinology Unit
University of Genova
Genoa, Italy
manuela.albertelli@unige.it

Manuela Avellino
ENETs Center of Excellence for
Neuroendocrine Tumours
Department of Cardiothoracic and
Respiratory Sciences, Surgical
Endoscopy Unit
University of Campania Luigi Vanvitelli
Naples, Italy

Albert Beckers
Endocrinology
CHU of Liège University of Liège
Liège, Belgium
albert.beckers@chu.ulg.ac.be

Carlo Bergaminelli
ENETs Center of Excellence
for Neuroendocrine Tumours
AORN Ospedali dei Colli, «A. Monaldi»
Naples, Italy

Antonella Bianco
ENETs Center of Excellence for
Neuroendocrine Tumours
AORN Ospedali dei Colli – Monaldi
Naples, Italy

Guido Biasco
Department of Experimental, Diagnostic
and Specialty Medicine
S.Orsola-Malpighi University Hospital
Bologna, Italy

Lisa Bodei
Memorial Sloan Kettering Cancer Center
New York, NY, USA

Laura A. Boos
Institute of Pathology
City Hospital Triemli
Zürich, Switzerland
Laura.Boos@triemli.zuerich.ch

Nicole Brighi
Department of Experimental,
Diagnostic and Specialty Medicine
S.Orsola-Malpighi University Hospital
Bologna, Italy

Luigi Camera
ENETs Center of Excellence for
Neuroendocrine Tumours
Department of Advanced Biomedical
Sciences, Section of Diagnostic Imaging
University of Naples Federico II
Naples, Italy

Davide Campana
Department of Medical
and Surgical Sciences
S.Orsola-Malpighi University Hospital
Bologna, Italy
davide.campana@unibo.it

Monica Capozzi
ENETs Center of Excellence
for Neuroendocrine Tumours
Istituto Nazionale Tumori
IRCCS – Fondazione «G. Pascale»
Naples, Italy

Marco Castellaneta
Department of Internal Medicine
Ospedale Evangelico Internazionale
Genoa, Italy

Federica Cavalcoli
Department of Endocrinology/Diabetes
Mater Misericordiae University Hospital
Dublin7, Ireland

Gastroenterology and Endoscopy Unit
Fondazione IRCCS Ca' Granda Ospedale
Maggiore Policlinico
Milan, Italy

David L. Chan
Odette Cancer Centre, Sunnybrook Health Sciences Centre
Toronto, Canada

Sydney Medical School
University of Sydney
Sydney, NSW, Australia

Mauro Cives
Department of Biomedical Sciences and Human Oncology, Section of Internal Medicine and Clinical Oncology
University of Bari «Aldo Moro»
Bari, Italy

Annamaria Colao
ENETs Center of Excellence
for Neuroendocrine Tumours
Department of Clinical Medicine and Surgery, University of Naples Federico II
Naples, Italy

Elisa Cosaro
Department of Medicine,
Section of Endocrinology
University of Verona
Verona, Italy

Niccolò Daddi
Thoracic Surgery Department
University of Bologna
Bologna, Italy
niccolo.daddi@unibo.it

Maria Vittoria Davì
Section of Endocrinology, Medicina Generale e Malattie Aterotrombotiche e Degenerative, Department of Medicine
University of Verona
Verona, Italy
mariavittoria.davi@ospedaleuniverona.it

Maria Laura del Basso de Caro
ENETs Center of Excellence
for Neuroendocrine Tumours
Department of Advanced Biomedical Sciences, Pathology Section
University of Naples Federico II
Naples, Italy
marialaura.delbasso@unina.it

Chiara De Divitiis
ENETs Center of Excellence
for Neuroendocrine Tumours
Istituto Nazionale Tumori
IRCCS – Fondazione "G. Pascale"
Naples, Italy
chiaradedivitiis@yahoo.it

Leonardo De Luca
ENETs Center of Excellence
for Neuroendocrine Tumours
Gastroenterology and Digestive Endoscopy Unit, Pellegrini Hospital
Naples, Italy

Maria Luisa De Rimini
ENETs Center of Excellence
for Neuroendocrine Tumours
Department of Health Services, Molecular and Tomographic Imaging
AORN Ospedali dei Colli – Monaldi
Naples, Italy
marialuisa.derimini@ospedalideicolli.it

Gaetano De Rosa
ENETs Center of Excellence
for Neuroendocrine Tumours
Department of Advanced Biomedical
Sciences, Pathology Section
University of Naples Federico II
Naples, Italy

Nicolina De Rosa
ENETs Center of Excellence for
Neuroendocrine Tumours
AORN Ospedali dei Colli – Monaldi
Naples, Italy

Silvana Del Vecchio
ENETs Center of Excellence
for Neuroendocrine Tumours
Department of Advanced Biomedical
Sciences, University of Naples Federico II
Naples, Italy

Gianfranco Delle Fave
Digestive and Liver Disease, Sapienza
University of Rome, Sant'Andrea Hospital
Rome, Italy

Elena Di Girolamo
ENETs Center of Excellence
for Neuroendocrine Tumours
Istituto Nazionale Tumori
IRCCS – Fondazione «G. Pascale»
Naples, Italy

Antonella Di Sarno
ENETs Center of Excellence for
Neuroendocrine Tumours
AORN Ospedali dei Colli – Monaldi
Naples, Italy

Diego Ferone
Endocrinology Unit, Department
of Internal Medicine and Medical
Specialties (DiMI)
University of Genova
Genoa, Italy
Center of Excellence for Biomedical
Research (CEBR); IRCCS AOU San
Martino-IST, University of Genova
Genoa, Italy
ferone@unige.it

George K. Dimitriadis
The Arden NET CoE, Warwickshire Institute
for the Study of Diabetes, Endocrinology
and Metabolism, University Hospitals of
Coventry and Warwickshire NHS Trust
Coventry, UK
g.dimitriadis@warwick.ac.uk

Eleonora Duregon
Departments of Oncology
University of Turin
Turin, Italy

Dario Fabbri
Department of Medical and
Surgical Sciences
S.Orsola-Malpighi University Hospital
Bologna, Italy

Antongiulio Faggiano
ENETs Center of Excellence for
Neuroendocrine Tumours
Department of Clinical Medicine and
Surgery, University of Naples Federico II
Naples, Italy
afaggian@unina.it

Massimo Falconi
Department of Pancreatic Surgery
San Raffaele Scientific Institute
Milan, Italy
falconi.massimo@hsr.it

Nicola Fazio
Unit of Gastrointestinal Medical Oncology
and Neuroendocrine Tumors
European Institute of Oncology
Milan, Italy
Nicola.fazio@ieo.it

Piero Ferolla
Department of Medical Oncology
University of Perugia
Perugia, Italy

Multidisciplinary NET Group, Umbria Regional Cancer Network
Perugia, Italy
pferolla@gmail.com

Pier Luigi Filosso
Department of Thoracic Surgery
University of Turin
Torino, Italy
pierluigi.filosso@unito.it

Rosa Fonti
ENETs Center of Excellence for Neuroendocrine Tumours
Institute of Biostructures and Bioimaging, National Research Council
Naples, Italy

Aoife Garrahy
Department of Endocrinology/Diabetes
Mater Misericordiae University Hospital
Dublin7, Ireland

Elia Guadagno
ENETs Center of Excellence for Neuroendocrine Tumours
Department of Advanced Biomedical Sciences, Pathology Section
University of Naples Federico II
Naples, Italy

Francesco Guerrera
Department of Thoracic Surgery
University of Turin
Torino, Italy

Per Hellman
Department of Surgical Sciences
Uppsala University
Uppsala, Sweden
per.hellman@surgsci.uu.se

Marie-Lise Jaffrain-Rea
Department of Applied Clinical Sciences and Biotechnology
University of L'Aquila
Pozzili, IS, Italy

Department of Neuroendocrinology
Neuromed IRCCS
Pozzili, IS, Italy
marielise.jaffrain@univaq.it

Gregory Kaltsas
Department of Pathophysiology
National & Kapodistrian University of Athens
Athens, Greece

Warwickshire Institute for the Study of Diabetes, Endocrinology and Metabolism, University Hospitals of Coventry and Warwickshire NHS Trust
Coventry, UK
gkaltsas@endo.gr

Mark Kidd
Wren Laboratories
Branford, CT, USA

Paul Komminoth
Institute of Pathology, City Hospital Triemli
Zürich, Switzerland
paul.komminoth@triemli.zuerich.ch

Beata Kos-Kudła
Division of Endocrinology, Department of Pathophysiology and Endocrinology
Medical University of Silesia
Katowice, Poland
beatakos@ka.onet.pl

Francesco Lassandro
ENETs Center of Excellence for Neuroendocrine Tumours
AORN Ospedali dei Colli – Monaldi
Naples, Italy

Marco Lupattelli
Department of Radiation Oncology
Perugia S.M. Misericordia Hospital
Perugia, Italy

Department of Medical Oncology
University of Perugia
Perugia, Italy

Anna Malczewska
Division of Endocrinology, Department of Pathophysiology and Endocrinology
Medical University of Silesia
Katowice, Poland

Caterina Marchiò
Department of Medical Sciences
University of Turin
Turin, Italy

Sara Massironi
Gastroenterology and Endoscopy Unit
Fondazione IRCCS Ca' Granda Ospedale Maggiore Policlinico
Milan, Italy
sara.massironi@policlinico.mi.it

Mauro Papotti
Departments of Oncology
University of Turin
Turin, Italy

Anatomia Patologica
University of Turin at Città della Salute Hospital
Torino, Italy
mauro.papotti@unito.it

Gennaro Mazzarella
Nuclear Medicine
AORN Ospedali dei Colli – Monaldi
Naples, Italy

Massimo Milione
Anatomic Pathology
Department of Pathology and Laboratory Medicine, IRCCS Foundation National Cancer Institute
Milan, Italy

Vincenzo Minotti
Department of Radiation Oncology
Perugia S.M. Misericordia Hospital
Perugia, Italy

Department of Medical Oncology
University of Perugia
Perugia, Italy

Multidisciplinary NET Group, Umbria Regional Cancer Network
Perugia, Italy

Roberta Modica
ENETs Center of Excellence for Neuroendocrine Tumours
Department of Clinical Medicine and Surgery, University of Naples Federico II
Naples, Italy
robertamodica@libero.it

Irvin M. Modlin
Yale University School of Medicine
New Haven, CT, USA

Francesca Muffatti
Department of Pancreatic Surgery
San Raffaele Scientific Institute
Milan, Italy

Pietro Muto
ENETs Center of Excellence for Neuroendocrine Tumours
Nuclear Medicine
AORN Ospedali dei Colli – Monaldi
Naples, Italy

Vincenzo Napolitano
ENETs Center of Excellence for Neuroendocrine Tumours
Department of Cardiothoracic and Respiratory Sciences
Surgical Endoscopy Unit
University of Campania Luigi Vanvitelli
Naples, Italy

Natalie Prinzi
Department of Medical Oncology
IRCCS Foundation National Cancer Institute
Milan, Italy

Elena Nazzari
Endocrinology Unit
University of Genova
Genoa, Italy

Olov Norlen
Department of Surgical Sciences
Uppsala University
Uppsala, Sweden

Kjell Öberg
Endocrine Oncology
Uppsala University Hospital
Uppsala, Sweden
kjell.oberg@medsci.uu.se

Alessandro Ottaiano
ENETs Center of Excellence for
Neuroendocrine Tumours
Istituto Nazionale Tumori
IRCCS – Fondazione «G. Pascale»
Naples, Italy

Nico Pagano
Department of Medical
and Surgical Sciences
S.Orsola-Malpighi University Hospital
Bologna, Italy

Francesco Panzuto
Digestive and Liver Disease, Sapienza
University of Rome, Sant'Andrea Hospital
Rome, Italy
francesco.panzuto@gmail.com

Stefano Partelli
Department of Pancreatic Surgery
San Raffaele Scientific Institute
Milan, Italy

Antonella Petrillo
ENETs Center of Excellence,
Multidisciplinary Group of Istituto
Nazionale Tumori, IRCCS – Fondazione
«G. Pascale»
Naples, Italy

Alessandro Piovesan
Division of Endocrinology
Città della Salute Hospital
Torino, Italy

Karolina Poczkaj
Division of Endocrinology
Department of Pathophysiology
and Endocrinology
Medical University of Silesia
Katowice, Poland

Francesco Puma
Department of Radiation Oncology
Perugia S.M. Misericordia Hospital
Perugia, Italy

Department of Medical Oncology
University of Perugia
Perugia, Italy

Multidisciplinary NET Group
Umbria Regional Cancer Network
Perugia, Italy

John K. Ramage
Department Gastroenterology
Hampshire Hospitals NHS trust
Aldermaston Rd Basingstoke,
Hants, UK

Kings Health Partners NET
centre of Excellence
London, UK

University of Winchester,
Sparkford Rd, Winchester, UK
John.ramage@hhft.nhs.uk

Luisella Righi
Departments of Oncology
University of Turin
Turin, Italy

Maria Rinzivillo
Digestive and Liver Disease, Sapienza
University of Rome, Sant'Andrea Hospital
Rome, Italy

Matteo Roffinella
Department of Thoracic Surgery
University of Turin
Torino, Italy

Roberta Elisa Rossi
Gastroenterology and Endoscopy Unit
Fondazione IRCCS Ca' Granda Ospedale
Maggiore Policlinico
Milan, Italy

Department of Pathophysiology
and Transplantation
Università degli Studi di Milano
Milan, Italy

Liliya Rostomyan
Endocrinology
CHU of Liège, University of Liège
Liège, Belgium

Manila Rubino
Unit of Gastrointestinal Medical Oncology
and Neuroendocrine Tumors
European Institute of Oncology
Milan, Italy

Alberto Sandri
Department of Thoracic Surgery
University of Turin
Torino, Italy

Eva Segelov
St. Vincent's Clinical School
University of New South Wales
Sydney, NSW, Australia

Anna Settembre
ENETs Center of Excellence
for Neuroendocrine Tumours
Endocrine Surgery
AORN Ospedali dei Colli – Monaldi
Naples, Italy

Franco Silvestris
Department of Biomedical Sciences and
Human Oncology, Section of Internal
Medicine and Clinical Oncology
University of Bari «Aldo Moro»
Bari, Italy

Simron Singh
Odette Cancer Centre, Sunnybrook Health
Sciences Centre
Toronto, Canada
simron.singh@sunnybrook.ca

Paolo Solidoro
Unit of Pulmonology
San Giovanni Battista Hospital
Torino, Italy

Rajaventhan Srirajaskanthan
Kings Health Partners
NET centre of Excellence
London, UK

Peter Stålberg
Department of Surgical Sciences
Uppsala University
Uppsala, Sweden

Salvatore Tafuto
ENETs Center of Excellence
for Neuroendocrine Tumours
Istituto Nazionale Tumori
IRCCS – Fondazione «G. Pascale»
Naples, Italy

Gianluca Tamagno
Department of Endocrinology/Diabetes
Mater Misericordiae University Hospital
Dublin7, Ireland
gianlucatamagno@tiscali.it

Valentina Tassi
Thoracic Surgery Department
University of Bologna
Bologna, Italy

Department of Radiation Oncology
Perugia S.M. Misericordia Hospital
Perugia, Italy

Department of Medical Oncology
University of Perugia
Perugia, Italy

Fabiana Tatangelo
ENETs Center of Excellence
for Neuroendocrine Tumours
Istituto Nazionale Tumori
IRCCS – Fondazione «G. Pascale»
Naples, Italy

Giovanni Vitale
Department of Clinical Sciences and
Community Health (DISCCO)
University of Milan
Milan, Italy

Laboratory of Endocrine and
Metabolic Research, Istituto
Auxologico Italiano IRCCS
Cusano Milanino, Italy
giovanni.vitale@unimi.it

Marco Volante
Departments of Oncology
University of Turin
Turin, Italy

Maria Chiara Zatelli
Section of Endocrinology & Internal
Medicine, Department of Medical
Sciences
University of Ferrara
Ferrara, Italy
ztlmch@unife.it

General Remarks

Contents

Epidemiology of Neuroendocrine Tumours: By Site of Tumour and by Geographical Area

Federica Cavalcoli, Aoife Garrahy, Marco Castellaneta, and Gianluca Tamagno

A. Colao et al. (eds.), *Neuroendocrine Tumors in Real Life*,
https://doi.org/10.1007/978-3-319-59024-0_1

Overview
Neuroendocrine tumours are a heterogeneous group of neoplasms arising from cells of the diffuse neuroendocrine system virtually located in every organ, most frequently in the digestive tract and the respiratory system. Although rare, the worldwide incidence of neuroendocrine tumours is rising and ranges from 3.24/100,000 in Northern Europe to 5.25/100,000 in the USA. However, data on the epidemiology of neuroendocrine tumours are still incomplete due to the heterogeneity of tumours and the lack of large population-based databases in many countries. From the available data, it appears that the epidemiological characteristics and the biological behaviour of neuroendocrine tumours depend significantly on the anatomical site of origin and the biological features of the tumour cells. Interestingly, the distribution according to the primary tumour site differs across geographical areas and reflects possible ethnic/genetic factors. This chapter summarizes the demographic and epidemiologic features of the neuroendocrine tumours, including a brief overview of the rarest neuroendocrine tumours arising at uncommon sites. A better understanding of the epidemiological trends of neuroendocrine tumours may help and direct the next steps of patient care through a more precise patient-targeted approach.

1.1 Introduction

Neuroendocrine tumours (NET) consist of a spectrum of rare and highly heterogeneous neoplasms with distinct functional and biological behaviour in relation to location, tumour size, and histological differentiation. NET arise from the neuroendocrine cells of the diffuse neuroendocrine system located in almost every organ [1]. The most common primary sites for NET are the gastroenteropancreatic system (about 70%) and the lungs (more than 25%), reflecting the high density of neuroendocrine cells in these organ systems [1, 2].

NET are usually divided into functioning and non-functioning forms [3]. Non-functioning NET frequently secrete pancreatic polypeptide, chromogranin A, neuron-specific enolase, neurotensin, and other peptides, but they do not usually produce specific hormonal syndromes. Functioning NET produce specific hormones that can be responsible for different clinical syndromes. Thus, functioning NET are further classified based on their specific functional behaviour and synthetic products (e.g. carcinoid syndrome, insulinomas, gastrinomas). Functioning NET are usually detected earlier due to the presence of typical hormonal syndromes, while non-functioning forms are more often detected in advanced stage of disease due to mass effect (jaundice, pain, intestinal obstruction, or palpable masses) [4–6].

NET are usually sporadic and often occur during adulthood or in the elderly. However, these tumours may also be multiple and can occur as part of several genetic syndromes such as multiple endocrine neoplasia type 1 (MEN1), von Hippel-Lindau (VHL) syndrome, neurofibromatosis type 1, and tuberous sclerosis, usually presenting in younger patients [7, 8]. Their frequency in the setting of these syndromes varies from very low (<1%) for carcinoid to high (80–100%) for pancreatic endocrine tumours

1

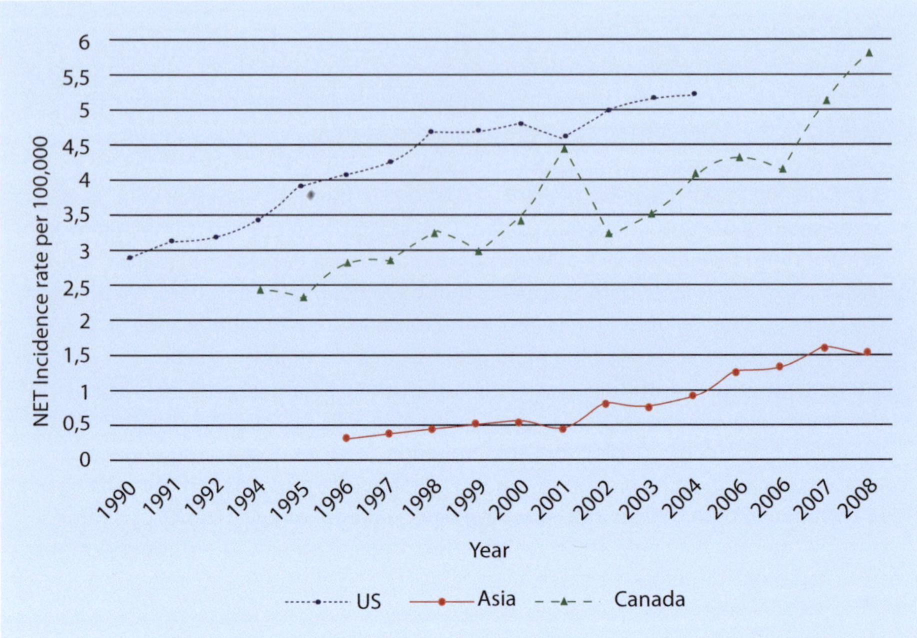

Fig. 1.1 NET incidence per geographical areas (References: for the USA, Yao et al. (2008) [2]; for Asia, Tsai et al. (2013) [14]; for Canada, Hallet et al. (2015) [13]

(insulinoma 5–20%, gastrinoma 25–30%, non-functioning tumour >50%) [9]. Patients with inherited syndromes typically present at a younger age, in most cases between 30 and 50 years of age [10]. A few cases of familial clustering, characterized by younger onset, have also been reported [11, 12].

Although NET are rare, based on the current medical literature, their worldwide incidence seems to have increased; current incidence rates range from 3.24/100,000 in North Europe [1] to 5.25/100,000 in USA [2]. In particular, in the SEER database, the annual age-adjusted incidence increased from 1.09/100,000 in 1973 to 5.25/100,000 in 2004 [2]. A similar significant increase over time has been reported from other authors in different geographical areas [13, 14] (Fig. 1.1). However, data on the epidemiology of NET appear incomplete due to the extreme heterogeneity of classification in different countries, different methods of patient identification, and the lack of large population-based databases in most countries. Moreover, NET distribution according to the primary site is different in the various geographical areas and reflects possible ethnic or genetic differences [1, 2, 13–16] (Fig. 1.2). These appear to be relevant considering that NET incidence, characteristics, and biological behaviour are highly heterogeneous depending on the specific site of origin.

Finally, several risk factors have been recognized in NET development. Family history of cancer appears to be the most relevant risk factor for NET at all investigated sites, followed by high BMI and diabetes mellitus. Cigarette smoking and alcohol consumption are also associated with increased risk of NET, especially for selected anatomical sites [17, 18]. In particular, cigarette smoking has been identified as a risk factor for small intestine,

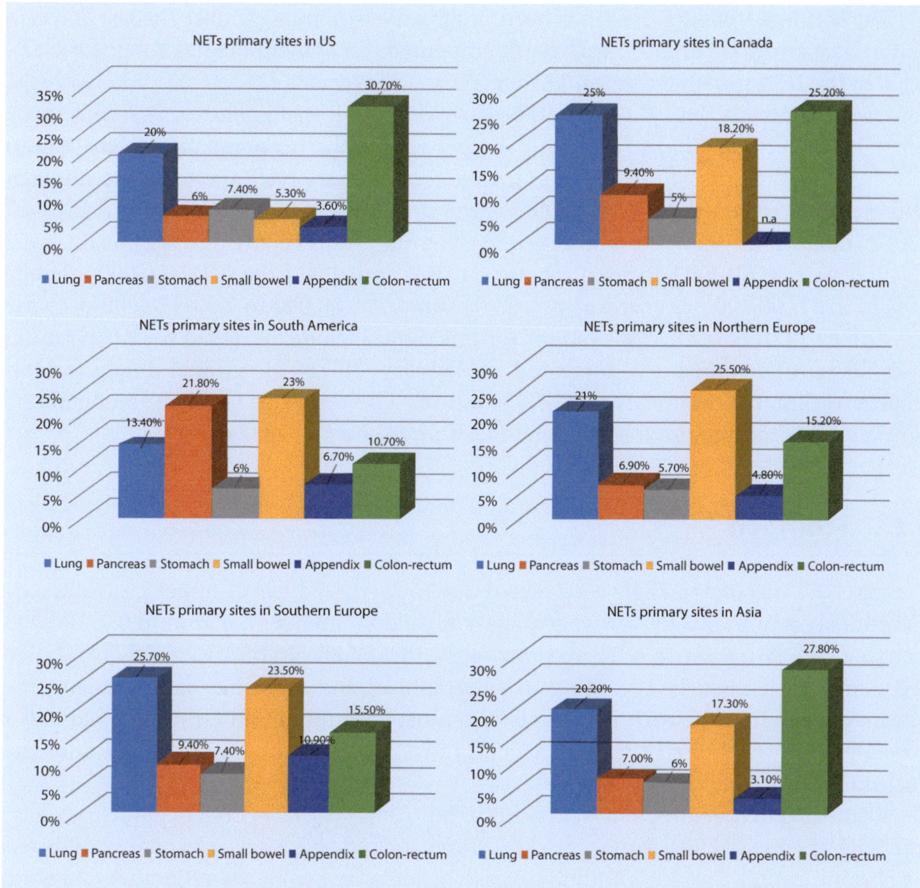

Fig. 1.2 Primary NET sites per geographical areas (References: for the USA, Yao et al. (2008) [2]; for Asia, Tsai et al. (2013) [14]; for Canada, Hallet et al. (2015) [13]; for South America, O'Connor et al. (2013) [17]; for Northern Europe, Hauso et al. (2008) [1], for Southern Europe, Caldarella et al. (2011) [18]

pancreas, and some types of bronchial NET, while alcohol intake represents a risk factor for rectum and pancreas NET. In general terms, the risk factors for gastrointestinal NET development appear to somehow overlap those predisposing to non-neuroendocrine cancers at the various sites of the respiratory and the gastroenteropancreatic tract [18]. A better knowledge of NET epidemiological data appears to be essential, and it may help clinicians in the diagnostic and therapeutic management of these patients.

1.2 Gastroenteropancreatic Neuroendocrine Tumours

Gastroenteropancreatic neuroendocrine tumours (GEP-NET) originate from the diffuse neuroendocrine cell system of the gastrointestinal tract and pancreas and represent 1–4% of all gastrointestinal neoplasms [2, 19, 20].

The incidence of GEP-NET has been progressively increasing over the last 30 years [2, 21]. Data from different series have documented this epidemiologic change for GEP-NET in the USA, South America, Europe, Asia, and Oceania [15, 20–22]. Interestingly, this trend contrasts with those of other gastrointestinal malignancies. A recent study reported an average annual increase of 4.4 per year in the US population from 1973 to 2009 [20]. In the same study, a greater increase for primary NET arising in the stomach and rectum is reported, while the incidence of primary appendiceal NET has decreased [20]. Similar results have been observed in a German study reporting a significant overall increase in GEP-NET incidence between 1976 and 2006 from 0.31/100,000 inhabitants to 2.27/100,000 per year for men and from 0.57/100,000 to 2.38/100,000 per year for women [23]. Possible explanations for this trend include increased use of screening and diagnostic endoscopy, increased availability of cross-sectional imaging, and improved clinician's awareness of NET. Moreover, a possible role for environmental factors such as proton pump inhibitors has been proposed [21, 23, 24].

1.2.1 Stomach

Gastric NET are increasingly recognized due to increased use of upper gastrointestinal endoscopy and biopsy. The yearly age-adjusted incidence is of around 0.2/100,000 per year [25, 26]. Gastric NET account for 5–14% of all NET; however their relative frequency varies widely according to geographical area. Recently an Austrian prospective study found gastric NET to be the most common of all GEP-NET [26]. In a Korean study, the stomach was the second most common site for GEP-NET after the rectum [27].

According to the European Neuroendocrine Tumor Society (ENET) guidelines, gastric NET are divided into three types [28]. Type-1 gastric NET occur in patients affected by chronic atrophic gastritis with hypergastrinaemia caused by the reduction of gastric acid secretion. Lesions are usually polypoid, mostly limited to the mucosa or submucosa, and located in atrophic oxyntic mucosa in the fundus [29]. Such neoplasms are mostly multiple (65% of cases) with a median diameter of 5 mm. They are usually benign and well-differentiated, with Ki-67 <1% (NET G1) [29]. Type-2 gastric NET develop in response to hypergastrinaemia resulting from the neoplastic secretion from gastrinomas [Zollinger-Ellison syndrome (ZES)], mostly in patients with MEN1 [30]. Type-3 gastric NET are sporadic, unrelated to hypergastrinaemia, and not associated to enterochromaffin-like cell hyperplasia and arise from a normal mucosa [31]. These tumours are usually solitary and poorly differentiated, with an elevated Ki-67 (NEC G3). Deep wall invasion, lymphatic invasion, or metastases can be present at the time of their diagnosis [32].

The main epidemiological characteristics of gastric NET are further detailed in ◘ Table 1.1. In recent years however, few cases of gastric NET not completely meeting the current classification criteria have been reported. A possible association with proton pump inhibitor therapy has also been suggested [33–35]. Mean age at presentation of gastric NET is 60–64 years in the USA and Europe [2, 12, 36] and slightly higher (67 years) in Taiwan [37]. In the USA, the incidence of gastric NET is higher in the Afro-Americans [2, 25].

Table 1.1 Main epidemiological characteristics of gastric NET according to the ENET classification [28]

Gastric neuroendocrine tumours	Type 1	Type 2	Type 3
Proportion among gastric NET	70–80%	5–6%	14–25%
Tumour characteristics	Often small (<1–2 cm), multiple in 65% of cases, polypoid in 78% of cases	Often small (<1–2 cm) and multiple, polypoid	Unique often large (>2 cm) Polypoid and ulcerated
Associated conditions	Chronic atrophic gastritis	Gastrinoma/MEN1	None
Metastases (%)	2–5	10–30	50–10
Tumour-related deaths (%)	0	<10	25–30

Most patients present with local disease and prognosis are usually good [25, 38]. In a recent prospective study, gastric NET have a benign behaviour in 68% of cases, uncertain in 12%, and a malignant behaviour in 20% of cases [26]. Overall, the incidence of malignant NET in the stomach was low, calculated as 0.08/100,000 per year.

Reported risk factors for gastric NET include a positive family history of cancer (especially other neuroendocrine neoplasms) and, according to a case-control study from the USA, history of diabetes mellitus [39].

1.2.2 Duodenum

Duodenal NET comprise up to 3% of all duodenal tumours and almost 3% of all NET tumours in the SEER (Surveillance, Epidemiology, and End Results) Registry [40, 41]. In 2015, Fitzgerald et al. [42] found a significant increase over the last three decades in the incidence of duodenal NET, from 0.027/100,000 in 1983 to 1.1/100,000 in 2010, representing an impressive fourfold increase.

Duodenal NET include functional (mainly gastrinomas and somatostatinomas) and non-functional NET, duodenal gangliocytic paragangliomas, and high-grade poorly differentiated NEC [40]. They may be sporadic or associated with familial syndrome, such as neurofibromatosis and multiple endocrine neoplasia type 1. Multiple tumours should raise the suspicion of an inherited syndrome [26]. Duodenal NET arise more frequently (90%) in the first and second part of the duodenum, while approximately 20% occur in the periampullary region [43]. They are characteristically small (mean, 1.2–1.5 cm) and >75% have a diameter of <2 cm [43, 44]. The majority of patients present with localized disease at the time of diagnosis, while regional lymph node metastases have been reported to occur in 10–60% of cases [2, 3, 42]. Liver metastases generally occur in <10% of all patients with duodenal NET [2, 43].

Overall duodenal NET have a favourable prognosis with a 5-year disease-specific survival ranging from 80% to 100% [42, 45, 46]. Whether duodenal NET should be treated by surgical resection or by endoscopic resection has not been fully established [43]. However postsurgical morbidity can be relevant especially in patients with other medical conditions that may increase the risk of surgical resection [43].

1.2.3 Small Bowel

Small bowel NET represent the most frequent primary site of all GEP-NET in some publications [2, 23, 47] and the second or third subgroups of GEP-NET in other series [26, 48]. Interestingly, in eastern Asia small bowel NET are much less common than in Western countries [37, 49].

The reported incidence of small bowel NET ranges between 0.32–0.33/100,000 in England and Japan [47, 49] and 0.67/100,000 in the USA [2] and up to 1.12/100,000 in North Europe [50]. Small bowel NET account for up to 30–50% of all small bowel neoplasms [26, 51], and similar to other neuroendocrine neoplasms, their incidence is on the rise, as demonstrated by recent epidemiological studies [52]. In an autopsy series, the incidence of small bowel NET is significantly higher than the clinical incidence, being 1.22:100, suggesting that the majority of small bowel NET may remain at an early stage for years [53].

The incidence rate of small bowel NET increases with age starting at age 40, reaching a peak at the eighth decade of life [24]. The mean age at diagnosis is between 59 and 65 years [53]. A slight male preponderance has been suggested in some studies [51, 54]; however these data has not been confirmed by other series [2, 47, 55]. As suggested by the SEER database findings, small bowel NET may have a different ethnic distribution being more frequent in Afro-Americans and less common in Asian patients [2].

The majority of small bowel NET are characterized by a low proliferation rate, G1 or G2, while G3 tumours are exceptionally rare. Despite the often low to intermediate proliferation rate, these tumours may present with loco-regional (36%) and/or distant metastases (48%) at the time of the diagnosis and, moreover, may be discovered at a relatively advanced disease stage possibly due to their indolent course [52]. The main prognostic factors for small bowel NET are TNM stage and histological grading, based on Ki-67 index [52]. Recently, it has been reported that the 5-year survival rate for jejunoileal NET is 100% for stages I and II, 97.1% for stage III, and 84.8% for stage IV [56]. In the same study, the grading-dependent 5-year survival rate for small bowel NET was 93.8% for G1, 83.0% for G2, and 50.0% for G3 [56].

1.2.4 Appendix

The incidence and the relative frequency of appendiceal NET are difficult to assess because of different classifications of these neoplasms, with the arbitrary inclusion or exclusion of some appendiceal tumour types in the NET register in the various countries. For example, in some registers the incidental, benignly behaving, sub-centimetre appendiceal NET are excluded [2, 22]. Furthermore, in some countries the NET of the appendix are included as part of all colon NET. Again, the goblet cell tumours of the appendix are inconsistently included or excluded in the various NET registers.

Overall, NET of the appendix are a relatively frequent subgroup of NET with an incidence of 0.15–0.6/100,000 per year [2]. However, they represent the least common NET subgroup in the SEER database (3.44%) in years 1973–2007, in Norway (4.8% of all NET) in years 1993–2004, and in Asia [1, 2, 22, 27, 37]. On the other hand, appendiceal NET are among the most frequent NET in other European series and comprise up to 38% of all GEP-NET in UK and in Spain [47, 57]. Part of this high geographical variability is probably due to recording differences.

Most appendiceal NET are asymptomatic and incidentally diagnosed on post-operative histopathological examination of resected appendectomy specimens with a rate of approximately 3–5/1000 appendix resections [58]. The prevalence of appendiceal NET has been reported to be related to the total number of appendectomies performed [59]. In last decades, an increase in appendiceal NET incidence has been observed probably because of a better knowledge by surgeons and pathologists. The median age of diagnosis is of 40–50 years with a higher prevalence in female patients. Appendiceal NET incidence rates in females are about twice those of males in Europe and in the USA [2, 60]. These gender differences could be related to the higher rates of appendectomies and gynaecological procedures in females [24]. The incidence of appendiceal NET in children is far lower than in the adult population, although appendiceal NET are the most common tumour of the gastrointestinal tract in children. The prognosis of appendiceal NET seems to be excellent in children [58, 61]. Some reports suggest the existence of ethnic differences, but data are still inconclusive [1, 2, 24]. However, malignant tumours seem to occur more frequently in the Caucasians as compared to other populations [58]. In general, the prognosis of appendiceal NET strongly depends on the TNM staging and grading. The prognosis is considered to be excellent for the low-stage tumours with 5-year survival rates of up to 100% [62]. Prognosis is less favourable for higher-stage tumours with 5-year survival rates ranging between 70% and 85% [63, 64].

A recent meta-analysis shows that the risk of occurrence of an appendiceal NET is higher among patients with history of other NET or tumours of the urinary tract, breast, or endocrine glands [18]. Interestingly, also a positive familial history for NET, tumours of nervous system, or endocrine gland neoplasms appears to be associated with the risk of occurrence of appendiceal NET [18].

1.2.5 Colon

The incidence of colon and rectum NET is difficult to assess, as registers variably reported data of colorectal, colon, and rectum NET either together or separately. Furthermore, appendiceal NET have been included with colorectal NET in some studies. For these reasons, comparisons among geographical areas are especially challenging.

Colon NET account for 4–7% of all NET in European and US series [2, 52]; a higher proportion (8%) has been reported in Asian series [65]. The incidence of colon NET in different countries is increasing. In the US SEER database, colon NET incidence has risen from approximately 0.02 to approximately 0.4/100,000 from 1973 to 2007 [22, 49]; similarly a fourfold increase has been reported in the UK [47]. On the other hand, a less marked increase in incidence rates has been observed in Norway [1]. Interestingly, in 2010 a report from Austria has demonstrated a particularly low incidence of colon NET of 0.06 [26].

In the USA, a slightly higher incidence of colon NET has been observed in the Afro-American ethnic group, while the lowest incidence was reported in the population of Asiatic ethnic origin [2]. As regards the gender, a slightly higher incidence was reported in males in the USA [1, 2], while a female predominance was observed in Europe [1, 12, 16].

Colon NET are often aggressive, poorly differentiated, and high in grade (G3), and they are often metastatic at the time of diagnosis (approximately 30–40%), possibly because of the later presentation due to the absence of early symptoms. The main sites of metastatic involvement are the liver, the lymph nodes, the mesentery, and the peritoneum. Overall survival at 5-year is roughly 43–50% [2].

A few studies have focused on the risk factors possibly involved in the development of the NET of the colon. It appears that the risk is significantly higher among patients with a parental history of NET (RR 2.78) [66].

1.2.6 Rectum

Rectal NET often present as an incidental finding at sigmoidoscopy or colonoscopy with an incidence of about 1:2500 examinations. From the latest SEER report, rectal NET have an incidence of 0.86/100,000 [2]. The incidence of rectal NET has been found to be on the rise probably due to expanding indications for lower gastrointestinal endoscopy and implementation of screening colonoscopy. For these reasons, rectal NET represent the most common gastrointestinal neuroendocrine neoplasm in Asian studies and in the SEER database in years 2000–2007 [2, 14, 22, 67].

Median age at diagnosis is of 56.2 years, lower than that reported for other gastrointestinal NET [68]. Rectal NET show a peculiar ethnic distribution. In the USA, the highest incidence was observed in Asians (OR 10), Afro-Americans (OR 1.96), and Hispanics (OR 2.6) [2, 69]. As regards to the gender distribution, a higher incidence in female patients has been reported in the USA (OR 1.20). On the contrary, Asian reports suggest a male prevalence (OR 1.92) [69, 70].

Rectal NEN are small, non-functioning, polypoid lesions located between 4 and 20 cm above the dentate line on the anterior or lateral rectal wall [71]. NET arising from the rectum are generally low to intermediate grade (G1 or G2), and distant metastases are rarely present at the time of diagnosis. Small rectal NET (<2 cm) rarely metastasize, and endoscopic or trans-anal excision is curative; however larger tumours may present a higher malignant potential, and metastases to the bone, lymph nodes, and liver have been reported [49]. Overall, the prognosis of rectal NET appears to be very good. In the USA, 5-year survival of patients with a rectal NET is up to 90% [22, 38, 68]. Similarly, a high 5-year survival rate has been reported in a patient series from Taiwan (86%) [37], while slightly lower survival rates have been observed in Norway (74%) and in Spain (64%) [1, 60].

The role of risk factors in the development of rectal NET has not been fully elucidated. There are conflicting data on the impact of cigarette smoking, alcohol consumption, obesity, and previous history or family history of NET [18]. As a matter of curiosity, a Korean study found low high-density lipoprotein-cholesterol levels to be an independent risk factor for rectal NET [70].

1.2.7 Pancreas

Pancreatic NET are a heterogeneous group of neoplasm with a reported incidence of almost 5/1000,000 year. They are relatively uncommon, accounting for only 1–2% of all pancreatic tumours [49, 72]. However, the incidence of pancreatic NET is on the rise in recent decades, both due to increased awareness of these neoplasms and the diffusion of highly sensitive and specific imaging techniques, such as computed tomography, functional imaging, and endoscopic ultrasound [24]. The American SEER database shows that the incidence of pancreatic NET had increased approximately fivefold in the past 30 years [2], and similar results have been reported in a number of other countries [23, 49].

Pancreatic NET are usually divided into functioning and non-functioning. In some recent series, 60–90% of pancreatic NET are non-functioning. These tumours are generally diagnosed at more advanced stages because of the absence of a clinical syndrome, and also their biological behaviour and slow growth can contribute to a delay in the onset of symptoms and, subsequently, in the diagnosis [73]. However, there is also an exponential increase in the incidental diagnosis of non-functioning pancreatic NET, probably due to the widespread use of high-quality imaging techniques [74, 75]. Functioning pancreatic NET are further subdivided according to clinical syndrome and their incidence. The more frequent are gastrinomas (0.5–21.5/1000,000 per year) and insulinomas (1–32/1000,000 per year), followed by VIPomas (0.05–0.2/1000,000 per year) and glucagonomas (0.01–0.1/1000,000 per year). Other functioning pancreatic NET, such as GRFomas, ACTHomas, and somatostatinomas, are indeed very rare, and their incidences have not been elucidated [73].

Insulinomas are the most common functioning NET of the pancreas and are characterized by hypoglycaemia due to inappropriate insulin secretion [76–78]. Less than 10% are malignant. There is an age-specific incidence peak in the fifth decade of life, and the incidence is slightly higher in women than in men. Approximately 10% are multiple, and approximately 5% are associated with MEN1 syndrome.

Gastrinomas account for up to 30% of all functioning pancreatic NET [76, 79]. According to the WHO 2010 classification, gastrinomas are usually G1–G2 NET, often with a diameter of about 1 cm, and may show local invasion and/or proximal lymph node metastases [80]. Liver metastases are reported in 22–35% of cases of pancreatic gastrinomas [81].

Rare functioning pancreatic NET represent less than 10% of all pancreatic NET, and the majority present with metastatic disease (40–90%) in the liver. Not enough data is currently available to give accurate estimates on survival. The average age at diagnosis is estimated to be 50–55 years, with equal gender distribution [81].

Most pancreatic NET occur as sporadic tumours, although a variable proportion of the different functioning pancreatic NET may occur in the setting of an inherited syndrome. MEN1 is the most important inherited condition responsible for 20–30% of gastrinomas. Non-functioning pancreatic NET have been reported to be more frequent in the setting of VHL disease, in which up to 17% of the patients can develop a pancreatic NET, in von Recklinghausen syndrome (neurofibromatosis 1), and in tuberous sclerosis [10].

According to the National Cancer Institute's SEER data in the USA, incidence of pancreatic NET is higher in males (male to female = 2:1), with an increasing incidence with age [82]. The peak incidence rate of pancreatic NET occurs in the sixth to eighth decade, and the median age of presentation is 60 years [2, 24, 48].

The overall survival in patients with a pancreatic NET is highly variable in different countries. Data from the SEER register show the lowest 5-year survival rate (27–38%) in comparison to the other GEP-NET. Such rate is even lower in patients with an already advanced stage of the tumour at the time of diagnosis [2, 22, 74]. Higher 5-year survival rates have been reported in Norway (43%), Italy (62%), and Spain (71–78%) [1, 16, 60].

As regards risk factors, alcohol intake has been associated with an increased risk of developing pancreatic NET with a OR of 2.44 for heavy alcohol drinkers [18]. Also a slight increased risk for tobacco smokers and obese patients has been observed in a recent meta-analysis [18]. Patients with pancreatic NET were more likely to report a personal history of diabetes and family history of other pancreatic NET or cancer (in particular sarcomas, oesophagus, gallbladder, stomach, and ovarian cancer) [18, 39, 74, 83]. Finally, in a large case-control study from Italy, a previous history of chronic pancreatitis was associated with an increased pancreatic NET risk [83].

1.3 Thoracic Neuroendocrine Tumours

1.3.1 Lung

Lung NET account for approximately 20–30% of all NET and 1–2% of all lung malignancies in adults [2, 68]. Overall, pulmonary NET are rare tumours with an incidence of 0.2–2.0/100,000 in both the USA and Europe. However, an impressive increase in prevalence of about 6% per year has been reported in the last 30 years [84]. The increase in prevalence appears to be mainly due to a better knowledge of pulmonary NET and the implementation of radiological and immunohistochemical techniques for the diagnosis [68].

Lung NET include typical carcinoid (TC), atypical carcinoid (AC), large cell neuroendocrine carcinoma (LCNEC), and small cell lung carcinoma (SCLC), the latter two being very rare.

Lung NET mostly occur in the fourth to sixth decades of life, with a median age at diagnosis of 64 years [2]. An earlier age at diagnosis (45 years) has been reported for TC. TC represents the most common primary lung neoplasm in children and late adolescents [85], and, in this setting, TC prevails over AC. As regards to the gender distribution, pulmonary NET present a slightly higher incidence in women over men [84]. There is a trend toward a higher prevalence in patients of Caucasian origin over those of African and other origins [1, 2, 84, 86].

Pulmonary NET are usually sporadic. They may also occur in the setting of MEN1 (up to 5% of patients had bronchial NET, usually TC with a smaller number of AC) [87, 88]. Moreover, rare familial cases have been reported [89, 90].

Published reports provide contrasting evidence regarding environmental risk factors associated with thoracic NET. A US case-control study identified a family history for cancer as the main prognostic factor for pulmonary NET, and the estimated OR for pulmonary NET was 2.40 for every positive family history of cancer with a higher risk carried by first-degree relatives. A Swedish study reported a slightly increased risk of developing PC (OR 2.60) in patients with a family history of NET [18]. Data on cigarette smoking are controversial; however it may be possible that smoking is associated with an overall increase in susceptibility to develop bronchial NET (OR 1.50). In contrast to that hypothesis, a few series have demonstrated that the majority of patients who develop bronchial NET have never been or are just light cigarette smokers [39, 91]. AC patients are more often current or former smokers than patients with TC [36, 91]. In contrast, it is well established that SCLC and LCNEC are associated with heavy smoking habit [92].

1.3.2 Thymus

Thymic NET are rare and account for approximately 2–5% of all thymic malignancies [93]. Data from the most recent SEER database showed an incidence for thymic NET of 0.02/100,000 population per year [94]. The median age at diagnosis is about 54 years with a male prevalence [94]. Up to 25% of thymic NET arise in patients affected by MEN1; on the other hand, 3–8% of patients with MEN1 develop a thymic NET [95]. Rarely, thymic NET may be found in MEN-2A patients [93]. Nearly all cases associated with MEN1 are men and smokers [94]. The clinical behaviour of these tumours closely correlates with the histologic degree of differentiation. The disease-free survival is 50% at 5 years and 9% at 10 years for well-differentiated tumours, 20% at 5 years and 0% at 10 years for moderately differentiated tumours, and 0% at 5 years for poorly differentiated tumours [96]. One-third of patients are asymptomatic, and the lesions may be discovered incidentally by imaging performed for other reasons or during MEN1 surveillance. Not infrequently, distant metastases are already detected at the time of diagnosis [97].

1.4 Other Sites

As already stated, NET arise from the neuroendocrine cells of the diffuse neuroendocrine system which is located in almost every organs, and, for this reason, a neuroendocrine neoplasm can virtually occur in any organs of the human body. Rare neuroendocrine tumours include a heterogeneous group of neoplasms with varying epidemiology and clinical behaviour, which are difficult to assess due to their extreme rarity and heterogeneous characteristics. In many cases, due to the low frequency of the rarest NET, reliable data on incidence and survival may be absent or limited. An additional issue affecting the epidemiological analysis of most of these rare tumours is represented by the lack of a homogeneous classification system and the use of multiple or non-specific denominations.

The group of non-neuroendocrine cancers carrying some degree of neuroendocrine differentiation and those which are primarily mixed neuroendocrine and non-neuroendocrine tumours fall out of this epidemiological picture since they are essentially not NET. Thus, they have not been considered here. The most important rare and ultra-rare sites for NET are listed in ◘ Table 1.2, and the gross epidemiological figures from the literature are shortly described below following the order of frequency.

1

Table 1.2 Anatomical sites of rare NET

Anatomical sites	Neuroendocrine tumour classification	Frequency
Bladder and urinary system	Small cell neuroendocrine carcinoma Large cell neuroendocrine carcinoma Well-differentiated neuroendocrine tumour Paraganglioma	0.14/100,000 [103]
Skin	Merkel cell carcinoma Small cell neuroendocrine carcinoma Neuroendocrine tumour/carcinoid Carcinomas with neuroendocrine differentiation (mixed)	1.78/100,000[a] [115]
Biliary tract	Neuroendocrine tumour G1 Neuroendocrine tumour G2 Neuroendocrine carcinoma (large or small cell)	0.12/100,000 [68]
Larynx	Typical carcinoid Atypical carcinoid Small cell neuroendocrine carcinoma Paraganglioma	~700 cases reported
Genital tract	Ovary Typical carcinoid Atypical carcinoid, Small cell neuroendocrine carcinoma Large cell neuroendocrine carcinoma Testes Not available	~500 cases reported
Liver	Neuroendocrine tumour G1 Neuroendocrine tumour G2 Neuroendocrine carcinoma (large or small cell)	~150 cases reported
Kidney	Not homogeneously defined	~100 cases reported
Brain	Not available	~5 cases
Heart	Not available	~3 cases reported

[a]Including all tumour subtypes

1.4.1 Urinary Tract

Neuroendocrine neoplasms of the urinary system are rare and comprise <1% of all urinary malignancies. The tumours tend to affect older men, and clinical presentation is reported to be similar to that of the more common invasive urothelial carcinoma [98]. The 2016 WHO classification recognizes four subtypes of neuroendocrine tumours of the urinary system, namely, small cell neuroendocrine carcinoma, large cell neuroendocrine carcinoma, well-differentiated neuroendocrine tumour, and paragangliomas [99].

Small cell carcinoma of the bladder usually affects patients over the age of 60 with a male predominance [100, 101]. Approximately 60% of patients have metastases at the time of diagnosis [102]. Large cell neuroendocrine carcinoma is usually high grade, biologically aggressive, and associated with poor prognosis. There is a male predominance and older age at presentation [103]. Primary well-differentiated NET of the bladder are very rare with approximately ten cases described in the literature. This rare neoplasm seems to have a favourable prognosis [103]; however regional or distant metastases have been reported in up to 25% of cases in previous reports [104]. Primary paraganglioma of the bladder is extremely rare and makes up less than 0.05% of all bladder malignancies [98]. The mean age at presentation is 45 years with slight higher incidence in women [105].

NET arising from the kidney are extremely uncommon. To date less than 100 cases have been reported in the literature. The mean age at diagnosis is 47 years (range, 13–68 years) with no gender differences [106, 107]. The most common symptoms are abdominal/flank pain, weight loss, and haematuria, and an abdominal mass could be noticed [108]. Symptoms related to carcinoid syndrome have been reported in approximately 13% of cases only [106]. Interestingly, an association between the occurrence of a renal NET and a patient background of horseshoe kidneys, renal teratoma, or polycystic kidney disease has been suggested [106]. Due to a small number of cases, the biological behaviour of renal NET is still undetermined. Although about 50% of renal NET present with local or distant metastatic disease at diagnosis, most patients are asymptomatic and seem to have a reasonably long survival. The most common metastatic sites include lymph nodes, the liver, bone, and lung [108, 109].

1.4.2 Skin

Primary cutaneous NET, including carcinomas, are very rare. In the World Health Organization blue books of skin tumours, there are no descriptions of primary neuroendocrine tumours except for Merkel cell carcinoma (MCC) of the skin [110]. The diagnosis of these lesions relies on structural, cytological, and immunohistochemical criteria, and they are usually divided into three major histologic groups: small cell neuroendocrine carcinomas, carcinoids/NET, and carcinomas with neuroendocrine differentiation (mixed type) [110].

Primary cutaneous NET (carcinoids) are very rare with approximately ten cases described in the literature [111]. Primary cutaneous NET usually affect patients in the sixth to ninth decades of life, with a mean age at presentation of 66 years [111]. These neoplasms have an equal gender distribution and predilection for the head and trunk region. They are localized in the dermis and usually have well-defined borders. Despite the small number of cases from which to draw definitive conclusions, information to date suggests that cutaneous NET may have a benign behaviour [112]. Small cell carcinoma of the skin or MCC is an uncommon neoplasm, typically affecting elderly patients [113]. The reported incidence is about 1500 cases per year in the USA and 1.78/100,000 in the UK. Incidence is apparently on the rise probably due to new pathological techniques and an increased population at risk

[114, 115]. MCC is usually located in the basal layer of the skin and occurs more frequently in the head-neck region and the limbs. The biological behaviour is usually aggressive with high mitotic index up to evidence of atypical mitoses [113]. Recent studies estimates of 5-year survival to be about 40% [116].

1.4.3 Biliary Tract

NET arising from the biliary tract are among the rarest primary sites of NET, accounting for 0.2–2% of all such malignancies [68]. Intra-hepatic biliary NET are exceedingly rare and only few cases have been reported [117, 118]. The gallbladder is an exceptionally infrequent site for NET accounting for 0.2% of all NET and only 2% of all gallbladder carcinomas. The age at presentation of gallbladder NET ranges from 38 to 81 years, and there is a higher incidence in women [119].

Extrahepatic biliary duct NET consist of tumours localized on left or right hepatic duct, common hepatic duct, cystic duct, or common bile duct. To date about 150 cases have been reported [120]. The most frequent sites are the common hepatic duct and the proximal common bile duct [120]. A recent review reported metastases to be present in about 30% of cases and that surgical resection is feasible in the large majority of NET [120]. A high prevalence of cholelithiasis (19.2%) in association with extrahepatic bile duct NET has been also observed, and this finding led to the hypothesis that cholelithiasis may be associated with NET pathogenesis [120].

Very rarely, NET may arise from the ampulla of Vater. To date about 105 cases have been reported, mostly as single case reports. Approximately 26% of all patients with NET tumours reported in the literature had neurofibromatosis [121]. The average age is 48.6 years and the gender ratio of female to male is 2.8:1 [122]. The most common symptoms at presentation are jaundice (53%), pain (24.6%), weight loss (3.7%), and acute pancreatitis (6.0%) [121]. Data on prognosis are scarce. However, an overall 5-year survival rate of 90% has been reported [121].

1.4.4 Larynx

Laryngeal NET are a rare heterogeneous group of neoplasms accounting for less than 1% of all laryngeal neoplasms. However, laryngeal NET have been recognized as the most common non-squamous type of neoplasms arising in this organ [123]. To date, more than 700 cases of laryngeal NET have been reported in the literature.

Laryngeal neuroendocrine neoplasms are divided into two broad categories based on their tissue of origin: epithelial and neural. The epithelial-derived tumours, neuroendocrine carcinomas, are then subclassified into three subtypes: typical carcinoids (well-differentiated neuroendocrine carcinomas, grade I), atypical carcinoids (moderately differentiated neuroendocrine carcinomas, grade II; large cell neuroendocrine carcinomas), and small cell neuroendocrine carcinomas (poorly differentiated neuroendocrine carcinoma, grade III). The neural-derived laryngeal NETs are represented by paragangliomas [124]. Atypical carcinoids are the most frequent of all laryngeal NETs, followed by small cell neuroendocrine carcinomas, paragangliomas, and typical carcinoid [123].

1.4.5 Genital Tract

It appears difficult to provide data on the epidemiology of neuroendocrine tumours of the genital tract as many neoplasms may manifest neuroendocrine differentiation and the classification of genital NET has not been fully established yet. The main primary sites for genital tract NET are the ovaries and the testes.

Neuroendocrine tumours in the ovary are rare and account for less than 1–2% of malignant ovarian neoplasms [125]. To date the nomenclature used is still that of the pulmonary classification systems: carcinoid, atypical carcinoid, small cell neuroendocrine carcinoma, and large cell neuroendocrine carcinoma [126]. Primary NET of the ovary account for less than 5% of all carcinoid tumours and for less than 0.1% of all ovarian neoplasms [68]. The median age of diagnosis is 55 years [127]. Most ovarian carcinoids are unilateral and early stage; cases presenting with carcinoid syndrome even in the absence of metastatic disease have been reported [127]. Prognosis is reported to be excellent for stage I disease, with greater than 90% survival [68]; however for women with more advanced disease, the prognosis is poor [127].

NET of the testes are rare and account for less than 1% of all testicular neoplasms [128]. More than 60 cases have been reported to date [129]. The age at presentation in the reported cases ranges from 10 to 83 years of age with a higher incidence in the fifth and sixth decade of life [130]. Most of the patients present with unilateral painless testicular mass. Carcinoid syndrome occurs in about 16% of cases [129]. Metastatic disease at the time of diagnosis has been reported in 11% of patients [131].

1.4.6 Liver

NET often metastasize to the liver [132–135], but NET arising primarily in the liver are extremely rare. To data, only few anecdotal cases have been reported [136–139], and the existence of this entity is still a matter of debate since the liver is the most common site of metastatic involvement of GEP-NET even when the primary tumour is very small and undetected [137]. In the reported cases, the mean age at presentation of patients with diagnosis of hepatic NET is greater than 40 years, with a slightly higher incidence in women [140].

In the literature, the large majority of patients with a diagnosis of hepatic NET present with resectable disease [141]. When feasible, the surgical resection should be taken into consideration, and the post-operative survival rate at 5 years is estimated at 74% with a recurrence rate of 18% [142].

1.4.7 Heart

Primary tumours of the heart are very rare, with an incidence of 0.0017–0.19% in unselected autopsy series [143]. Metastatic involvement of cardiac tissue from gastroenteropancreatic or bronchial NET, though rare, may occur more frequently than the development of a primary heart NET [144]. Only few cases of primary cardiac NET, including a carcinoma, have been reported [144–146].

1

Bibliography

1. Hauso O, Gustafsson BI, Kidd M, Waldum HL, Drozdov I, Chan AK et al (2008) Neuroendocrine tumor epidemiology: contrasting Norway and North America. Cancer 113(10):2655–2664. doi:10.1002/cncr.23883. PubMed PMID: 18853416
2. Yao JC, Hassan M, Phan A, Dagohoy C, Leary C, Mares JE et al (2008) One hundred years after "carcinoid": epidemiology of and prognostic factors for neuroendocrine tumors in 35,825 cases in the United States. J Clin Oncol 26(18):3063–3072. doi:10.1200/JCO.2007.15.4377. PubMed PMID: 18565894
3. Klöppel G, Perren A, Heitz PU (2004) The gastroenteropancreatic neuroendocrine cell system and its tumors: the WHO classification. Ann N Y Acad Sci 1014:13–27. PubMed PMID: 15153416
4. Tamagno G, Sheahan K, Skehan SJ, Geoghegan JG, Fennelly D, Collins CD et al (2013) Initial impact of a systematic multidisciplinary approach on the management of patients with gastroenteropancreatic neuroendocrine tumor. Endocrine 44(2):504–509. doi:10.1007/s12020-013-9910-5. PubMed PMID: 23471696
5. Modlin IM, Oberg K, Chung DC, Jensen RT, de Herder WW, Thakker RV et al (2008) Gastroenteropancreatic neuroendocrine tumours. Lancet Oncol 9(1):61–72. doi:10.1016/S1470-2045(07)70410-2. PubMed PMID: 18177818
6. Warner RR (2005) Enteroendocrine tumors other than carcinoid: a review of clinically significant advances. Gastroenterology 128(6):1668–1684. PubMed PMID: 15887158
7. Duerr EM, Chung DC (2007) Molecular genetics of neuroendocrine tumors. Best Pract Res Clin Endocrinol Metab 21(1):1–14. doi:10.1016/j.beem.2006.12.001. PubMed PMID: 17382262
8. Toumpanakis CG, Caplin ME (2008) Molecular genetics of gastroenteropancreatic neuroendocrine tumors. Am J Gastroenterol 103(3):729–732. doi:10.1111/j.1572-0241.2007.01777.x. PubMed PMID: 18341492
9. Ramage JK, Davies AH, Ardill J, Bax N, Caplin M, Grossman A et al (2005) Guidelines for the management of gastroenteropancreatic neuroendocrine (including carcinoid) tumours. Gut 54(Suppl 4):iv1–i16. doi:10.1136/gut.2004.053314. PubMed PMID: 15888809; PubMed Central PMCID: PMCPMC1867801
10. Jensen RT, Berna MJ, Bingham DB, Norton JA (2008) Inherited pancreatic endocrine tumor syndromes: advances in molecular pathogenesis, diagnosis, management, and controversies. Cancer 113(7 Suppl):1807–1843. doi:10.1002/cncr.23648. PubMed PMID: 18798544; PubMed Central PMCID: PMCPMC2574000
11. Maioli M, Ciccarese M, Pacifico A, Tonolo G, Ganau A, Cossu S et al (1992) Familial insulinoma: description of two cases. Acta Diabetol 29(1):38–40. PubMed PMID: 1520905
12. Hemminki K, Li X (2001) Incidence trends and risk factors of carcinoid tumors: a nationwide epidemiologic study from Sweden. Cancer 92(8):2204–2210. PubMed PMID: 11596039
13. Hallet J, Law CH, Cukier M, Saskin R, Liu N, Singh S (2015) Exploring the rising incidence of neuroendocrine tumors: a population-based analysis of epidemiology, metastatic presentation, and outcomes. Cancer 121(4):589–597. doi:10.1002/cncr.29099. PubMed PMID: 25312765
14. Tsai HJ, Wu CC, Tsai CR, Lin SF, Chen LT, Chang JS (2013) The epidemiology of neuroendocrine tumors in Taiwan: a nation-wide cancer registry-based study. PLoS One 8(4):e62487. doi:10.1371/journal.pone.0062487. PubMed PMID: 23614051; PubMed Central PMCID: PMCPMC3632554
15. O'Connor JM, Marmissolle F, Bestani C, Pesce V, Belli S, Dominichini E et al (2014) Observational study of patients with gastroenteropancreatic and bronchial neuroendocrine tumors in Argentina: results from the large database of a multidisciplinary group clinical multicenter study. Mol Clin Oncol 2(5):673–684. doi:10.3892/mco.2014.332. PubMed PMID: 25054030; PubMed Central PMCID: PMCPMC4106663
16. Caldarella A, Crocetti E, Paci E (2011) Distribution, incidence, and prognosis in neuroendocrine tumors: a population based study from a cancer registry. Pathol Oncol Res 17(3):759–763. doi:10.1007/s12253-011-9382-y. PubMed PMID: 21476126
17. Kaerlev L, Teglbjaerg PS, Sabroe S, Kolstad HA, Ahrens W, Eriksson M et al (2002) The importance of smoking and medical history for development of small bowel carcinoid tumor: a European population-based case-control study. Cancer Causes Control 13(1):27–34. PubMed PMID: 11899115
18. Leoncini E, Carioli G, La Vecchia C, Boccia S, Rindi G (2016) Risk factors for neuroendocrine neoplasms: a systematic review and meta-analysis. Ann Oncol 27(1):68–81. doi:10.1093/annonc/mdv505. PubMed PMID: 26487581

19. Lepage C, Bouvier AM, Faivre J (2013) Endocrine tumours: epidemiology of malignant digestive neuroendocrine tumours. Eur J Endocrinol 168(4):R77–R83. doi:10.1530/EJE-12-0418. PubMed PMID: 23349330
20. Mocellin S, Nitti D (2013) Gastrointestinal carcinoid: epidemiological and survival evidence from a large population-based study (n = 25 531). Ann Oncol 24(12):3040–3044. doi:10.1093/annonc/mdt377. PubMed PMID: 24050954
21. Fitzgerald TL, Hickner ZJ, Schmitz M, Kort EJ (2008) Changing incidence of pancreatic neoplasms: a 16-year review of statewide tumor registry. Pancreas 37(2):134–138. doi:10.1097/MPA.0b013e318163a329. PubMed PMID: 18665072
22. Lawrence B, Gustafsson BI, Chan A, Svejda B, Kidd M, Modlin IM (2011) The epidemiology of gastroenteropancreatic neuroendocrine tumors. Endocrinol Metab Clin N Am 40(1):1–18, vii. doi: 10.1016/j.ecl.2010.12.005. PubMed PMID: 21349409
23. Scherübl H, Streller B, Stabenow R, Herbst H, Höpfner M, Schwertner C et al (2013) Clinically detected gastroenteropancreatic neuroendocrine tumors are on the rise: epidemiological changes in Germany. World J Gastroenterol 19(47):9012–9019. doi:10.3748/wjg.v19.i47.9012. PubMed PMID: 24379626; PubMed Central PMCID: PMCPMC3870554
24. Fraenkel M, Kim MK, Faggiano A, Valk GD (2012) Epidemiology of gastroenteropancreatic neuroendocrine tumours. Best Pract Res Clin Gastroenterol 26(6):691–703. doi:10.1016/j.bpg.2013.01.006. PubMed PMID: 23582913
25. Modlin IM, Lye KD, Kidd M (2004) A 50-year analysis of 562 gastric carcinoids: small tumor or larger problem? Am J Gastroenterol 99(1):23–32. Epub 2003/12/23. PubMed PMID: 14687136
26. Niederle MB, Hackl M, Kaserer K, Niederle B (2010) Gastroenteropancreatic neuroendocrine tumours: the current incidence and staging based on the WHO and European neuroendocrine tumour society classification: an analysis based on prospectively collected parameters. Endocr Relat Cancer 17(4):909–918. doi:10.1677/erc-10-0152. Epub 2010/08/13. PubMed PMID: 20702725
27. Cho MY, Kim JM, Sohn JH, Kim MJ, Kim KM, Kim WH et al (2012) Current trends of the incidence and pathological diagnosis of Gastroenteropancreatic neuroendocrine tumors (GEP-NET) in Korea 2000-2009: multicenter study. Cancer Res Treat 44(3):157–165. doi:10.4143/crt.2012.44.3.157. PubMed PMID: 23091441; PubMed Central PMCID: PMCPMC3467418
28. Delle Fave G, Kwekkeboom DJ, Van Cutsem E, Rindi G, Kos-Kudla B, Knigge U et al (2012) ENET consensus guidelines for the management of patients with gastroduodenal neoplasms. Neuroendocrinology 95(2):74–87. doi:10.1159/000335595. PubMed PMID: 22262004
29. Rindi G, Arnold R, Bosman F, Capella C, Kilmstra D, Kloppel G (2010) Nomenclature and classification of neuroendocrine neoplasms of the digestive system. In: Bosman FT (ed) WHO classification of Tumours of the digestive system. IARC Press, Lyon, pp 13–14
30. Lehy T, Cadiot G, Mignon M, Ruszniewski P, Bonfils S (1992) Influence of multiple endocrine neoplasia type 1 on gastric endocrine cells in patients with the Zollinger-Ellison syndrome. Gut 33(9):1275–1279. Epub 1992/09/01. PubMed PMID: 1358767; PubMed Central PMCID: PMC1379501
31. Rindi G, Azzoni C, La Rosa S, Klersy C, Paolotti D, Rappel S et al (1999) ECL cell tumor and poorly differentiated endocrine carcinoma of the stomach: prognostic evaluation by pathological analysis. Gastroenterology 116(3):532–542. Epub 1999/02/25. PubMed PMID: 10029611
32. Modlin IM, Lye KD, Kidd M (2003) Carcinoid tumors of the stomach. Surg Oncol 12(2):153–172. Epub 2003/08/30. PubMed PMID: 12946486
33. Cavalcoli F, Zilli A, Conte D, Ciafardini C, Massironi S (2015) Gastric neuroendocrine neoplasms and proton pump inhibitors: fact or coincidence? Scand J Gastroenterol 50(11):1397–1403. doi:10.3109/00365521.2015.1054426. PubMed PMID: 26059834
34. Waldum HL, Qvigstad G (2007) Proton pump inhibitors and gastric neoplasia. Gut 56(7):1019–1020; author reply 20. doi: 10.1136/gut.2006.116434. PubMed PMID: 17566032; PubMed Central PMCID: PMCPMC1994369
35. Lahner E, Pilozzi E, Esposito G, Galli G, Annibale B (2014) Gastric carcinoid in the absence of atrophic body gastritis and with low Ki67 index: a clinical challenge. Scand J Gastroenterol 49(4):506–510. doi:10.3109/00365521.2013.878381. PubMed PMID: 24417768
36. Faggiano A, Ferolla P, Grimaldi F, Campana D, Manzoni M, Davì MV et al (2012) Natural history of gastro-entero-pancreatic and thoracic neuroendocrine tumors. Data from a large prospective and retrospective Italian epidemiological study: the NET management study. J Endocrinol Investig 35(9):817–823. doi:10.3275/8102. PubMed PMID: 22080849

37. Li AF, Hsu CY, Li A, Tai LC, Liang WY, Li WY et al (2008) A 35-year retrospective study of carcinoid tumors in Taiwan: differences in distribution with a high probability of associated second primary malignancies. Cancer 112(2):274–283. doi:10.1002/cncr.23159. PubMed PMID: 18008361
38. Maggard MA, O'Connell JB, Ko CY (2004) Updated population-based review of carcinoid tumors. Ann Surg 240(1):117–122. PubMed PMID: 15213627; PubMed Central PMCID: PMCPMC1356383
39. Hassan MM, Phan A, Li D, Dagohoy CG, Leary C, Yao JC (2008) Risk factors associated with neuroendocrine tumors: a U.S.-based case-control study. Int J Cancer 123(4):867–873. doi:10.1002/ijc.23529. PubMed PMID: 18491401
40. O'Toole D, Delle Fave G, Jensen RT (2012) Gastric and duodenal neuroendocrine tumours. Best Pract Res Clin Gastroenterol 26(6):719–735. doi:10.1016/j.bpg.2013.01.002. PubMed PMID: 23582915
41. Jensen RT, Rindi G, Arnold R, Lopes JM, Brandi ML, Bechstein WO et al (2006) Well-differentiated duodenal tumor/carcinoma (excluding gastrinomas). Neuroendocrinology 84(3):165–172. doi:10.1159/000098008. PubMed PMID: 17312376
42. Fitzgerald TL, Dennis SO, Kachare SD, Vohra NA, Zervos EE (2015) Increasing incidence of duodenal neuroendocrine tumors: incidental discovery of indolent disease? Surgery 158(2):466–471. doi:10.1016/j.surg.2015.03.042. PubMed PMID: 26013986
43. Hoffmann KM, Furukawa M, Jensen RT (2005) Duodenal neuroendocrine tumors: classification, functional syndromes, diagnosis and medical treatment. Best Pract Res Clin Gastroenterol 19(5):675–697. doi:10.1016/j.bpg.2005.05.009. PubMed PMID: 16253893
44. Soga J (2003) Carcinoids and their variant endocrinomas. An analysis of 11842 reported cases. J Exp Clin Cancer Res 22(4):517–530. PubMed PMID: 15053292
45. Mullen JT, Wang H, Yao JC, Lee JH, Perrier ND, Pisters PW, et al (2005) Carcinoid tumors of the duodenum. Surgery 138(6):971–977; discussion 7–8. doi: 10.1016/j.surg.2005.09.016. PubMed PMID: 16360380
46. Untch BR, Bonner KP, Roggin KK, Reidy-Lagunes D, Klimstra DS, Schattner MA, et al (2014) Pathologic grade and tumor size are associated with recurrence-free survival in patients with duodenal neuroendocrine tumors. J Gastrointest Surg 18(3):457–462; discussion 62–3. doi: 10.1007/s11605-014-2456-x. PubMed PMID: 24448999
47. Ellis L, Shale MJ, Coleman MP (2010) Carcinoid tumors of the gastrointestinal tract: trends in incidence in England since 1971. Am J Gastroenterol 105(12):2563–2569. doi:10.1038/ajg.2010.341. PubMed PMID: 20823835
48. Ploeckinger U, Kloeppel G, Wiedenmann B, Lohmann R (2009) Centers roGN. The German NET-registry: an audit on the diagnosis and therapy of neuroendocrine tumors. Neuroendocrinology 90(4):349–363. doi:10.1159/000242109. PubMed PMID: 19776553
49. Ito T, Sasano H, Tanaka M, Osamura RY, Sasaki I, Kimura W et al (2010) Epidemiological study of gastroenteropancreatic neuroendocrine tumors in Japan. J Gastroenterol 45(2):234–243. doi:10.1007/s00535-009-0194-8. PubMed PMID: 20058030
50. Landerholm K, Falkmer S, Järhult J (2010) Epidemiology of small bowel carcinoids in a defined population. World J Surg 34(7):1500–1505. doi:10.1007/s00268-010-0519-z. PubMed PMID: 20237925
51. Lepage C, Bouvier AM, Manfredi S, Dancourt V, Faivre J (2006) Incidence and management of primary malignant small bowel cancers: a well-defined French population study. Am J Gastroenterol 101(12):2826–2832. doi:10.1111/j.1572-0241.2006.00854.x. PubMed PMID: 17026561
52. Niederle B, Pape UF, Costa F, Gross D, Kelestimur F, Knigge U et al (2016) ENET consensus guidelines update for neuroendocrine neoplasms of the jejunum and ileum. Neuroendocrinology 103(2):125–138. doi:10.1159/000443170. PubMed PMID: 26758972
53. Berge T, Linell F (1976) Carcinoid tumours. Frequency in a defined population during a 12-year period. Acta Pathol Microbiol Scand A 84(4):322–330. PubMed PMID: 961424
54. Bergestuen DS, Aabakken L, Holm K, Vatn M, Thiis-Evensen E (2009) Small intestinal neuroendocrine tumors: prognostic factors and survival. Scand J Gastroenterol 44(9):1084–1091. doi:10.1080/00365520903082432. PubMed PMID: 19572232
55. Garcia-Carbonero R, Sorbye H, Baudin E, Raymond E, Wiedenmann B, Niederle B et al (2016) ENET consensus guidelines for high-grade Gastroenteropancreatic neuroendocrine tumors and neuroendocrine carcinomas. Neuroendocrinology 103(2):186–194. doi:10.1159/000443172. PubMed PMID: 26731334

56. Jann H, Roll S, Couvelard A, Hentic O, Pavel M, Müller-Nordhorn J et al (2011) Neuroendocrine tumors of midgut and hindgut origin: tumor-node-metastasis classification determines clinical outcome. Cancer 117(15):3332–3341. doi:10.1002/cncr.25855. PubMed PMID: 21246527
57. Alsina M, Marcos-Gragera R, Capdevila J, Buxó M, Ortiz RM, Barretina P et al (2011) Neuroendocrine tumors: a population-based study of incidence and survival in Girona Province, 1994-2004. Cancer Epidemiol 35(6):e49–e54. doi:10.1016/j.canep.2011.05.011. PubMed PMID: 21840785
58. Pape UF, Niederle B, Costa F, Gross D, Kelestimur F, Kianmanesh R et al (2016) ENET consensus guidelines for neuroendocrine neoplasms of the appendix (excluding goblet cell carcinomas). Neuroendocrinology 103(2):144–152. doi:10.1159/000443165. PubMed PMID: 26730583
59. Doede T, Foss HD, Waldschmidt J (2000) Carcinoid tumors of the appendix in children--epidemiology, clinical aspects and procedure. Eur J Pediatr Surg 10(6):372–377. doi:10.1055/s-2008-1072394. PubMed PMID: 11215778
60. Garcia-Carbonero R, Capdevila J, Crespo-Herrero G, Díaz-Pérez JA, Martínez Del Prado MP, Alonso Orduña V et al (2010) Incidence, patterns of care and prognostic factors for outcome of gastroenteropancreatic neuroendocrine tumors (GEP-NET): results from the National Cancer Registry of Spain (RGETNE). Ann Oncol 21(9):1794–1803. doi:10.1093/annonc/mdq022. PubMed PMID: 20139156
61. Boxberger N, Redlich A, Böger C, Leuschner I, von Schweinitz D, Dralle H et al (2013) Neuroendocrine tumors of the appendix in children and adolescents. Pediatr Blood Cancer 60(1):65–70. doi:10.1002/pbc.24267. PubMed PMID: 22887869
62. In't Hof KH, van der Wal HC, Kazemier G, Lange JF (2008) Carcinoid tumour of the appendix: an analysis of 1,485 consecutive emergency appendectomies. J Gastrointest Surg 12(8):1436–1438. doi:10.1007/s11605-008-0545-4. PubMed PMID: 18521695; PubMed Central PMCID: PMCPMC2491701
63. McCusker ME, Coté TR, Clegg LX, Sobin LH (2002) Primary malignant neoplasms of the appendix: a population-based study from the surveillance, epidemiology and end-results program, 1973-1998. Cancer 94(12):3307–3312. doi:10.1002/cncr.10589. PubMed PMID: 12115365
64. McGory ML, Maggard MA, Kang H, O'Connell JB, Ko CY (2005) Malignancies of the appendix: beyond case series reports. Dis Colon Rectum 48(12):2264–2271. doi:10.1007/s10350-005-0196-4. PubMed PMID: 16258711
65. Shebani KO, Souba WW, Finkelstein DM, Stark PC, Elgadi KM, Tanabe KK et al (1999) Prognosis and survival in patients with gastrointestinal tract carcinoid tumors. Ann Surg 229(6):815–821. discussion 22-3. PubMed PMID: 10363895; PubMed Central PMCID: PMCPMC1420828
66. Hiripi E, Bermejo JL, Sundquist J, Hemminki K (2009) Familial gastrointestinal carcinoid tumours and associated cancers. Ann Oncol 20(5):950–954. doi:10.1093/annonc/mdn706. PubMed PMID: 19150948
67. Ramage JK, De Herder WW, Delle Fave G, Ferolla P, Ferone D, Ito T et al (2016) ENET consensus guidelines update for colorectal neuroendocrine neoplasms. Neuroendocrinology 103(2):139–143. doi:10.1159/000443166. PubMed PMID: 26730835
68. Modlin IM, Lye KD, Kidd M (2003) A 5-decade analysis of 13,715 carcinoid tumors. Cancer 97(4):934–959. doi:10.1002/cncr.11105. PubMed PMID: 12569593
69. Taghavi S, Jayarajan SN, Powers BD, Davey A, Willis AI (2013) Examining rectal carcinoids in the era of screening colonoscopy: a surveillance, epidemiology, and end results analysis. Dis Colon Rectum 56(8):952–959. doi:10.1097/DCR.0b013e318291f512. PubMed PMID: 23838863
70. Jung YS, Yun KE, Chang Y, Ryu S, Park JH, Kim HJ et al (2014) Risk factors associated with rectal neuroendocrine tumors: a cross-sectional study. Cancer Epidemiol Biomark Prev 23(7):1406–1413. doi:10.1158/1055-9965.EPI-14-0132. PubMed PMID: 24813818
71. Caplin M, Sundin A, Nillson O, Baum RP, Klose KJ, Kelestimur F et al (2012) ENET consensus guidelines for the management of patients with digestive neuroendocrine neoplasms: colorectal neuroendocrine neoplasms. Neuroendocrinology 95(2):88–97. doi:10.1159/000335594. PubMed PMID: 22261972
72. Pape UF, Böhmig M, Berndt U, Tiling N, Wiedenmann B, Plöckinger U (2004) Survival and clinical outcome of patients with neuroendocrine tumors of the gastroenteropancreatic tract in a german referral center. Ann N Y Acad Sci 1014:222–233. PubMed PMID: 15153439
73. Falconi M, Eriksson B, Kaltsas G, Bartsch DK, Capdevila J, Caplin M, et al (2016) ENET Consensus Guidelines Update for the Management of Patients with Functional Pancreatic Neuroendocrine Tumors and Non-Functional Pancreatic Neuroendocrine Tumors. Neuroendocrinology 103(2):153–171. doi: 10.1159/000443171. PubMed PMID: 26742109; PubMed Central PMCID: PMCPMC4849884

74. Halfdanarson TR, Rabe KG, Rubin J, Petersen GM (2008) Pancreatic neuroendocrine tumors (PNET): incidence, prognosis and recent trend toward improved survival. Ann Oncol 19(10):1727–1733. doi:10.1093/annonc/mdn351. PubMed PMID: 18515795; PubMed Central PMCID: PMCPMC2735065
75. Lee LC, Grant CS, Salomao DR, Fletcher JG, Takahashi N, Fidler JL et al (2012) Small, nonfunctioning, asymptomatic pancreatic neuroendocrine tumors (PNET): role for nonoperative management. Surgery 152(6):965–974. doi:10.1016/j.surg.2012.08.038. PubMed PMID: 23102679
76. Metz DC, Jensen RT (2008) Gastrointestinal neuroendocrine tumors: pancreatic endocrine tumors. Gastroenterology 135(5):1469–1492. doi:10.1053/j.gastro.2008.05.047. PubMed PMID: 18703061; PubMed Central PMCID: PMCPMC2612755
77. Oberg K (2010) Pancreatic endocrine tumors. Semin Oncol 37(6):594–618. doi:10.1053/j.seminoncol.2010.10.014. PubMed PMID: 21167379
78. Tamagno G, O'Shea D (2012) Anatomical localization of insulinomas: still a need to combine a set of diagnostic procedures. Hormones (Athens) 11(4):483–487. PubMed PMID: 23422772
79. Jensen RT, Niederle B, Mitry E, Ramage JK, Steinmuller T, Lewington V et al (2006) Gastrinoma (duodenal and pancreatic). Neuroendocrinology 84(3):173–182. doi:10.1159/000098009. PubMed PMID: 17312377
80. Gibril F, Jensen RT (2005) Advances in evaluation and management of gastrinoma in patients with Zollinger-Ellison syndrome. Curr Gastroenterol Rep 7(2):114–121. PubMed PMID: 15802099
81. Jensen RT, Cadiot G, Brandi ML, de Herder WW, Kaltsas G, Komminoth P et al (2012) ENET consensus guidelines for the management of patients with digestive neuroendocrine neoplasms: functional pancreatic endocrine tumor syndromes. Neuroendocrinology 95(2):98–119. doi:10.1159/000335591. PubMed PMID: 22261919; PubMed Central PMCID: PMCPMC3701449
82. Capelli P, Fassan M, Scarpa A (2012) Pathology – grading and staging of GEP-NET. Best Pract Res Clin Gastroenterol 26(6):705–717. doi:10.1016/j.bpg.2013.01.003. PubMed PMID: 23582914
83. Capurso G, Falconi M, Panzuto F, Rinzivillo M, Boninsegna L, Bettini R et al (2009) Risk factors for sporadic pancreatic endocrine tumors: a case-control study of prospectively evaluated patients. Am J Gastroenterol 104(12):3034–3041. doi:10.1038/ajg.2009.466. PubMed PMID: 19690522
84. Caplin ME, Baudin E, Ferolla P, Filosso P, Garcia-Yuste M, Lim E et al (2015) Pulmonary neuroendocrine (carcinoid) tumors: European neuroendocrine tumor society expert consensus and recommendations for best practice for typical and atypical pulmonary carcinoids. Ann Oncol 26(8):1604–1620. doi:10.1093/annonc/mdv041. PubMed PMID: 25646366
85. Dishop MK, Kuruvilla S (2008) Primary and metastatic lung tumors in the pediatric population: a review and 25-year experience at a large children's hospital. Arch Pathol Lab Med 132(7):1079–1103. doi:10.1043/1543-2165(2008)132[1079:PAMLTI]2.0.CO;2. PubMed PMID: 18605764
86. de Jong WK, Schaapveld M, Blaauwgeers JL, Groen HJ (2008) Pulmonary tumours in the Netherlands: focus on temporal trends in histology and stage and on rare tumours. Thorax 63(12):1096–1102. doi:10.1136/thx.2007.095067. PubMed PMID: 18678702
87. Sachithanandan N, Harle RA, Burgess JR (2005) Bronchopulmonary carcinoid in multiple endocrine neoplasia type 1. Cancer 103(3):509–515. doi:10.1002/cncr.20825. PubMed PMID: 15611976
88. Ferolla P, Daddi N, Urbani M, Semeraro A, Ribacchi R, Giovenali P et al (2009) Tumorlets, multicentric carcinoids, lymph-nodal metastases, and long-term behavior in bronchial carcinoids. J Thorac Oncol 4(3):383–387. doi:10.1097/JTO.0b013e318197f2e7. PubMed PMID: 19247084
89. De Giorgi U, Fanini F, Amadori D, Cancellieri A, Fiorentini G, Poletti V et al (2011) Tumorlets in familial history of bronchopulmonary carcinoid. J Thorac Oncol 6(9):1613–1614. doi:10.1097/JTO.0b013e318221f54f. PubMed PMID: 21849858
90. Oliveira AM, Tazelaar HD, Wentzlaff KA, Kosugi NS, Hai N, Benson A et al (2001) Familial pulmonary carcinoid tumors. Cancer 91(11):2104–2109. PubMed PMID: 11391591
91. Beasley MB, Thunnissen FB, Brambilla E, Hasleton P, Steele R, Hammar SP et al (2000) Pulmonary atypical carcinoid: predictors of survival in 106 cases. Hum Pathol 31(10):1255–1265. doi:10.1053/hupa.2000.19294. PubMed PMID: 11070119
92. Travis WD, World Health Organization, International Agency for Research on Cancer, International Association for the Study of Lung Cancer, International Academy of Pathology (2004) Pathology and genetics of tumours of the lung, pleura, thymus, and heart. IARC Press, Lyon, p 344
93. Chaer R, Massad MG, Evans A, Snow NJ, Geha AS (2002) Primary neuroendocrine tumors of the thymus. Ann Thorac Surg 74(5):1733–1740. PubMed PMID: 12440652

94. Gaur P, Leary C, Yao JC (2010) Thymic neuroendocrine tumors: a SEER database analysis of 160 patients. Ann Surg 251(6):1117–1121. doi:10.1097/SLA.0b013e3181dd4ec4. PubMed PMID: 20485130
95. Gibril F, Chen YJ, Schrump DS, Vortmeyer A, Zhuang Z, Lubensky IA et al (2003) Prospective study of thymic carcinoids in patients with multiple endocrine neoplasia type 1. J Clin Endocrinol Metab 88(3):1066–1081. doi:10.1210/jc.2002-021314. PubMed PMID: 12629087
96. Moran CA, Suster S (2000) Neuroendocrine carcinomas (carcinoid tumor) of the thymus. A clinicopathologic analysis of 80 cases. Am J Clin Pathol 114(1):100–110. doi:10.1309/3PDN-PMT5-EQTM-H0CD. PubMed PMID: 10884805
97. Lausi PO, Refai M, Filosso PL, Ruffini E, Oliaro A, Guerrera F et al (2014) Thymic neuroendocrine tumors. Thorac Surg Clin 24(3):327–332. doi:10.1016/j.thorsurg.2014.05.007. PubMed PMID: 25065934
98. Bostwick DG, Cheng L (2014) Urologic surgical pathology, 3rd edn. Elsevier/Saunders, Philadelphia. ix, 966 pages p
99. Moch H, Cubilla AL, Humphrey PA, Reuter VE, Ulbright TM (2016) The 2016 WHO classification of Tumours of the urinary system and male genital organs-part a: renal, penile, and testicular Tumours. Eur Urol 70(1):93–105. doi:10.1016/j.eururo.2016.02.029. PubMed PMID: 26935559
100. Shatagopam K, Kaimakliotis HZ, Cheng L, Koch MO (2015) Genitourinary small cell malignancies: prostate and bladder. Future Oncol 11(3):479–488. doi:10.2217/fon.14.277. PubMed PMID: 25675127
101. Eliyakin N, Postaci H, Baskin Y, Kozacioğlu Z (2015) Small cell carcinoma of the urinary bladder: KIT and PDGFRA gene mutations. Rare Tumors 7(4):5982. doi:10.4081/rt.2015.5982. PubMed PMID: 26788274; PubMed Central PMCID: PMCPMC4703920
102. Zheng X, Liu D, Fallon JT, Zhong M (2015) Distinct genetic alterations in small cell carcinoma from different anatomic sites. Exp Hematol Oncol 4:2. doi:10.1186/2162-3619-4-2. PubMed PMID: 25937998; PubMed Central PMCID: PMCPMC4417281
103. Kouba E, Cheng L (2016) Neuroendocrine tumors of the urinary bladder according to the 2016 World Health Organization classification: molecular and clinical characteristics. Endocr Pathol 27(3):188–199. doi:10.1007/s12022-016-9444-5. PubMed PMID: 27334654
104. Murali R, Kneale K, Lalak N, Delprado W (2006) Carcinoid tumors of the urinary tract and prostate. Arch Pathol Lab Med 130(11):1693–1706. doi:10.1043/1543-2165(2006)130[1693:CTOTUT]2.0.CO;2. PubMed PMID: 17076534
105. Henderson SJ, Kearns PJ, Tong CM, Reddy M, Khurgin J, Bickell M et al (2015) Patients with urinary bladder paragangliomas: a compiled case series from a literature review for clinical management. Urology 85(4):e25–e29. doi:10.1016/j.urology.2014.11.006. PubMed PMID: 25618559
106. Romero FR, Rais-Bahrami S, Permpongkosol S, Fine SW, Kohanim S, Jarrett TW (2006) Primary carcinoid tumors of the kidney. J Urol 176(6 Pt 1):2359–2366. doi:10.1016/j.juro.2006.07.129. PubMed PMID: 17085102
107. Hansel DE, Epstein JI, Berbescu E, Fine SW, Young RH, Cheville JC (2007) Renal carcinoid tumor: a clinicopathologic study of 21 cases. Am J Surg Pathol 31(10):1539–1544. doi:10.1097/PAS.0b013e318042d596. PubMed PMID: 17895755
108. Jeung JA, Cao D, Selli BW, Clapp WL, Oliai BR, Parwani AV et al (2011) Primary renal carcinoid tumors: clinicopathologic features of 9 cases with emphasis on novel immunohistochemical findings. Hum Pathol 42(10):1554–1561. doi:10.1016/j.humpath.2010.12.019. PubMed PMID: 21496872
109. Canacci AM, MacLennan GT (2008) Carcinoid tumor of the kidney. J Urol 180(5):2193. doi:10.1016/j.juro.2008.08.011. PubMed PMID: 18804792
110. LeBoit PE, International Agency for Research on Cancer, World Health Organization, International Academy of Pathology, European Organization for Research on Treatment of Cancer, UniversitätsSpital Zürich, Departement Pathologie (2006) Pathology and genetics of skin tumours. IARC Press, Lyon. 355 p
111. Jedrych J, Pulitzer M (2014) Primary carcinoid tumor of the skin: a literature review. Int J Surg Pathol 22(2):129–135. doi:10.1177/1066896913516672. PubMed PMID: 24401190
112. Eloy-Garcia Carrasco C, Benguigui Benadiva J, Martinez Garcia S, Sanz Trelles A, Palacios S (2006) Atypical primary carcinoid tumour of the skin. J Cutan Pathol 33(Suppl 2):32–34. doi:10.1111/j.1600-0560.2006.00502.x. PubMed PMID: 16972951

113. Frigerio B, Capella C, Eusebi V, Tenti P, Azzopardi JG (1983) Merkel cell carcinoma of the skin: the structure and origin of normal Merkel cells. Histopathology 7(2):229–249. PubMed PMID: 6852784
114. Lemos B, Nghiem P (2007) Merkel cell carcinoma: more deaths but still no pathway to blame. J Invest Dermatol 127(9):2100–2103. doi:10.1038/sj.jid.5700925. PubMed PMID: 17700621
115. Goon PK, Greenberg DC, Igali L, Levell NJ (2016) Merkel cell carcinoma: rising incidence in the east of England. J Eur Acad Dermatol Venereol. doi:10.1111/jdv.13828. PubMed PMID: 27515234
116. Lemos BD, Storer BE, Iyer JG, Phillips JL, Bichakjian CK, Fang LC et al (2010) Pathologic nodal evaluation improves prognostic accuracy in Merkel cell carcinoma: analysis of 5823 cases as the basis of the first consensus staging system. J Am Acad Dermatol 63(5):751–761. doi:10.1016/j.jaad.2010.02.056. PubMed PMID: 20646783; PubMed Central PMCID: PMCPMC2956767
117. Gembala RB, Arsuaga JE, Friedman AC, Radecki PD, Ball DS, Hartman GG et al (1993) Carcinoid of the intrahepatic ducts. Abdom Imaging 18(3):242–244. PubMed PMID: 8508084
118. Jiménez R, Beguiristain A, Ruiz-Montesinos I, Villar F, Medrano MA, Garnateo F et al (2008) Intrahepatic biliary carcinoid. Am J Clin Oncol 31(5):521–522. doi:10.1097/01.coc.0000224492.61906.76. PubMed PMID: 18838892
119. Modlin IM, Kidd M, Latich I, Zikusoka MN, Shapiro MD (2005) Current status of gastrointestinal carcinoids. Gastroenterology 128(6):1717–1751. PubMed PMID: 15887161
120. Michalopoulos N, Papavramidis TS, Karayannopoulou G, Pliakos I, Papavramidis ST, Kanellos I (2014) Neuroendocrine tumors of extrahepatic biliary tract. Pathol Oncol Res 20(4):765–775. doi:10.1007/s12253-014-9808-4. PubMed PMID: 24917351
121. Hatzitheoklitos E, Büchler MW, Friess H, Poch B, Ebert M, Mohr W et al (1994) Carcinoid of the ampulla of Vater. Clinical characteristics and morphologic features. Cancer 73(6):1580–1588. PubMed PMID: 8156484
122. Hartel M, Wente MN, Sido B, Friess H, Büchler MW (2005) Carcinoid of the ampulla of Vater. J Gastroenterol Hepatol 20(5):676–681. doi:10.1111/j.1440-1746.2005.03744.x. PubMed PMID: 15853978
123. Ferlito A, Silver CE, Bradford CR, Rinaldo A (2009) Neuroendocrine neoplasms of the larynx: an overview. Head Neck 31(12):1634–1646. doi:10.1002/hed.21162. PubMed PMID: 19536850
124. Barnes L, UniversitätsSpital Zürich, Departement Pathologie, International Academy of Pathology, World Health Organization, International Agency for Research on Cancer (2005) Pathology and genetics of head and neck tumours. IARC Press, Lyon. 430 p
125. Gardner GJ, Reidy-Lagunes D, Gehrig PA (2011) Neuroendocrine tumors of the gynecologic tract: a Society of Gynecologic Oncology (SGO) clinical document. Gynecol Oncol 122(1):190–198. doi:10.1016/j.ygyno.2011.04.011. PubMed PMID: 21621706
126. Rouzbahman M, Clarke B (2013) Neuroendocrine tumors of the gynecologic tract: select topics. Semin Diagn Pathol 30(3):224–233. doi:10.1053/j.semdp.2013.06.007. PubMed PMID: 24144291
127. Davis KP, Hartmann LK, Keeney GL, Shapiro H (1996) Primary ovarian carcinoid tumors. Gynecol Oncol 61(2):259–265. doi:10.1006/gyno.1996.0136. PubMed PMID: 8626144
128. Ulbright TM, Amin MB, Young RH, Armed Forces Institute of Pathology (U.S.), Universities Associated for Research and Education in Pathology (1999) Tumors of the testis, adnexa, spermatic cord, and scrotum. Armed Forces Institute of Pathology : Available from the American Registry of Pathology, Armed Forces Institute of Pathology, Washington, D.C.. 385 p
129. Stroosma OB, Delaere KP (2008) Carcinoid tumours of the testis. BJU Int 101(9):1101–1105. doi:10.1111/j.1464-410X.2007.07360.x. PubMed PMID: 18190641
130. Wang WP, Guo C, Berney DM, Ulbright TM, Ubright TM, Hansel DE et al (2010) Primary carcinoid tumors of the testis: a clinicopathologic study of 29 cases. Am J Surg Pathol 34(4):519–524. doi:10.1097/PAS.0b013e3181d31f33. PubMed PMID: 20351489
131. Sutherland RS, Wettlaufer JN, Miller GJ (1992) Primary carcinoid tumor of the testicle: a case report and management schema. J Urol 148(3):880–882. PubMed PMID: 1512846
132. Rossi RE, Massironi S, Spampatti MP, Conte D, Ciafardini C, Cavalcoli F et al (2012) Treatment of liver metastases in patients with digestive neuroendocrine tumors. J Gastrointest Surg 16(10):1981–1992. doi:10.1007/s11605-012-1951-1. PubMed PMID: 22829240
133. Pavel M, Baudin E, Couvelard A, Krenning E, Öberg K, Steinmüller T et al (2012) ENET consensus guidelines for the management of patients with liver and other distant metastases from neuroendocrine neoplasms of foregut, midgut, hindgut, and unknown primary. Neuroendocrinology 95(2):157–176. doi:10.1159/000335597. PubMed PMID: 22262022

134. Strosberg JR, Cheema A, Kvols LK (2011) A review of systemic and liver-directed therapies for metastatic neuroendocrine tumors of the gastroenteropancreatic tract. Cancer Control 18(2):127–137. PubMed PMID: 21451455
135. Mazzaferro V, Pulvirenti A, Coppa J (2007) Neuroendocrine tumors metastatic to the liver: how to select patients for liver transplantation? J Hepatol 47(4):460–466. doi:10.1016/j.jhep.2007.07.004. PubMed PMID: 17697723
136. Iwao M, Nakamuta M, Enjoji M, Kubo H, Fukutomi T, Tanabe Y et al (2001) Primary hepatic carcinoid tumor: case report and review of 53 cases. Med Sci Monit 7(4):746–750. PubMed PMID: 11433205
137. Touloumis Z, Delis SG, Triantopoulou C, Giannakou N, Avgerinos C, Dervenis C (2008) Primary hepatic carcinoid; a diagnostic dilemma: a case report. Cases J 1(1):314. doi:10.1186/1757-1626-1-314. PubMed PMID: 19014620; PubMed Central PMCID: PMCPMC2596793
138. Mima K, Beppu T, Murata A, Otao R, Miyake K, Okabe H et al (2011) Primary neuroendocrine tumor in the liver treated by hepatectomy: report of a case. Surg Today 41(12):1655–1660. doi:10.1007/s00595-011-4497-z. PubMed PMID: 21969201
139. Kim JM, Kim SY, Kwon CH, Joh JW, Park JB, Lee JH et al (2013) Primary hepatic neuroendocrine carcinoma. Korean J Hepatobiliary Pancreat Surg 17(u):34–37. doi:10.14701/kjhbps.2013.17.1.34. PubMed PMID: 26155210; PubMed Central PMCID: PMCPMC4304509
140. Yang K, Cheng YS, Yang JJ, Jiang X, Guo JX (2015) Primary hepatic neuroendocrine tumor with multiple liver metastases: a case report with review of the literature. World J Gastroenterol 21(10):3132–3138. doi:10.3748/wjg.v21.i10.3132. PubMed PMID: 25780316; PubMed Central PMCID: PMCPMC4356938
141. Fenwick SW, Wyatt JI, Toogood GJ, Lodge JP (2004) Hepatic resection and transplantation for primary carcinoid tumors of the liver. Ann Surg 239(2):210–219. doi:10.1097/01.sla.0000109155.89514.42. PubMed PMID: 14745329; PubMed Central PMCID: PMCPMC1356214
142. Miura K, Shirasawa H (1988) Primary carcinoid tumor of the liver. Am J Clin Pathol 89(4):561–564. PubMed PMID: 3354510
143. Bakaeen FG, Reardon MJ, Coselli JS, Miller CC, Howell JF, Lawrie GM, et al (2003) Surgical outcome in 85 patients with primary cardiac tumors. Am J Surg 186(6):641–647; discussion 7. PubMed PMID: 14672772
144. Guajardo-Salinas GE, Anaya-Ayala JE, Rice DC, Moran CA, Reardon MJ (2013) Primary high-grade neuroendocrine carcinoma of the heart. Tex Heart Inst J 40(1):71–74. PubMed PMID: 23466749; PubMed Central PMCID: PMCPMC3568293
145. Gibril F, Curtis LT, Termanini B, Fritsch MK, Lubensky IA, Doppman JL et al (1997) Primary cardiac gastrinoma causing Zollinger-Ellison syndrome. Gastroenterology 112(2):567–574. PubMed PMID: 9024311
146. Carmona P, Lázaro J, Llagunes J, Cánovas S (2012) Primary cardiac neuroendocrine carcinoma and minimally invasive cardiac surgery. Asian Cardiovasc Thorac Ann 20(6):721–723. doi:10.1177/0218492312440265. PubMed PMID: 23284120

Pathological Classification: GEP, TNET, and Rare Forms

Maria Laura Del Basso De Caro, Elia Guadagno, and Gaetano De Rosa

A. Colao et al. (eds.), *Neuroendocrine Tumors in Real Life*,
https://doi.org/10.1007/978-3-319-59024-0_2

Overview

Pathological classification of neuroendocrine tumors is based mainly on proliferative activity in both gastrointestinal tract (GEP-NETs) and thorax. Ki67 has been introduced as the mainstay of grading in the 2010 WHO classification of GEP-NETs, with the definition of three grades of malignancy, depending on whether the value is ≤2%, 3–20%, and >20%, respectively, in case of well-differentiated NET, moderately differentiated NET, or neuroendocrine carcinoma (NEC). A recent matter of debate is whether dividing or not high-grade NEC into two subgroups on the basis of both morphologic differentiation and proliferation rate. According to 2015 WHO, thoracic neuroendocrine tumors are classified into typical carcinoid, atypical carcinoid, large-cell neuroendocrine carcinoma, and small-cell neuroendocrine carcinoma on the base of mitotic activity and the presence/absence of necrosis. More information have been acquired on preneoplastic lesions and mixed forms.

Less extensive is the knowledge of neuroendocrine neoplasms in uncommon sites (urinary system and male genital organs, female genital organs, breast, head and neck, and skin).

2.1 Gastroenteropancreatic Neuroendocrine Neoplasms (GEP-NEN)

The concept of neuroendocrine cell has evolved over time together with the definition of neuroendocrine tumors (NET). These arise from diffuse neuroendocrine system (DNS), including the pituitary gland, C cells of the thyroid, parathyroid glands, the endocrine pancreas, gastrointestinal neuroendocrine cells, adrenal medullary tissue, and other scattered neuroendocrine cells of the skin and bronchi, with common embryologic, morphologic, and functional features [1]. Neuroendocrine is the interaction between the endocrine and the nervous system.

The gastrointestinal tract is the largest «organ» that makes part of the diffuse neuroendocrine system. In the pancreas most neuroendocrine cells form well-circumscribed nests, called islets of Langerhans, while a few are scattered in the main pancreatic and larger interlobular ducts. Gastroenteropancreatic neuroendocrine neoplasms tumors (GEP-NEN) represent heterogeneous tumors due to the extreme variety of the cells from which they originate [2].

2.1.1 Classification and Immunohistochemistry

GEP-NEN are classified according to the 2010 *WHO Classification of Tumours of the Digestive System* [3]. They are distinguished into neuroendocrine tumors (Grade 1 and Grade 2) and neuroendocrine carcinoma (Grade 3). Histological diagnosis is made on tissue taken from core biopsy or surgical specimen. Cytological sample cannot be always considered suitable for diagnosis. Diagnosis is based primarily on the observation of morphologic features (nested growth pattern, granular eosinophilic cytoplasm, and «salt and pepper» chromatin) (▫ Fig. 2.1), and then it is confirmed by immunohistochemical techniques (chromogranin A and synaptophysin are the most specific

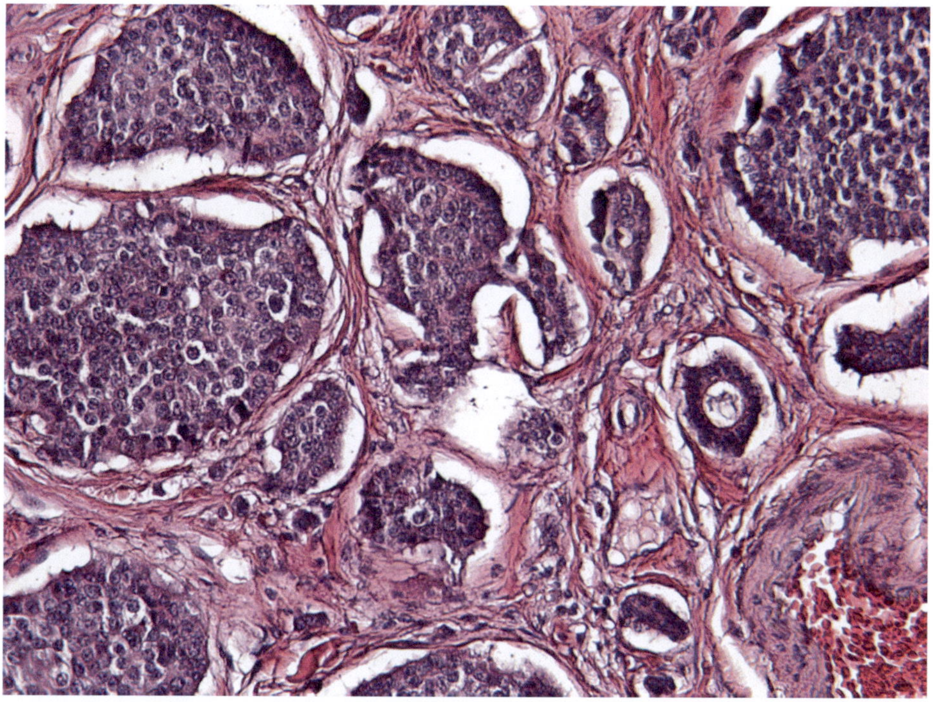

Fig. 2.1 Ileal NET G1: neoplastic cells arranged in nests, with «salt and pepper» chromatin and granular eosinophilic cytoplasm. Hematoxylin and eosin stain, 20× magnification

neuroendocrine markers; not recommended because unspecific, NSE, i.e., neuron specific enolase, and CD56) [4] (Fig. 2.2). The presence of more pleomorphic nuclei and a more diffuse pattern is suggestive of a higher grade of differentiation. The 2010 WHO classification establishes the grade of NEN differentiation on the basis of the Ki67 proliferation index that is calculated in the areas with the highest number of labeled cells (hot spot) and of the mitotic activity (Fig. 2.3).

Grading criteria for GEP-NEN are as follows:

Definition

- NET G1: mitotic count <2/ 10 high power fields (HPF) and/or ≤2% Ki67 index
- NET G2: mitotic count 2–20/10 HPF and/or 3–20% Ki67 index
- NEC G3: mitotic count >20/ 10 HPF and/or >20% Ki67 index → small-cell carcinoma/ large-cell neuroendocrine carcinoma

Immunohistochemistry is useful also in identifying the primary site in case of metastatic well-differentiated neuroendocrine tumor [5].

TTF1 [6, 7] is expressed in most pulmonary carcinoids (however, some high-grade NEC can aberrantly express it) [8, 9]; CDX2 (Fig. 2.4) is specific of intestinal, appendiceal, and, to a lesser extent, pancreatic origin [58, 59, 62]; islet 1 and PAX8 are observed mainly in pancreatic and rectal NET [10–11]. CK7 and CK20 are of limited utility [12].

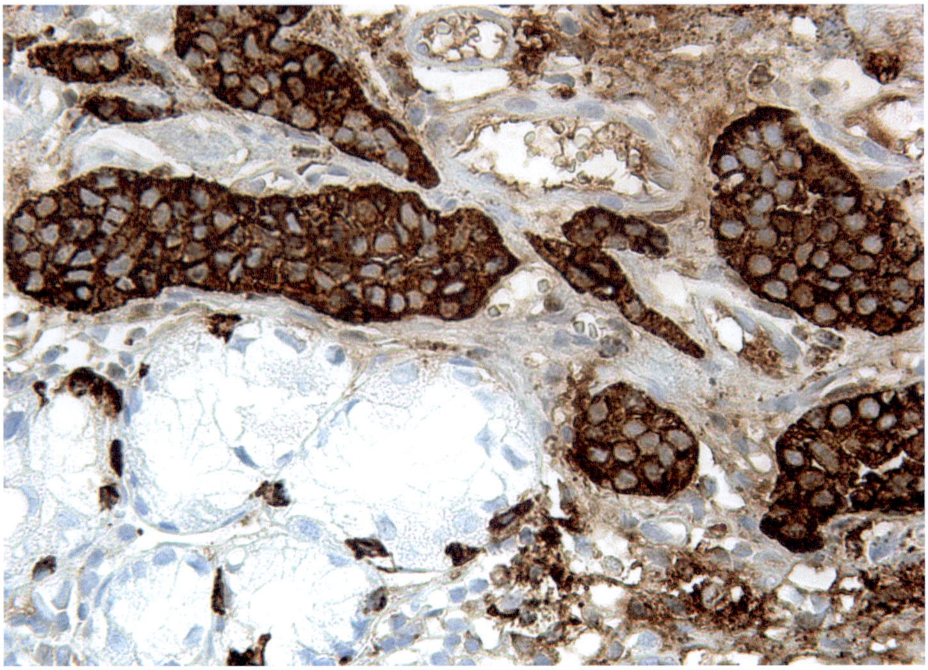

Fig. 2.2 Gastric NET G1: strong cytoplasmic immunoreactivity for chromogranin evident in neoplastic nests. 40× magnification

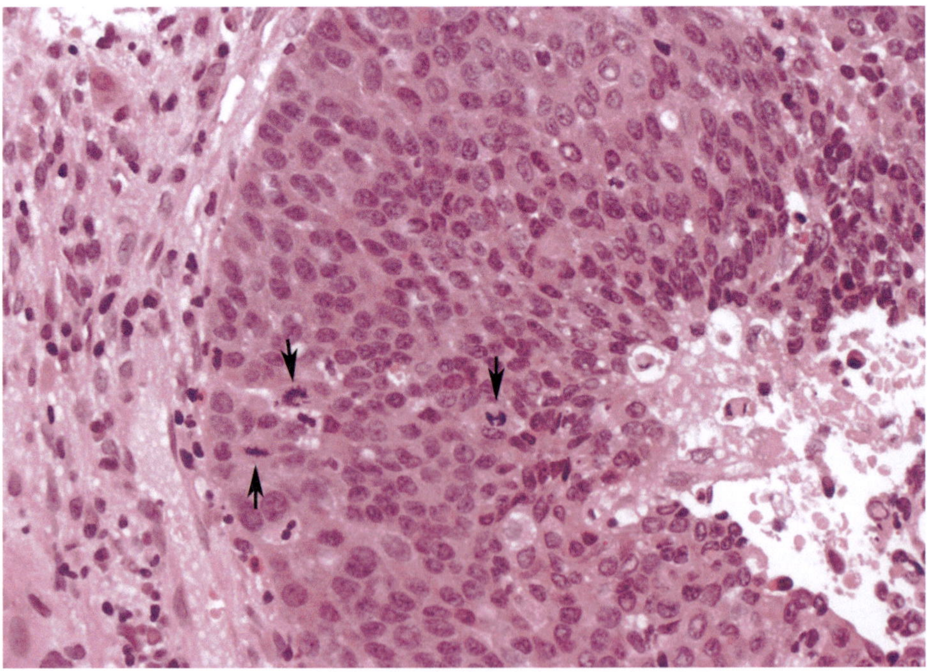

Fig. 2.3 Neuroendocrine carcinoma, showing high mitotic rate (*arrows*). Hematoxylin and eosin stain, 40× magnification

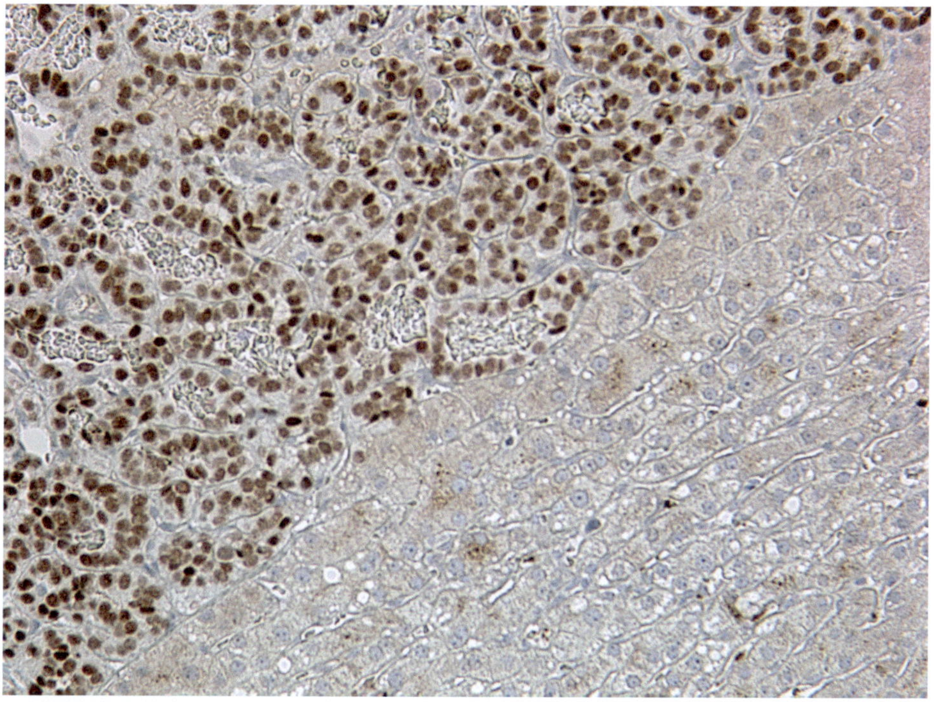

Fig. 2.4 Liver metastasis from ileal NET G1: strong and diffuse nuclear CDX2 reactivity. 20× magnification

2.1.2 Grading: Ki67 and Mitotic Index

Mitotic count is invalidated by high interobserver variability for which it is considered not so reproducible. Furthermore, it is difficult to discriminate between true mitosis and its mimics. Mitosis-specific marker, phosphorylate histone H3(PHH3), has been tested in NET, and it showed to have a practical impact by reducing time and improving interobserver reproducibility [13].

Ki67 protein is a nuclear cellular marker for proliferation, and it is detected during all active phases of cell cycle (G1, S, G2, and M), absent in resting cells (G0). Ki67 and MIB-1 monoclonal antibodies are directed against different epitopes of the same antigen. MIB-1 is preferred for clinical use (to determine the Ki67 labeling index, L.I.), because of its good performances displayed on formalin-fixed paraffin-embedded tissues. It was shown that mitotic activity is decreased by the delay in fixation so that grading by Ki67 is usually higher than by mitosis [14]. When mitotic count and Ki67 L.I. are discordant, it is recommended to assign the higher grade, but specific data justifying this approach do not exist. Some authors consider Ki67 L.I. a more reliable, reproducible, and valuable prognostic marker [15].

Controversies exist on what to count and on how to make Ki67 count. Only strong dark-brown nuclear staining is recommended by most authors to be counted (Fig. 2.5) [16]. Three Ki67 counting methodologies have been compared in terms of

2

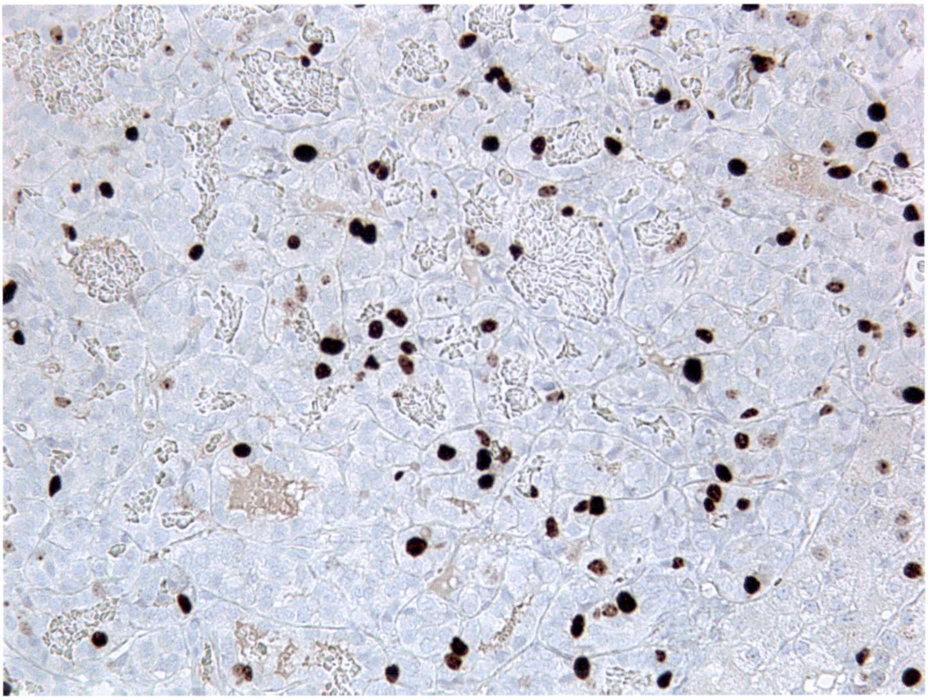

Fig. 2.5 NET G2: Ki67 proliferative index with a 15% L.I. in a hot spot area. 20× magnification

costs, impact on turnaround time, and reproducibility: «eye-balled,» automated counting by image analyzer, manual eye counting (count of Ki67 positive cells/500–2000 tumor cells in a «hot spot» area), and manual count of camera-captured/camera-printed image [17]. In this analysis, camera-captured/camera-printed image resulted in the most practical methodology because of its low cost/benefit ratio and high reproducibility. However, it takes longer than eye balling, which is considered the most unreliable technique.

A relevant issue is that Ki67-LI may vary during the disease course, including from primary to metastasis, from primary to recurrence, or during progression. This evidence needs to be taken into consideration for the decision making of monitoring and treatment [18].

2.1.3 G3 Neuroendocrine Carcinoma (G3-NEC)

G3 NEC are characterized by the presence of large nests or sheets of neoplastic cells with the interposition of «geographic chart» necrosis (Fig. 2.6). They are divided into small- and large-cell subtypes, depending on cell size (small/medium for the former and large for the latter) and cellular morphology (round/oval, sometimes hyperchromatic nuclei with an inconspicuous nucleolus and scant cytoplasm in the former, round nuclei

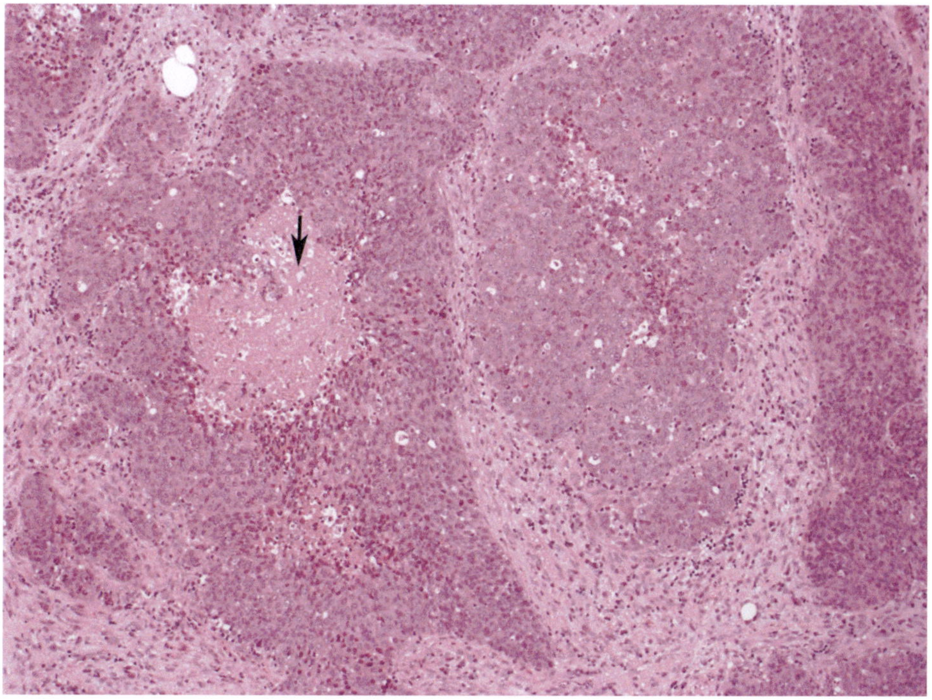

Fig. 2.6 Large-cell NEC: necrosis (*arrow*) is a feature of this neoplasm. Hematoxylin and eosin stain, 20× magnification

with an evident nucleolus and abundant eosinophilic cytoplasm in the latter). Although these peculiar morphologic features, in case of positive neuroendocrine staining, the diagnosis of NEC actually relies on the evidence of high mitotic count (>20/10HPF) and/or high proliferation index (Ki67 > 20%). Accordingly, well- to moderately differentiated tumors with high proliferation rate (mitotic count >20/10 HPF and/or >20% Ki67 index) are included in the group of NEC. Well-differentiated NEC are tumors composed predominantly of cells with minimal pleomorphism and lacking extensive necrosis.

A recent matter of debate is whether dividing or not high-grade NEC into two subgroups on the basis of both morphologic differentiation and proliferation rate. It was shown that well-differentiated NEC had a worse overall survival than NET G2, but they were prognostically better than poorly differentiated NEC [19, 20]. Furthermore, the NORDIC study [21] showed that gastrointestinal-NEC with a Ki67 proliferation index <55% were less responsive to platinum-based chemotherapy.

Given the considerable differences in treatment strategies that are available in the field of pancreatic neuroendocrine neoplasms, some attempts to make the diagnosis of high-grade NEN more accurate have been made [22, 23]. Some authors [22] recommend to make a thorough examination of pathology material, searching for an additional component of lower grade (NET G1 or G2) in the same or in another previous specimen, in order to make a diagnosis of NET G3, i.e., well-differentiated neuroendocrine tumor with high-grade progression. Furthermore, also a diversified molecular profile has been identified for these two categories. Overall, on this regard further studies are needed.

2.1.4 Mixed Forms

In the 2010 WHO classification of tumors of the digestive tract, mixed exocrine-endocrine tumors are called mixed adenoneuroendocrine carcinoma (MANEC); they are tumors composed by a mixture of epithelial (adenocarcinoma or, rarely, squamous cell carcinoma) and neuroendocrine malignancies, with each component representing at least 30% of the lesion. However, in the digestive tract, there is a wide spectrum of combinations of exocrine and endocrine components, ranging from adenoma or carcinoma with interspersed neuroendocrine cells on the one end to classical neuroendocrine tumors with focal exocrine component on the other end [24, 25]. For this reason some authors suggest to replace the term MANEC with MANEN which stands for mixed adenoneuroendocrine neoplasms.

In case of MANEC, it was shown that the predominant tumor component in primary tumor was a prognostic factor and could predict tumor emboli and liver metastases pathology [26]. This finding may be of support in deciding the appropriate treatment strategy [26].

2.1.5 Preneoplastic Lesions

Sequential changes from hyperplasia to neoplasm can be observed in NET, especially in case of familial genetic syndromes. In gastric disease, this sequence is well described. Gastric NETs are categorized into three subtypes: type I, associated with autoimmune chronic atrophic gastritis, involving mainly the corpus-fundus; type II, occurring in MEN1 and Zollinger-Ellison syndrome; and type III, sporadic. Type I and II NET may be preceded by enterochromaffin-like (ECL) cell hyperplasia. In the former the loss of parietal cells, due to the autoimmune reaction against the gastric mucosa, provokes achlorhydria that stimulates antral and duodenal gastrin production. Hypergastrinemia, together with growth factors (TGF-β and b-FGF) and the anti-apoptotic Bcl2 protein, has a trophic effect on ECL cells. In MEN1 hypergastrinemia is caused by gastrin-producing NET [27, 28].

ECL cell hyperplasia refers to the presence of more than five cells/gland, at least two linear chains/mm (linear), or one micronodule less than 150 μm/mm (micronodular) (◘ Fig. 2.7). The enlargement and fusion of micronodules, microinvasion of the lamina propria, or nodules associated with newly formed stroma are features of dysplasia, a high predictor of developing neoplasia [29, 30]. The evidence of invasion of the submucosa or a size larger than 0.5 mm is indicative of neoplasm (microcarcinoid or microtumor in case of nodule < 5 mm).

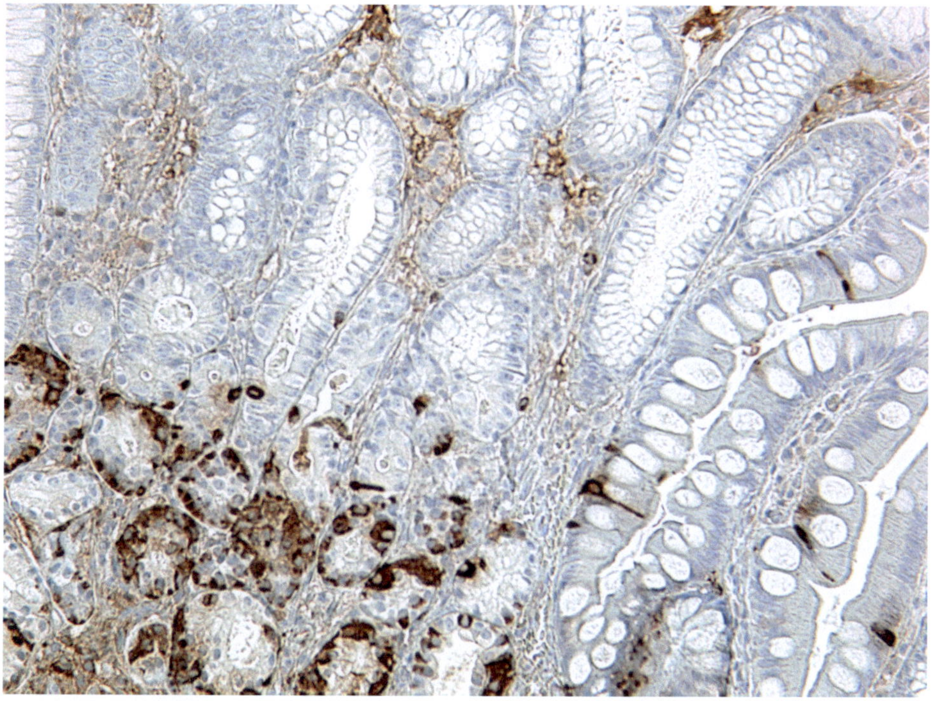

Fig. 2.7 Linear and micronodular ECL cell hyperplasia, highlighted by chromogranin staining. On the right, intestinal metaplasia is present. 20× magnification

2.2 Thoracic Neuroendocrine Tumors (TNET)

2.2.1 Classification and Immunohistochemistry

The new 2015 WHO classification [31] on neuroendocrine neoplasms of the lung and the thymus did not introduce Ki67 as diagnostic criteria. It retained the terminology of carcinoid, respectively, for well- and moderately differentiated neuroendocrine tumors and of large-cell and small-cell neuroendocrine carcinoma for high-grade neuroendocrine neoplasms.

Grading criteria are as follows:

- *Typical carcinoid*: carcinoid morphology and <2 mitoses/ 2mm^2, no necrosis, and ≥0.5 cm (Fig. 2.8).
- *Atypical carcinoid*: carcinoid morphology and 2–10 mitoses/2 mm^2 and/or necrosis (often punctuate) or both.
- *Large-cell neuroendocrine carcinoma*: neuroendocrine morphology (organoid nesting, trabecular growth, rosette-like structures, and peripheral palisading patterns), high mitotic rate (>10 mitoses/2mm^2), necrosis (often in large zones), typical cytology (large-sized cells with vesicular nuclear chromatin and frequent central

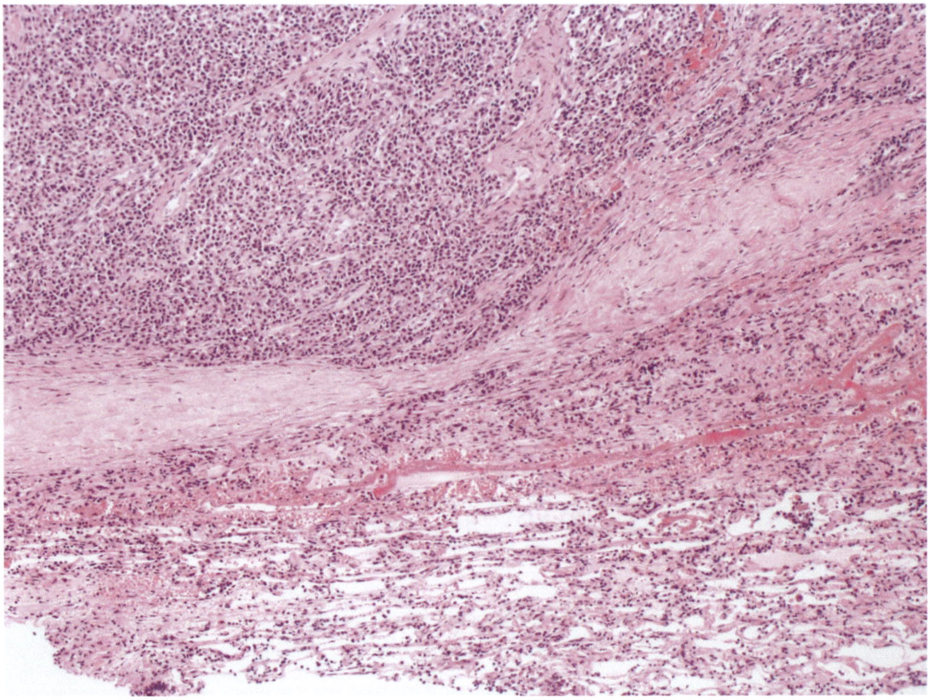

Fig. 2.8 Typical carcinoid of the lung. Hematoxylin and eosin stain, 10× magnification

nucleolus and abundant cytoplasm) (Fig. 2.9), and immunoreactivity for at least one neuroendocrine marker (CD56, chromogranin, synaptophysin) in more than 10% of neoplastic cells.

- *Small-cell neuroendocrine carcinoma*: small-sized cells (less than the diameter of three small lymphocytes), scant cytoplasm, nuclei with granular nuclear chromatin (Fig. 2.10), high mitotic rate (>10 mitoses/2mm^2), and frequent necrosis. Diagnosis may be based only on morphology but immunohistochemistry may be required: they show reactivity to cytokeratins, with either dot-like or diffuse staining pattern, to neuroendocrine markers (CD56 is the most sensitive marker but also less specific so that it should be interpreted in presence of a morphologic context; synaptophysin may diffusely stain; chromogranin A can be focal) [32], and to TTF1 (90–95%) [33]. Negative high-molecular-weight cytokeratins.

This scheme is suitable for surgical specimens.

Since many therapeutic advances [34, 35, 36] have taken place in the lung cancer field, nowadays diagnosis on bioptic tissue needs to be always more accurate. However, in bioptic specimens, neuroendocrine markers (CD56, chromogranin, and/or synaptophysin) are recommended only in case of neuroendocrine morphology. The presence of immunohistochemical neuroendocrine differentiation in cases with adenocarcinoma or squamous cell carcinoma morphology is prognostically and therapeutically irrelevant [37, 38].

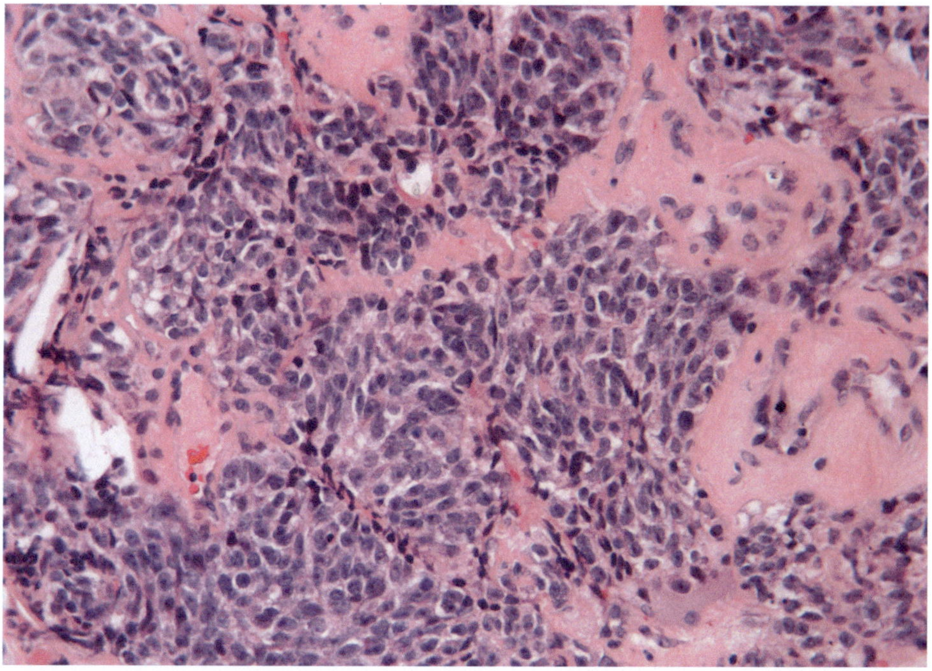

Fig. 2.9 Large-cell NEC of the lung: large-sized cells with vesicular nuclear chromatin and frequent central nucleolus and abundant cytoplasm. Hematoxylin and eosin stain, 20× magnification

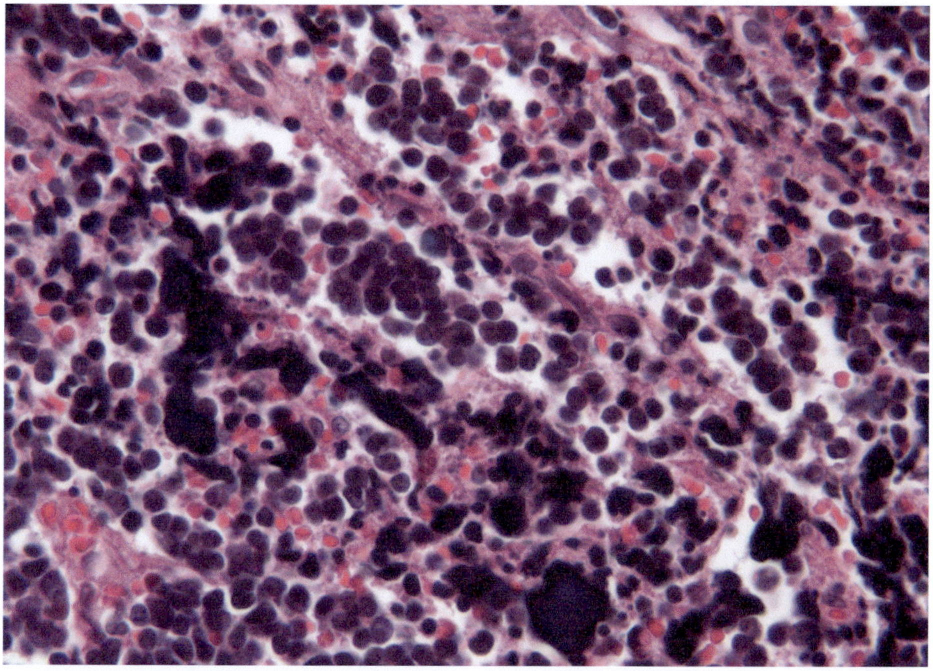

Fig. 2.10 Small-cell NEC of the lung: small-sized cells (less than the diameter of three small lymphocytes), scant cytoplasm, nuclei with granular nuclear chromatin. Hematoxylin and eosin stain, 63× magnification

2.2.2 Grading System

Controversial issues have been raised on the clinical utility of a four-tier classification for pulmonary neuroendocrine neoplasms, because of its poor reproducibility and lack of prognostic efficacy [39]. Furthermore, epidemiologic, clinical, and genetic data [40] favor a three-tier pathology classification scheme (G1–3). Studies have been conducted to define a prognostic grading system [41], based on Ki67 L.I. (with cutoffs specific to this site), mitotic count, and necrosis. Encouraging results have been achieved, but the utility of Ki67 as additional diagnostic parameter in lung NEN was not established. However, Ki67 plays an important role in the differential diagnosis between carcinoid and small-cell carcinoma, in case of crushed biopsies: the former is a low (Ki67 < 5%) while the latter is a high (>50%) [42] proliferating neoplasm.

Lack of reproducibility is mainly due to difficulties encountered in recognizing mitoses and necrosis [43] and great variability observed in assessing cell size [44].

2.2.3 Preneoplastic Lesions

Diffuse idiopathic pulmonary neuroendocrine cell hyperplasia (DIPNECH) is a generalized proliferation of pulmonary neuroendocrine cells. It is a rare condition, usually an incidental radiological finding, or the final evolution of chronic obstructive complaints. The minority of patients with this condition may develop typical and rarely atypical carcinoid, never small-cell carcinoma nor large-cell neuroendocrine carcinoma.

Microscopically, pulmonary neuroendocrine cells may form small groups or a monolayer in the mucosa or they may invade the basal lamina to form tumorlets. The latter are distinguished from small carcinoid tumors because of their irregular, infiltrative margins, a conspicuously fibrotic stroma, and the size ≤5 mm in diameter [45].

2.2.4 Mixed Forms

Neither the typical nor the atypical carcinoid is observed in combination with other neoplasms. Combined small-cell or large-cell neuroendocrine carcinoma is an admixture with non-small-cell components (without indication of percentage), as adenocarcinoma, squamous cell carcinoma, large-cell carcinoma, and, less often, spindle-cell carcinoma or giant-cell carcinoma. A combination of small-cell and large-cell neuroendocrine carcinoma (only if it represents at least 10% of the tumor) can also be observed.

2.3 Neuroendocrine Neoplasms in Rare Sites

The knowledge of neuroendocrine neoplasms in uncommon sites is much less extensive than in gastroenteropancreatic tract and in the thorax. Diagnostic difficulties may arise because of the different morphologies shown in each site [46].

2.3.1 Urinary System and Male Genital Organs

Prostate

In the 2016 WHO classification of tumors of the urinary system and male genital organs [47], a new morphological classification of prostate cancer with neuroendocrine differentiation (NED) has been issued.

Five categories have been identified:

- *Usual prostate adenocarcinoma with NED*, showed by immunohistochemistry (synaptophysin, chromogranin, or CD56). However, the use of neuroendocrine markers in routine diagnostics is not recommended.
- *Adenocarcinoma with Paneth cell-like NED* that is characterized by the presence of cells with eosinophilic cytoplasmic granules expressing neuroendocrine markers. This morphology does not impact on prognosis [48]. Therefore, applying the Gleason score to these foci does not accurately reflect their clinical behavior.
- *Well-differentiated neuroendocrine tumor (carcinoid)*, extremely rare, never associated with concomitant adenocarcinoma of the prostate, immunopositive for neuroendocrine markers, and negative for PSA. All these features allow the differential diagnosis with carcinoid-like adenocarcinoma that behaves like ordinary prostate cancer.
- *Small-cell neuroendocrine carcinoma* that represents the most frequent prostatic NEN and whose classic morphology is identical to its pulmonary counterpart. It may be pure (50–60%) or mixed with prostate acinar adenocarcinoma. An intermediate cell-type variant [49] is contemplated, composed of cells with slightly more open chromatin and visible small nucleoli. On immunohistochemistry it shows positivity to neuroendocrine markers (synaptophysin, chromogranin, and CD56) in 90% of cases, focal to PSA in 17–25% of cases and to TTF1 in >50%. One half of prostatic SCC harbor a TMPRSS2-ERG gene fusion [50]: this may aid in the differential diagnosis with small-cell neuroendocrine carcinoma of other sites.
- *Large-cell neuroendocrine carcinoma*, rare and really aggressive, especially in pure form [51].

Bladder

- *Small-cell neuroendocrine carcinoma*, accounting for <1% of malignant bladder tumors. Almost always invasive at the level of muscularis propria, it can be diagnosed only with morphology and when it represents most of the tumor (it may be combined with a minor component of urothelial or squamous carcinoma, adenocarcinoma, or sarcoma). Reactivity to neuroendocrine markers is not always present (30–100% of cases). The immunophenotype has been extensively studied: cytokeratin 7+ (60%), cytokeratin 20−, uroplakin III−, cytokeratin 34βe12 + (40%), EMA+ (78%), cytokeratin CAM5.2+ (dot-like in 60%), p53 overexpressed (52%), TTF1+ (40%), and c-Kit (40%).
- *Large-cell neuroendocrine carcinoma*, rare and aggressive.
- *Carcinoid*, often presenting as polypoid lesions at cystoscopy. The morphology exhibited is like in other more typical sites. A peculiarity is that it may have a pseudoglandular pattern and may be associated with cystitis cystica and cystitis glandularis.

- *Paraganglioma*, clinically manifesting with the triad of sustained or paroxysmal hypertension, intermittent gross hematuria, and «micturition attacks.» Neoplastic cells (chromogranin A+, synaptophysin+, vimentin+, GATA3+, and cytokeratins-) [52] are arranged in nests (Zellballen), delimited by sustentacular cells (S100+). Malignant forms can be observed in 20% of cases.

Kidney

Neuroendocrine neoplasms of the kidney may span from the well-differentiated to the high-grade form:

- *Small-cell neuroendocrine carcinoma* is believed by some to be derived from metaplastic changes of urothelial high-grade neoplasms [53].
- *Large-cell neuroendocrine carcinoma*: only a few cases have been described [54, 55].
- *Carcinoid and atypical carcinoid*: often associated with renal congenital abnormalities or with metaplasia induced by chronic inflammation [56]. Morphology is almost always like elsewhere. Age > 40 years, size >4 cm, absence of congenital malformations, and Ki67 proliferation index >1% [57] have been identified as possible negative prognostic factors.

Testis

Included in the chapter of «Germ Cell Tumors Unrelated to Germ Cell Neoplasia In Situ,» carcinoids represent the only type of NE neoplasm that is mentioned in the current WHO testicular tumor classification [47]. It can occur as pure primary carcinoid (65–78%), or within a teratoma, or associated with epidermoid or dermoid cysts or as a metastasis (often from ileal tumor). In case of pure carcinoid, the ruling out of a metastatic process (10%) is mandatory, through extensive sampling of the organ, which can also expose any possible residual or stigmata (scar) of a coexisting or previous teratoma. Bilateral involvement, multifocality, vascular invasion, or extratesticular spread argues in favor of a metastasis. Testicular carcinoids are immunoreactive with neuroendocrine markers and keratin cocktails but are negative to CD30, OCT4, CDX2, TTF1, and c-kit.

Atypical carcinoids (with pleomorphism and necrosis and/or 2–10 mitoses/10HPF) are more often associated to metastases [58].

2.3.2 Female Genital Organs

Cervix

In this site the recommended [59] terminology for neuroendocrine neoplasms is similar to that used in the gastrointestinal tract, consisting of low-grade neuroendocrine tumors (grade 1/carcinoid and grade 2/atypical carcinoid) and high-grade neuroendocrine carcinomas (grade 3/small-cell or large-cell neuroendocrine carcinomas).

Low-Grade NET Unlike GEP-NETs, this diagnosis is still based on the degree of nuclear atypia, mitotic activity, and the presence or not of small foci of necrosis. No cutoff for Ki67 has been established.

High-Grade NEC Small-cell NEC is the most prevalent form of neuroendocrine neoplasm in this site. Besides neuroendocrine markers (chromogranin, synaptophysin, and CD56), it usually expresses cytokeratins, carcinoembryonic antigen, EMA, TTF1, and p16 (not specific of cervical primitiveness as HPV) [60]. Large-cell NEC, whose morphology is like elsewhere, can also have focal glandular differentiation [61].

Endometrium

Carcinoid Extremely rare (only two cases reported in literature).

Small-Cell NEC It shows a morphological conformity to other sites, and it may coexist with other high-grade malignancies, conferring a biphasic morphology that can erroneously be mistaken for a carcinosarcoma.

Large-Cell NEC Rare. Evidence of at least two neuroendocrine markers in >20% of neoplastic cells may aid in the differential diagnosis with a poorly differentiated endometrioid adenocarcinoma [62].

Ovary and Fallopian Tubes

Carcinoid is the most frequent ovarian neuroendocrine neoplasm, and it is often associated with teratoma (85%). Four subtypes are recognized (which may be present in combination or combined with other ovarian tumors):

- Insular: the most common (26–53%), composed of small acini or solid nests, arranged within a fibrous stroma, and with dense eosinophilic secretions that can also undergo psammomatous calcification
- Trabecular (23–29%): ribbons and parallel trabeculae of neoplastic cells surrounded by fibrous stroma
- Strumal: similar to the insular type but associated with struma ovarii
- Mucinous: rare (it may be associated with mature cystic teratoma, mucinous adenocarcinoma, mucinous borderline tumor, borderline Brenner tumor, and other carcinoids)

The differential diagnosis with metastasis (mostly from the gastrointestinal tract) is based mainly on clinicopathological features (unilaterality, lack of multinodular growth, early stage, presence of teratomatous elements, and size <3 cm are all elements in favor of a primitive form). Immunohistochemistry is not critical, since CDX2 is expressed in both primary and metastatic ovarian carcinoids. CK20, CK7, TTF1, and PAX8 are variably expressed, considering that the tumor may arise from teratomatous elements [63].

Vagina

High-grade NEC is the only form of neuroendocrine neoplasms that has rarely been described in this site. Small-cell NEC may be associated with both squamous cell carcinoma and adenocarcinoma. A rare form of Merkel cell phenotype [64] has been described. Small-cell variant of squamous cell carcinoma (p63+) and basaloid carcinoma (CK 34βE12 +) are two possible differential diagnoses. Extremely rare is paraganglioma [65].

Vulva

Most of vulvar neuroendocrine neoplasms are Merkel cell carcinomas. A diagnostic feature is the detection of a CK20 dot-like immunoreactivity [66].

2.3.3 Breast

NEC is a special histotype of breast cancer, with the same morphology observed elsewhere and the evidence of expression of neuroendocrine markers in more than 50% of neoplastic cells. Three entities have been identified [67]:

- *NET*, well differentiated: the exclusion of the possibility of a metastasis is essential before any other diagnostic hypotheses; carcinoid from gastrointestinal site (CDX2+) metastatic to the breast is common in both men and women [68].
- *NEC*, poorly differentiated/small-cell neuroendocrine carcinoma: the coexistence of an in situ component and a strong expression of estrogen receptor (ER) may aid in the diagnosis of primitiveness. They usually display reactivity to ER, progesterone receptor (PR), GCDFP15, CK7, Cam 5.2, bcl-2, and E-cadherin [69] and are negative to Her2. Small-cell carcinomas of the breast may be TTF1 positive (20% of cases) [70], and ER and PR may be expressed in pulmonary NET [71]. Rarely, there may be coincidental focal squamous differentiation [72].
- Invasive breast carcinoma with *NED*: up to 30% of non-special-type carcinomas of the breast and in two special-type carcinomas (mucinous, hypercellular variant, and solid papillary, in both the invasive and in situ components).

2.3.4 Head and Neck

Sinonasal Cavities

According to the 2005 WHO [73] classification of tumors of the sinonasal cavities, four main categories of neuroendocrine neoplasms may be identified: typical and atypical carcinoids, small-cell carcinoma, and NEC not otherwise specified (NEC-NOS). Its differential diagnosis is first of all with sinonasal undifferentiated carcinoma (SNUC) and then with all neoplasms expressing neuroendocrine markers (olfactory neuroblastoma, paraganglioma, pituitary adenoma, or metastases) [46].

Larynx

Matter of debate is the existence of large-cell neuroendocrine carcinoma in the larynx. The current WHO classification system categorizes neuroendocrine neoplasms into typical and atypical carcinoid, small-cell carcinoma/neuroendocrine type, combined small-cell carcinoma (with adenocarcinoma, squamous cell carcinoma, etc.), and paraganglioma. Therefore, cases showing >10 mitoses/10 HPF and prominent necrosis are diagnosed as atypical carcinoids, at most as moderately differentiated NEC, a variant of atypical carcinoid. Furthermore, the latter is more aggressive (5-year survival rate of 48%) than the pulmonary counterpart (5-year survival rate of 58%), probably because of those cases that should be classified as large-cell NEC of the larynx [74]. Morphology and clinical data are essential in making this diagnosis. Immunohistochemistry is of little aid: neither CK7, TTF1, nor calcitonin (often positive) is useful in the differential diagnosis with a metastasis from lung or thyroid.

Middle Ear

In this site the term adenoma and carcinoid may be used interchangeably. This is a tumor with mixed exocrine and neuroendocrine components. It may show glandular, trabecular, solid, infiltrating, or organoid pattern. Its immunophenotype consists of reactivity to CK7, CK5/6, chromogranin, synaptophysin, and p63. Negative is smooth muscle actin. S100 protein has been rarely reported [75]. The main differential diagnosis is with paraganglioma (CK- and S100+ sustentacular cells).

2.3.5 Skin

Merkel cell carcinoma is the term used for a cutaneous carcinoma expressing neuroendocrine markers and showing aggressive behavior. It may also be found as a nodal primary (often in inguinal lymph nodes). Ultraviolet light exposure and polyomavirus have been shown as etiological factors [76–78].

Dot-like immunohistochemical reactivity to CK20 is a diagnostic feature. Prognostic accuracy is improved by lymph node examination because of the treatment implications of microscopic nodal involvement [79].

Bibliography

1. Guadagno E, Del Basso De Caro M, Insabato L (2016) An update on the pathology of neuroendocrine tumors. Front Biosci (Scholar Ed) 8:1–12
2. Kim JY, Hong SM (2016) Recent updates on neuroendocrine Tumors from the gastrointestinal and Pancreatobiliary tracts. Arch Pathol Lab Med 140:437–448
3. Rindi G, Arnold R, Bosman FT, Capella C, Klimstra DS, Kloppel G, Komminoth P, Solcia E (2010) In: Bosman FT, Carneiro F, Hruban H et al (eds) Nomenclature and classification of neuroendocrine neoplasms of the digestive system. In: WHO classification of tumors of the digestive system. IARC Press, Lyon
4. Janson ET, Sorbye H, Welin S et al (2014) Nordic guidelines 2014 for diagnosis and treatment of gastroenteropancreatic neuroendocrine neoplasms. Acta Oncol 53:1284–1297
5. Koo J, Dhall D (2015) Problems with the diagnosis of metastatic neuroendocrine neoplasms. Which diagnostic criteria should we use to determine tumor origin and help guide therapy? Semin Diagn Pathol 32:456–468
6. Saqi A, Alexis D, Remotti F et al (2005) Usefulness of CDX2 and TTF-1 in differentiating gastrointestinal from pulmonary carcinoids. Am J Clin Pathol 123:394–404
7. Srivastava A, Hornick JL (2009) Immunohistochemical staining for CDX-2, PDX-1, NESP-55, and TTF-1 can help distinguish gastrointestinal carcinoid tumors from pancreatic endocrine and pulmonary carcinoid tumors. Am J Surg Pathol 33:626–632
8. Deshpande V, Fernandez-del Castillo C, Muzikansky A et al (2004) Cytokeratin 19 is a powerful predictor of survival in pancreatic endocrine tumors. Am J Surg Pathol 28:1145–1153
9. Viale G, Doglioni C, Gambacorta M et al (1992) Progesterone receptor immunoreactivity in pancreatic endocrine tumors. An immunocytochemical study of 156 neuroendocrine tumors of the pancreas, gastrointestinal and respiratory tracts, and skin. Cancer 70:2268–2277

10. Schmitt AM, Riniker F, Anlauf M et al (2008) Islet 1 (Isl1) expression is a reliable marker for pancreatic endocrine tumors and their metastases. Am J Surg Pathol 32:420–425
11. Koo J, Mertens RB, Mirocha JM et al (2012) Value of islet 1 and PAX8 in identifying metastatic neuroendocrine tumors of pancreatic origin. Mod Pathol 25:893–901
12. Bellizzi AM (2013) Assigning site of origin in metastatic neuroendocrine neoplasms: a clinically significant application of diagnostic immunohistochemistry. Adv Anat Pathol 20:285–314
13. Voss SM, Riley MP, Lokhandwala PM et al (2015) Mitotic count by phosphohistone H3 immunohistochemical staining predicts survivaland improves interobserver reproducibility in well-differentiated neuroendocrine tumors of the pancreas. Am J Surg Pathol 39:13–24
14. Cross SS, Start RD, Smith JH (1990) Does delay in fixation affect the number of mitotic figures in processed tissue? J Clin Pathol 43:597–599
15. McCall CM, Shi C, Cornish TC et al (2013) Grading of well-differentiated pancreatic neuroendocrine tumors is improved by the inclusion of both Ki67 proliferative index and mitotic rate. Am J Surg Pathol 37:1671–1677
16. Reid MD, Balci S, Saka B et al (2014) Neuroendocrine tumors of the pancreas: current concepts and controversies. Endocr Pathol 25:65–79
17. Reid MD, Bagci P, Ohike N et al (2016) Calculation of the Ki67 index in pancreatic neuroendocrine tumors: a comparativeanalysis of four counting methodologies. Mod Pathol 29:93
18. Singh S, Hallet J, Rowsell C et al (2014) Variability of Ki67 labeling index in multiple neuroendocrine tumors specimens over the course of the disease. Eur J Surg Oncol 40:1517–1522
19. Vélayoudom-Céphise FL, Duvillard P, Foucan L et al (2013) Are G3 ENETS Neuroendocrine neoplasms heterogeneous? Endocr Relat Cancer 20:649–657
20. Basturk O, Yang Z, Tang LH et al (2015) The high-grade (WHO G3) pancreatic neuroendocrine tumor category is morphologically and biologically heterogenous and includes both well differentiated and poorly differentiated neoplasms. Am J Surg Pathol 39:683–690
21. Sorbye H, Welin S, Langer SW et al (2013) Predictive and prognostic factors for treatment and survival in 305 patients with advanced gastrointestinal neuroendocrine carcinoma (WHO G3): the NORDIC NEC study. Ann Oncol 24:152–160
22. Tang LH, Basturk O, Sue JJ et al (2016) A practical approach to the classification of WHO grade 3 (G3) well-differentiated neuroendocrine tumor (WD-NET) and poorly differentiated neuroendocrine carcinoma (PD-NEC) of the pancreas. Am J Surg Pathol 40:1192–1202
23. Hijioka S, Hosoda W, Mizuno N et al (2015) Does the WHO 2010 classification of pancreatic neuroendocrine neoplasms accurately characterize pancreatic neuroendocrine carcinomas? J Gastroenterol 50:564–572
24. Volante M, Rindi G, Papotti M (2006) The grey zone between pure (neuro)endocrine and non(neuro) endocrine tumours: a comment on concepts and classification of mixed exocrine-endocrine neoplasms. Virchows Arch 449:499–506
25. La Rosa S, Marando A, Sessa F et al (2012) Mixed Adenoneuroendocrine carcinomas (MANECs) of the gastrointestinal tract: An Update. Cancers (Basel) 4:11–30
26. Chen MH, Kuo YJ, Yeh YC et al (2015) High neuroendocrine component is a factor for poor prognosis in gastrointestinal high-grade malignant mixed adenoneuroendocrine neoplasms. J Chin Med Assoc 78:454–459
27. Delle Fave G, Marignani M, Corleto VD et al (2002) Progression of gastric enterochromaffin-like cells growth in Zollinger-Ellison syndrome and atrophic body gastritis patients. Dig Liver Dis 34:270–278
28. Klöppel G, Anlauf M, Perren A (2007) Endocrine precursor lesions of gastroenteropancreatic neuroendocrine tumors. Endocr Pathol 18:150–155
29. Annibale B, Azzoni C, Corleto VD et al (2001) Atrophic body gastritis patients with enterochromaffin-like cell dysplasia are at increased risk for the development of type I gastric carcinoid. Eur J Gastroenterol Hepatol 13:1449–1456
30. Vanoli A, La Rosa S, Luinetti O et al (2013) Histologic changes in type a chronic atrophic gastritis indicating increased risk of neuroendocrine tumor development: the predictive role of dysplastic and severely hyperplastic enterochromaffin-like cell lesions. HumPathol 44:1827–1837
31. Brambilla E, Beasley MB, Austin JHM et al (2015) Neuroendocrine tumours. In: WHO classification of tumors of the lung, pleura, thymus and heart. Eds: Travis WD, Brambilla E, burke AP et al. IARC Press, Lyon

32. Wick MR (2000) Immunohistology of neuroendocrine and neuroectodermal tumors. Semin Diagn Pathol 17:194–203
33. Sturm N, Rossi G, Lantuejoul S et al (2002) Expression of thyroid transcription factor-1 in the spectrum of neuroendocrine cell lung proliferations with special interest in carcinoids. Hum Pathol 33:175–182
34. Mitsudomi T, Morita S, Yatabe Y et al (2010) Gefitinib versus cisplatin plus docetaxel in patients with non-small-cell lung cancer harbouring mutations of the epidermal growth factor receptor (WJTOG3405): an open label, randomised phase 3 trial. Lancet Oncol 11:121–128
35. Mok TS, Wu YL, Thongprasert S et al (2009) Gefitinib or carboplatin-paclitaxel in pulmonary adenocarcinoma. N Engl J Med 361:947–957
36. Rosell R, Carcereny E, Gervais R et al (2012) Erlotinib versus standard chemotherapy as first-line treatment for European patients with advanced EGFR mutation-positive non-small-cell lung cancer (EURTAC): a multicentre, open-label, randomised phase 3 trial. Lancet Oncol 13:239–246
37. Travis WD, Brambilla E, Noguchi M et al (2013) Diagnosis of lung cancer in small biopsies and cytology: implications of the 2011 International Association for the Study of Lung Cancer/American Thoracic Society/European Respiratory Society classification. Arch Pathol Lab Med 137: 668–684
38. Ionescu DN, Treaba D, Gilks CB et al (2007) Nonsmall cell lung carcinoma with neuroendocrine differentiation--an entity of no clinical or prognostic significance. Am J Surg Pathol 31:26–32
39. Sterlacci W, Fiegl M, Hilbe W et al (2009) Clinical relevance of neuroendocrine differentiation in non-small cell lung cancer assessed by immunohistochemistry: a retrospective study on 405 surgically resected cases. Virchows Arch 455:125–132
40. Asamura H, Kameya T, Matsuno Y et al (2006) Neuroendocrine neoplasms of the lung: a prognostic spectrum. J Clin Oncol 24:70–76
41. Pelosi G, Hiroshima K, Mino-Kenudson M (2014) Controversial issues and new discoveries in lung neuroendocrine tumors. Diagn Histopathol 20:392–397
42. Rindi G, Klersy C, Inzani F et al (2013) Grading the neuroendocrine tumors of the lung: an evidence-based proposal. Endocr Relat Cancer 21:1–16
43. Pelosi G, Rodriguez J, Viale G (2005) Typical and atypical pulmonary carcinoid tumor overdiagnosed as small-cell carcinoma on biopsy specimens: a major pitfall in the management of lung cancer patients. Am J Surg Pathol 29:179–187
44. Ha SY, Han J, Kim WS et al (2012) Interobserver variability in diagnosing high-grade neuroendocrine carcinoma of the lung and comparing it with the morphometric analysis. Korean J Pathol 46:42–47
45. Rizvi SM, Goodwill J, Lim E et al (2009) The frequency of neuroendocrine cell hyperplasia in patients with pulmonary neuroendocrine tumours and non-neuroendocrine cell carcinomas. Histopathology 55:332–337
46. Guadagno E, De Rosa G, Del Basso De Caro M (2016) Neuroendocrine tumours in rare sites: differences in nomenclatureand diagnostics-arare and ubiquitous histotype. J Clin Pathol 69: 563–574
47. Epstein JI, Amin MB, Evans AJ et al (2016) Tumours of the prostate. Neuroendocrine tumours. In: Moch H, Humphrey PA, Ulbright TM et al (eds) WHO classification of tumours of the urinary system and male genital organs. IARC press, Lyon
48. Tamas EF, Epstein JI (2006) Prognostic significance of paneth cell-like neuroendocrine differentiation in adenocarcinoma of the prostate. Am J Surg Pathol 30:980–985
49. Wang W, Epstein JI (2008) Small cell carcinoma of the prostate. A morphologic and immunohistochemical study of 95 cases. Am J Surg Pathol 32:65–71
50. Guo CC, Dancer JY, Wang Y et al (2011) TMPRSS2-ERG gene fusion in small cell carcinoma of the prostate. Hum Pathol 42:11–17
51. Evans AJ, Humphrey PA, Belani J et al (2006) Large cell neuroendocrine carcinoma of prostate: a clinicopathologic summary of 7 cases of a rare manifestation of advanced prostate cancer. Am J Surg Pathol 30:684–693
52. So JS, Epstein JI (2013) GATA3 expression in paragangliomas: a pitfall potentially leading to misdiagnosis of urothelial carcinoma. Mod Pathol 26:1365–1370

53. La Rosa S, Bernasconi B, Micello D et al (2009) Primary small cell neuroendocrine carcinoma of the kidney: morphological, immunohistochemical, ultrastructural, and cytogenetic study of a case and review of the literature. Endocr Pathol 20:24–34
54. Lane BR, Chery F, Jour G et al (2007) Renal neuroendocrine tumours: a clinicopathological study. BJU Int 100:1030–1035
55. Wann C, John NT, Kumar RM (2014) Primary renal large cell neuroendocrine carcinoma in a young man. J Clin Diagn Res 8:ND08–ND09
56. Romero FR, Rais-Bahrami S, Permpongkosol S et al (2006) Primary carcinoid tumors of the kidney. J Urol 176:2359–2366
57. Aung PP, Killian K, Poropatich CO et al (2013) Primary neuroendocrine tumors of the kidney: morphological and molecular alterations of an uncommon malignancy. Hum Pathol 44:873–880
58. Reyes A, Moran CA, Suster S et al (2003) Neuroendocrine carcinomas (carcinoid tumor) ofthe testis. A clinicopathologic and immunohistochemical study of ten cases. Am J Clin Pathol 120:182–187
59. Colgan TJ, Kim I, Hirschowitz L et al (2014) Neuroendocrine tumors. In: Kurman RJ, Carcangiu ML, Herrington CS et al (eds) WHO classification of tumors of the female reproductive organs, 4th edn. IARC Press, Lyon, pp 196–198
60. Ishida GM, Kato N, Hayasaka T et al (2004) Small cell neuroendocrine carcinomas of the uterine cervix: a histological, immunohistochemical, and molecular-genetic study. Int J Gynecol Pathol 23:366–372
61. Cui S, Lespinasse P, Cracchiolo B et al (2001) Large cell neuroendocrine carcinoma of the cervix associated with adenocarcinoma in situ: evidence of a common origin. Int J Gynecol Pathol 20: 311–312
62. Bartosch C, Manuel Lopes J, Oliva E (2011) Endometrial carcinomas: a review emphasizing overlapping and distinctive morphological and immunohistochemical features. Adv Anat Pathol 18: 415–437
63. Chun YK (2015) Neuroendocrine Tumors of the female reproductive tract: a literature review. J Pathol Transl Med 49:450–461
64. Khurana A, Gupta G, Gupta M et al (2013) Primary neuroendocrine carcinoma of the vagina with coexistent atypical vaginal adenosis: a rare entity. J Cancer Res Ther 9:328–330
65. Cai T, Li Y, Jiang Q et al (2014) Paraganglioma of the vagina: a case report and review of the literature. Onco Targets Ther 7:965–968
66. Hierro I, Blanes A, Matilla A et al (2000) Merkel cell (neuroendocrine) carcinoma of the vulva. A case report with immunohistochemical and ultrastructural findings and review of the literature. Pathol Res Pract 196:503–509
67. Bussolati G, Badve S (2012) Carcinomas with neuroendocrine features. In: Lakhani SR, Ellis IO, Schnitt SJ et al (eds) World Health Organization classification of tumours of the breast. IARC Press, Lyon, pp 62–63
68. O'Donnell ME, McCavert M, Carson J et al (2009) Non-epithelial malignancies and metastatic tumours of the breast. Ulster Med J 78:105–112
69. Shin SJ, DeLellis RA, Ying L et al (2000) Small cell carcinoma of the breast: a clinicopathologic and immunohistochemical study of nine patients. Am J Surg Pathol 24:1231–1238
70. Christie M, Chin-Lenn L, Watts MM et al (2010) Primary small cell carcinoma of the breast with TTF-1 and neuroendocrine marker expressing carcinoma in situ. Int J Clin Exp Pathol 3:629–633
71. Sica G, Wagner PL, Altorki N et al (2008) Immunohistochemical expression of estrogenand progesterone receptors in primary pulmonary neuroendocrine tumors. Arch Pathol Lab Med 132: 1889–1895
72. Mečiarová I, Sojáková M, Mego M et al (2016) High-grade neuroendocrine carcinoma of the breast With Focal squamous differentiation. Int J Surg Pathol. pii: 1066896916656444
73. Perez-Ordonez B (2005) Neuroendocrine tumors. In: Barnes L, Eveson JW, Reichart P et al (eds) World Health Organization classification of tumours. Pathology angenetics. Head and neck tumours. IARC Press, Lyon, pp 26–27
74. Lewis JS, Spence DC, Chiosea S et al (2010) Large cell neuroendocrine carcinoma of the larynx: definition of an entity. Head Neck Pathol 4:198–207
75. Torske KR, Thompson LD (2002) Adenoma versus carcinoid tumor of the middle ear: a study of 48 cases and review of the literature. Mod Pathol 15:543–555

76. Feng H, Shuda M, Chang Y, Moore PS (2008) Clonal integration of a polyomavirus in human Merkel cell carcinoma. Science 319:1096–1100
77. Mogha A, Fautrel A, Mouchet N, Guo N, Corre S, Adamski H, Watier E, Misery L, Galibert MD (2010) Merkel cell polyomavirus small T antigen mRNA level is increased following *in vivo* UV-radiation. PLoS One 5(7):e11423
78. Moshiri AS, Nghiem P (2014) Milestones in the staging, classification, and biology of Merkel cell carcinoma. J Natl Compr Cancer Netw 12:1255–1262
79. Lemos BD, Storer BE, Iyer JG, Phillips JL, Bichakjian CK, Fang LC, Johnson TM, Liegeois-Kwon NJ, Otley CC, Paulson KG, Ross MI, Yu SS, Zeitouni NC, Byrd DR, Sondak VK, Gershenwald JE, Sober AJ, Nghiem P (2010) Pathologic nodal evaluation improves prognostic accuracy in Merkel cell carcinoma: analysis of 5823 cases as the basis of the first consensus staging system. J Am Acad Dermatol 63:751–756

The Molecular Biology of NET: Current Status and Evaluation of Biomarkers for Prediction and Prognosis

Mark Kidd, Diego Ferone, Manuela Albertelli, Elena Nazzari, Lisa Bodei, and Irvin M. Modlin

A. Colao et al. (eds.), *Neuroendocrine Tumors in Real Life*,
https://doi.org/10.1007/978-3-319-59024-0_3

3

Overview

Neuroendocrine neoplasms (NEN) represent a heterogeneous group of neoplasia that are ubiquitous in location, exhibit protean symptomatology, and have ill-defined pathobiology. Clinical challenges include but are not limited to the general inability to establish an early diagnosis as well as the lack of a predictably effective management strategy. While clinical guidelines are useful and serve as a template for consensus-based thought, there is a paucity of scientific and mechanistic data necessary to accurately guide optimal management.

The most relevant criteria for prognostic stratification include differentiation and proliferation-based grading, according to the 2010 WHO classification of the digestive system and 2015 WHO for thoracic tumors. Differentiation allows the identification of two distinct prognostic groups: well-differentiated (WD, also named neuroendocrine tumors, NETs) and poorly differentiated (PD, known as neuroendocrine carcinoma, NEC) neoplasms. The outcome (survival – either short-term progression or longer term demise) depends on the cell of origin, the organ of origin, histopathological grading, and the variety of treatment protocols including surgery, that have been undertaken. These, for the most part, represent descriptive criteria since little is known of the molecular biology of the neoplasia.

The mechanisms of tumor development remain unidentified as are the potential drivers of the mutational phenotype. While factors that influence proliferation (e.g., TGFβ, EGF, and somatostatin) and angiogenesis (e.g., VEGF) have been identified, the mechanisms underlying metastasis and target organ tropism remain to be demarcated. Delineation of the somatostatin pathway has driven the development of diagnostics using somatostatin receptor-targeted imaging (either [111]Indium-Octreoscan or [68] Gallium-SSA-PET). Therapies have also evolved via targeting somatostatin receptors with drugs or isotopes (peptide receptor radiotherapy). Genomic and molecular biological analyses have, however, been less enlightening. Activating mutations are rarely identified and NEN disease is a tumor suppressor-driven disease. Epigenetic modifications frequently occur particularly in bronchopulmonary and pancreatic NETs. Most promising is the strategy of transcriptional profiling and network-based analyses to define the cellular toolkit and identify how a normal cell may transform, proliferate, and metastasize. Such techniques have also recently been leveraged for the development of multianalyte diagnostic tools which have facilitated more accurate molecular pathologic delineations of neuroendocrine disease.

Current knowledge of the molecular topography of neuroendocrine neoplasia is limited and represents a vast dark room illuminated by random lights – some of which are only reflections. Elucidation of the molecular machinery of NETs is inseparable from any possibility of rational or meaningful progress in the management of this disease.

3.1 Introduction

NENs represent numerous different tumors whose only commonality is their neuroendocrine cellular origin (◘ Table 3.1) [1–9]. Anatomically these lesions arise from diverse neuroendocrine cells which comprise the diffuse neuroendocrine system of the lungs,

Table 3.1 Heterogeneity and diversity in neuroendocrine neoplasms

Tumor	Putative cell of origin	Localization	Secretory products	Secretory regulation	Proliferative regulation	Omics-based analyses	Mutations
Bronchopulmonary	Clara or Kulchitsky cell	Bronchial epithelia	Serotonin	–	–	Transcriptome, LOH, exome, miRNome	*ARID1*, *PSIP1*
Small intestinal NEN	Enterochromaffin (EC)	Entire GI tract	Serotonin, substance P, guanylin, melatonin	Immune (e.g., IL1β), mechanical (e.g., ATP), neural (e.g., adrenaline) Somatostatin (PKA, MAPK)	TGFβ, EGFR (RAS/RAF/MAPK, GL1/snail)	Transcriptome, LOH, exome, miRNome	*CDKN1B*
Nonfunctional pancreatic	Precursor (ductal) cell or omnipotent stem cell	Pancreas	None defined	Calcium-dependent	Growth factors (e.g., VEGF) PI_3K, AKT, mTOR	Transcriptome, LOH, Exome, miRNome	*MEN-1*, *DAXX*, *ATRX*
Colorectal NEN	L, EC	Colon - rectum	GLP-1, PYY, NPY	Nutrient sensing[a]	EC: ATM	EC: Transcriptome, LOH, Exome, miRNome	–
ECLoma (types I-III)	Enterochromaffin-like (ECL)	Gastric fundus	Histamine	Gastrin, muscarinic, vagal (PI_3K/DAG/Calcium signaling) Somatostatin	Gastrin, PACAP, histamine, EGFR (MAPK)	Transcriptome, LOH	None (type II: *MEN-1*)

(continued)

Table 3.1 (continued)

Tumor	Putative cell of origin	Localization	Secretory products	Secretory regulation	Proliferative regulation	Omics-based analyses	Mutations
Gastrinoma	Gastrin (G)	Gastric antrum and duodenum, pancreas	Gastrin	Environmental (amino acids, tastants, calcium, pH), mechanical, vagal, (PKA, MAPK, calcium signaling) Somatostatin	IGF-1	Transcriptome, LOH	*MEN-1*
CCKoma	I	Duodenum	CCK	Environmental (amino and fatty acids), vagal	–	–	–
GIPoma	K	Duodenum, jejunum	GIP	Nutrient sensing[a]	–	–	–
Insulinoma	Beta	Pancreas	Insulin	GIP, GLP-1, Leptin, Somatostatin (depolarization calcium)	mTOR	Transcriptome, LOH, exome	*YY1*
Glucagonoma	Alpha	Pancreas	Glucagon	GIP, GLP-1, Somatostatin (depolarization calcium)	–	Transcriptome, LOH	*MEN-1*

Somatostatinoma	Delta	Pancreas	Somatostatin	–	Src Family kinases PI_3K-mTOR, MEK	–	*NF-1*
Somatostatinoma	Delta (D)	Duodenum	Somatostatin	–	Src Family kinases PI_3K-mTOR, MEK	–	–
Ghrelinoma	Ghrelin (gr)	Entire GI tract	Ghrelin	β1-adrenergic receptor	–	–	–
PPoma	Pancreatic polypeptide (PP)	Pancreas	PP	–	–	–	–
VIPoma	Vasoactive intestinal peptide (VIP)	Entire GI tract (pancreas, adrenal)	VIP	–	–	–	–

CCK cholecystokinin, *GIP* gastric inhibitory peptide, *GLP-1* glucagon-like peptide 1, *PYY* polypeptide YY (tyrosine, tyrosine), *NPY* neuropeptide Y (tyrosine), *PP* pancreatic polypeptide, *LOH* loss of heterozygosity, *ATM* ataxia telangiectasia-mutated kinase, *YY1* Yin Yang 1 transcriptional repressor

— No data

[a]Signaling pathways associated with nutrient sensing are poorly characterized

gastrointestinal tract, and pancreas. Functionally, each may produce a variety of biologically active amines and peptides. Clinical presentation depends on the site of the primary tumor and functionality which reflects the spectrum of bioactive agents produced by an individual lesion.

Archaic classifications have simplistically grouped NENs into nonfunctioning tumors (no hormone-related clinical features) and functioning tumors, which exhibit symptomatology referable to the production of bioactive agents (amines/peptides). Although functioning tumors cause distinct clinical syndromes, individual symptoms are often not recognized as syndromic of a disease [10]. Moreover, most NENs are nonfunctioning and present features that may include nonspecific symptoms of mass effect, such as pain (which may be intermittent and present for many years) due to local tumor invasion. In the gut, bowel obstruction, nausea, and vomiting, anemia due to blood loss occur while in the bronchopulmonary system cough, hemoptysis, or recurrent pneumonitis are prevalent [10]. It is uncommon and often a late feature of the disease for all these symptoms to be present. Conversely, nonfunctioning NENs are usually asymptomatic. As a consequence of the protean symptomatology, the often paroxysmal nature of the symptomatology and the confusion with prosaic complaints the diagnosis may be often delayed (5–7 years on average) with a consequent increase in synchronous or metachronous metastatic disease.

Diagnosis occurs at an advanced stage, with distant metastases (usually hepatic) in about 50–85% of patients [10–12]. A high index of suspicion is needed to identify patients, and diagnosis is often made as an incidental finding at surgery or during radiological assessment. At a genesis level, very little is known in regard to transformation and the genetics thereof. Given the data regarding germline mutations in tumor suppressor genes (MEN-1, VHL, NF2-kindred) and the alterations at the same gene loci in sporadic NETs of thoracic and pancreatic NETs, a two-hit etiology may be presumed. Nothing is known regarding tumors at other sites or the mechanisms that drive a second hit. In addition, very little is known about the role of environmental factors, except perhaps achlorhydria and gastrin overproduction. The molecular basis by which transformation from a naïve cell type to a neoplastic phenotype occurs is a key unresolved issue [13]. Proliferation also differs in each system, and tumor behavior can range from almost complete indolence to unregulated growth with aggressive invasion and metastases to different sites including liver and bone. While a variety of proliferative regulatory systems have been defined, somatostatin receptors currently appear to be only receptors that may exhibit some degree of proliferative inhibition irrespective of tumor type. The degree of proliferative regulation varies considerably, is not predictable pretreatment, and is most effective in well-differentiated lesions [14, 15]. Tumors are highly vascularized, and activation of angiogenesis, typically through expression of factors like VEGF, is another common feature. The mechanisms driving vascular remodeling are shared with other neoplasia and reflect standard hypoxia-related volumetric adaptive events [16]. Metastasis, as a component of the natural history of NET, is poorly understood. Although it is often related to size, this paradigm is not invariant since 50% of small bowel NET exhibit liver metastases even when they are <1 cm in size. The basis of the initiation and maintenance of metastatic disease remains to be defined. It is almost certain that such a propensity needs to be defined in terms of not only the tumor itself, but also components of the neoplastic microenvironment, particularly the immune system [17]. Nevertheless, it is apparent that tumors (even at the same site) are not biologically equal and have different propensities and abilities to metastasize. While the liver is the most common metastatic receptor organ, a subset ~20% of tumors also metastasize to bone and lungs [18]. The molecular mechanisms that define whether a metastatic cell will display a particular liver, lung or bone tropism remain to be defined.

3.2 Genesis, Proliferation, Angiogenesis, and Metastasis

A. *Genesis*: At a cellular level, NETs are generally thought to represent a malignant transformation of either a terminally differentiated neuroendocrine cell or a precursor/stem cell. The mechanism of these events is largely unknown. At a genetic level, activating mutations are infrequent or largely unknown, in NETs [19]. Most neuroendocrine neoplasms arise in a sporadic manner. It is postulated that damage to early, neuroendocrine precursor cell types leads to the development of higher grade or poorly differentiated neuroendocrine carcinomas (NECs). More well-differentiated, lower grade tumors are considered to develop from later stage or partially differentiated cells (◘ Fig. 3.1).

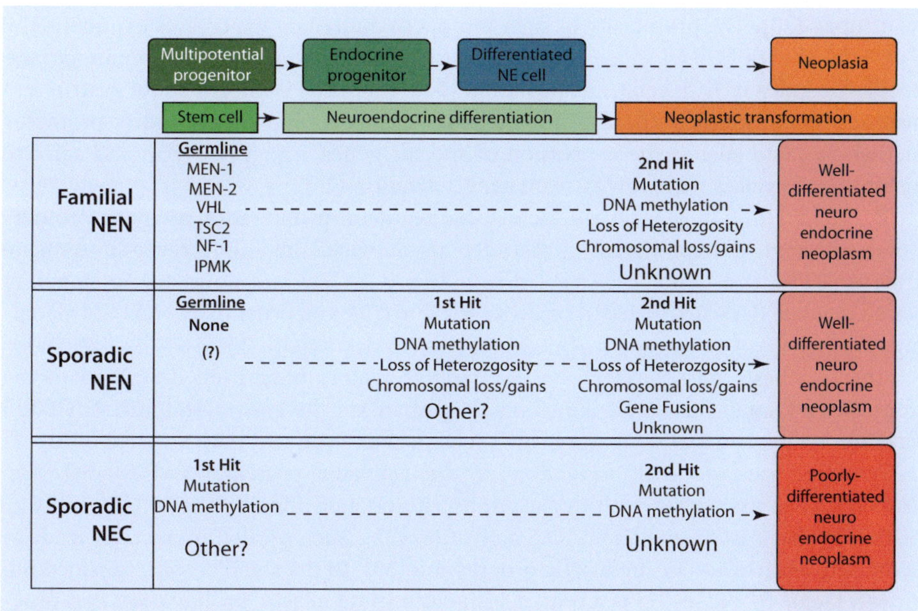

◘ **Fig. 3.1** Etiopathogenesis of NEN. Putative transformative events leading to the development of neuroendocrine neoplasia. Well-differentiated NETs develop in inherited/familiar tumors of the stomach and pancreas (gastric Type II, pancreatic NETs, lung [all MEN-1-related]) as a consequence of either a second hit – perhaps due to a second mutation or loss of expression through methylation (e.g., loss of ARID/SPIP at a promoter site or chromosomal losses. Somatic mutation-related tumors, the most common type, likely occur due to environmentally mediated damage at a committed neuroendocrine precursor stage. A second hit is required that may involve DNA methylation changes due to alterations in the epigenome. The specific timing when this occurs, either during neuroendocrine differentiation or once a cell is terminally committed to a neuroendocrine phenotype, is not currently known. It is postulated that if damage occurs at an early stage, e.g., in a multipotential progenitor [135], poorly differentiated neuroendocrine carcinomas are the consequence. The latter tumors exhibit a completely different genetic etiopathogenesis to well-differentiated neoplasia. «Other» refers to an as yet undefined molecular biological mechanism(s).

The mechanisms for «damage» are not known but are considered sufficient as a second hit or spontaneous mutation/loss of heterozygosity in critical genes, e.g., germline MEN1 [20]. The reasons why only certain sites develop tumors, e.g., lung and pancreas, despite a germline mutation suggest either the existence of exogenous causative factors or an inherent cellular susceptibility, e.g., in epigenetic programing. The latter, e.g., alterations in histone acetylation or chromosomal methylation, likely occurs at loci that make the cells susceptible to transformation and the development of neoplasia. By way of example, disruption of epigenetic regulators can result in altered gene function and eventually malignancy, via modification in DNA methylation, histone discharge, inappropriate nucleosome positioning, and miRNA expression [21]. This is supported by the observation of menin mutations associated with NETs. Indeed, menin is part of a histone methyltransferase complex associated with $p27^{Kip1}$ and $p18^{Ink4c}$ promoters to methylate histone H3. Its deficiency results in downregulation of $p27^{Kip1}$ and $p18^{Ink4c}$. Histone H3 methylation is reduced in islet tumors from MEN1 mutant mice that rapidly develop pituitary tumors [22]. The only known environmental factor associated with NET development is gastrin. NETs in the stomach, especially enterochromaffin-like (ECL) cell-derived tumors, are associated with hypergastrinemia in the background of mucosal atrophy [23]. The propensity of such tumors to malignancy increases exponentially if associated with MEN-I suggesting an important relationship between menin and the neoplastic index of ECL cell transformation [24]. Very little is known about gastrin and histone modifications, although this hormone has been shown to modify promoter methylation and silence the expression of specific genes, e.g., TFF1 [25], and activate histone deacetylases with downstream gene activation [26].

B. *Proliferation*: In general, the factors that regulator proliferation are poorly understood, although several signaling cascades are activated including receptor tyrosine kinases (RTK) and G protein-coupled receptors (GPCRs) and downstream signaling which regulate RAS/RAF/MAPK or PI_3K/ AKT/mTOR and potentially NOTCH signaling [27–29].

The two best characterized pro-proliferative factors have been described in the stomach and small bowel. In the stomach, gastrin via the cholecystokinin 2 (CCK_2) receptor is the principal regulator of ECL-cell proliferation via MAPK-activated signal transduction cascade with induction of the activator protein-1 (AP-1) [30, 31]. Proliferation is associated with fos/jun transcription activation by the MAPK pathway (ERK1/2) after gastrin-mediated RAS activation [32]. Such proliferation rarely leads to neoplastic progression or metastatic progression [33]. In the small bowel, transforming growth factor-β1 (TGF-β1) is a potent stimulator of neoplastic proliferation and functions to decrease expression of the SMAD family member 4 (SMAD4) with concomitant increased expression of the inhibitor of SMAD nuclear translocation, SMAD7 [34]. TGF-β1 downregulates P21 transcription and increases expression of c-Myc, resulting in phosphorylation and cross-activation of the ERK1/2 signaling pathway. This lead to downstream activation of malignancy-defining genes such as MTA1 (metastasis associated 1). Once transformed into a neoplastic metastatic phenotype, these tumors are characterized by a loss of responsiveness to TGF-β1 [34]. Other factors noted to play a role in proliferation include HER1 (EGFR, epidermal growth factor receptor) which is expressed in the majority (>80%) of small intestinal and rectal tumors [35]. Elevated EGFR copy number has been noted in about 40% [36]. Many of these relationships may, however, represent correlatable epiphenomena associated with neoplastic transformation rather than mechanistic events in the process.

Inhibitors of proliferation are better understood. This typically refers to the presence and activation of somatostatin receptors [37]. Somatostatin receptor activation inhibits adenyl cyclase decreasing [cAMP]i and thus downregulating PKA. K^+ and Ca^{2+} channels can be activated resulting in transmembrane Ca^{2+} influx inhibition and a reduction in $[Ca^{2+}]$i. Specific protein phosphatases, e.g., serine/threonine, are activated leading to the inhibition of exocytosis and Ca^{2+} and K^+ channels. In addition, intracellular tyrosine phosphatases are regulated that directly inhibit proliferation through antagonism of pro-phosphatase signaling pathways [14, 15, 38, 39].

C. *Angiogenesis*: Tumors are highly vascular due to the synthesis and secretion of pro-angiogenic factors, including VEGF. This growth factor and its receptor are associated with angiogenesis and prognosis [40, 41]. VEGF is well documented to stimulate angiogenesis during tumor development. VEGFR1–3 signaling promotes both physiological and pathological angiogenesis and lymphangiogenesis [42]. VEGF receptors are expressed in ~50% of tumors [43]; this receptor signals via the PI_3K/AKT/mTOR pathway and regulates TGFβ and CTGF (CCN2) expression. These are involved in both metastasis and the development of fibrosis [44]. At a clinical level, a variety of studies have identified that targeting these pathways may extend PFS in certain patient groups, e.g., pancreatic [45–47] but also that angiogenic-related growth factor expression may be useful for identifying patients who respond to therapeutic targeting. Rigorous mechanistic investigation is, however, still required to confirm these observations.

D. *Metastasis*: Defining and delineating the drivers of and the molecular basis of metastatic dissemination remain a formidable challenge. A variety of studies have investigated models that are able, in part, to elucidate early metastatic outgrowth (in the absence of mutations) of a subset of stem-like cancer cells [48]. Metastatic dissemination (similar to other cancers) requires a sequence of events that include the loss of cellular adhesion, invasive behavior including intravascular and extravascular migration, circulatory survival, and subsequent transvascular «emigration» followed by proliferative colonization at distant sites, e.g., liver.

One of the few characterized pathways is the loss of E-cadherin expression and function, associated with disruption of E-cadherin junctions and increased cell motility, as well as invasiveness [49]. E-cadherin loss has been identified in gastric NETs which resulted in lymph node metastasis but not with local invasion or distant metastasis [50]. In a separate study, cytoplasmic/nuclear β-catenin staining was observed in the majority of gastrointestinal NETs, and a mutant β-catenin (S37A) was identified in almost 40% [51]. Survival rates are typically reduced in tumors expressing high SNAIL1 (a member of the Snail superfamily of zinc finger transcription factors) protein levels, a cytoplasmic E-cadherin pattern, reduced N-cadherin expression, and loss of E-cadherin/β-catenin adhesion complex integrity at the cell membrane [52]. Another important effector is the matrix metalloproteinase (MMP)/tissue inhibitor of metalloproteinase (TIMP) system. Differences in the expression of MMP/TIMP between benign and malignant lesions have been recorded [53], while MMP activity in cancer cells prior to extravascular metastasis has been observed [54]. The expression of MMP2 in pancreatic NETs characterized a more malignant phenotype, while a weak expression of MMP9 indicated a less invasive one [55]. Upregulation of Src family kinases (SFK) has been recorded in pancreatic NETs, but higher expression is predominantly observed in primary lesions compared with metastases [56, 57]. Since activation of SFK during cell adhesion may stimulate the mTOR pathway, studies of its inhibition have reported a delay in cell adhesion, as well as an impaired migration and colonization processes [57]. A model of NET stem cells has provided the evidence that Src inhibition may result in a marked reduction of tumor growth, identifying this system as a potential anti-metastasis target [58].

Thus, angiogenesis may be regarded as representative of a crucial step in malignant transformation, cancer growth, and tumor progression. Its extensive study in NETs has identified some clinically useful targets. Among these, VEGF expression, as noted, is a prognostic factor and a target for therapeutic agents [59]. One theoretical benefit of targeting VEGF – and related pathways – is that this limits metastatic dissemination.

3.3 Insights from Molecular Genetic Analyses

While the majority (>90%) of NENs are sporadic [10], there are five well-described independent autosomal dominant-inherited syndromes that exhibit a percentage of mutations. These include multiple endocrine neoplasia (MEN) types 1 and 2, which are the most common forms, von Hippel-Lindau (VHL) disease, von Recklinghausen disease or neurofibromatosis (NF1), tuberous sclerosis (TSC), and Carney complex (CNC). These all exhibit tumor suppressor genes that require a «second hit» for penetrance and tumors associated with these genetic loci are typically restricted to the lung, stomach, and pancreas [19]. More recently inositol polyphosphate multikinase (IPMK) has been identified as a hereditary component in one small bowel NET family [60]. At this time, genotype–phenotype correlations that are likely to be clinically relevant to management or outcomes of the disease are rare for these mutations (◘ Fig. 3.2).

Exome sequencing: DNA sequencing has been reported for lung, pancreatic, and small bowel NETs. In lung, a very low mutation rate and a nonsmoking mutation pattern (i.e., no loss of p53, few G → T transversions) consistent with the absence of a nicotine-driven etiopathogenesis have been observed [61]. MEN-1 is the most common germline mutation (~5%), while sporadic alterations have been identified in *MEN-1*, *PSIP1*, and *ARID1* [61]. In a separate study comparing NETs with large and small cell carcinomas [62], MEN-1 mutations were confirmed to occur exclusively in NET, while mutations in chromatin-remodeling genes, including those encoding histone modifiers and members of SWI-SNF complexes, occurred at similar rates in both NETs (~45%) and carcinomas (~55%), suggesting epigenetic modification (and common environmental factors other than nicotine) as the principal drivers of lung neuroendocrine neoplasia. As noted, *TP53* and *RB1* mutations were rare events in NET [62]. Interestingly, PI_3K/AKT/mTOR pathway mutations were significantly enriched only in carcinomas [62].

In the pancreas, exome sequencing has not identified any novel gene activator mutations. The commonest mutations occur in MEN1 (~45–75%). Inactivation of *MEN-1* in gene *knock-out/knock-in* studies identifies that one of the consequences of menin loss is an uncoupling of endocrine cell cycle progression from environmental cues such as glucose, leading to islet cell proliferation [63]. A second area of importance is that menin functions as a subunit of MLL1/MLL2-containing histone methyltransferase complexes that trimethylates histone H3 at lysine 4 (H3K4me3), identifying a role in

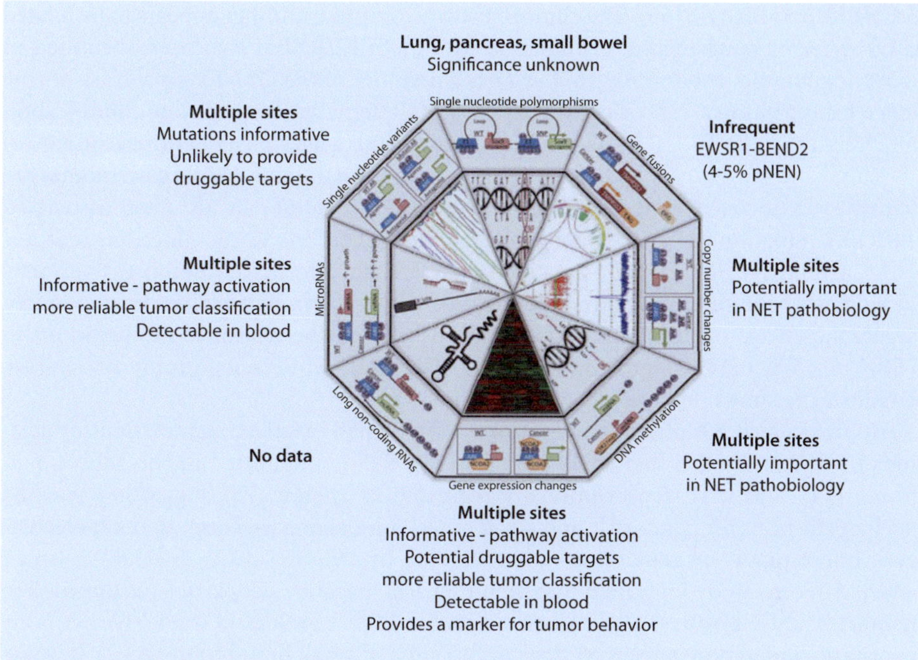

Fig. 3.2 Evaluation of the genetic topography of NEN and relationship to pathobiology. The best characterized tumors at a molecular genetic level include neuroendocrine neoplasia of the lung, pancreas, and small bowel. SNPs (single nucleotide polymorphisms) have been identified, the significance of them are unknown. Gene fusions are infrequently identified, but ~5% of sporadic pancreatic NEN may exhibit a novel fusion in EWSR1-BEND2. Copy number changes through chromosomal loss (deletion) or gain (or amplification) occur in all NEN and tend to occur more frequently in well-differentiated tumors. DNA methylation and alterations at specific promoter sites, e.g., VHL, are key features of the NEN landscape. Gene expression changes are the best characterized feature that defines this neoplasia. Studies have identified pathway activation, e.g., growth factor signaling and potentially druggable pathways, e.g., PI_3K/AKT. mRNA can be used to better and more reliably classify tumors. More recently, specific gene expression assays can be detected in the circulation as used as surrogate biomarkers of tumor behavior. While there is no published data about lncRNAs, small RNAs/miRNA have been identified. These are informative about pathway activity, have used as a classifier in lung neoplasia (including carcinoma), and can be detected in blood. Single nucleotide variants (including mutations) have been identified. Mutations per se are informative but provide a limited understanding of molecular pathogenesis. These are not currently druggable (Figure adapted for NEN from Spans et al [136])

epigenetic regulation of these tumors [64]. Other genes identified as mutated in sporadic tumors include alpha thalassemia/mental retardation syndrome X-linked (ATRX: 18%) and death domain-associated protein (DAXX: 25%) and occasionally genes in the AKT pathway (15%) [20]. Both *ATRX* and *DAXX* (both encode proteins involved in chromatin remodeling) are associated with activation of alternative lengthening of telomeres. A decreased expression is associated with chromosome instability and correlates with tumor stage and metastasis, a reduced time of relapse-free survival, and a decrease in survival [65]. More recently, a subset of patients has been identified with MUTYH inactivation (linked to instability), and a proportion of tumors has germline mutations in CHEK2 and BRAC2 [66]. The clinical relevance of these findings appears to be related to DNA repair mechanisms. A mutation in YY1 (T372R) has also been identified in ~30% of sporadic insulinomas [67]. YY1 is a member of the GLI-Kruppel class of zinc finger transcriptional repressors linked to mTOR signaling and histone modification [68]. Clinically, the T372R mutation is associated with a later onset of tumors [67].

Pancreatic tumors can be divided based on mutational status. While gastrinomas are exclusively associated with *MEN1* aberrations [69], insulinomas are often associated with *YY1* mutation [67] and glucagonomas with mutations in the glucagon receptor [70]. Currently, *MEN1*-mutation status is not clinically informative but might be a useful biomarker for guiding treatment decision-making if an agent can be developed that targets the effects of this tumor suppressor. Moreover, the relevance of alterations in ATRX, DAXX, mTOR signaling [71], and YY1 [72], while scientifically of interest, remains to be shown to have any clinical utility.

Approximately 8% of small bowel tumors have small inactivating insertions or deletions in *CDKN1B* (also known as $p27^{KIP1}$) [73]. P27 is implicated in the MEN4 syndrome [74], and it is transcriptionally regulated by menin [75] suggesting that the mechanistic basis for pancreatic and small bowel tumors may be coupled at a molecular level. Interestingly, no mutations were identified in *MEN1*, *DAXX*, or *ATRX* in small bowel. A recent study identified that menin or P27-negative neoplasms (as opposed to menin/P27-dual-positive) was associated with a high histological grade, lymph node metastasis, and a more advanced stage in foregut and small bowel tumors. P27 loss was significantly associated with a decreased survival and was an independent factor for poor overall survival. Somatic variants of unknown significance have been identified in small bowel tumors, some of which occur in cancer-related genes including FGFR2, HOOK3, EZH2, MLF1, CARD11, VHL, NONO, FANCD2, and BRAF [76]. Whether these SNVs have functional implications or reflect non-informative, biologically «silent» SNPs are unknown. Based upon the current scientific evidence, it is likely that many of these observations are epiphenomena and may ultimately have no mechanistic relation to the biology of the tumor.

The potential role of genomic instability: The two major types of genomic instability are microsatellite instability (MSI) and chromosomal instability (CIN). Both are related to mutations in DNA repair gene system, genes that are not typically mutated in NET [19]. As anticipated, studies have not identified consistent evidence for MSI in pancreatic tumors [77, 78] or in small bowel tumors [77–80]. One small study, however, suggested that this phenotype could occur in ~10% pf pancreatic tumors [81].

In contrast, CIN and aneuploidy are well-described phenomena in both pancreatic and small bowel tumors as well as in tumors of the lung, appendix, colon, and rectum. In lung tumors, aneuploidy occurs most frequently in the atypical histopathological variant of these tumors and is related to tumor size [82]. Typically, CIN includes alterations, and deletion of chromosome 11q (containing the MEN1 tumor suppressor gene) which occurs at a high frequency in lung NETs [83]. MEN-1 mutation occurs in 18% and LOH at 11q13 in 36% of sporadic lung NET [84]. Deletion of 11q is the most frequently observed alteration; it is less frequently lost in typical than atypical carcinoids and may represent a marker of progression [84]. As such, aneuploidy is a prognostic factor [85].

In pancreatic tumors, chromosomal losses are more frequently observed than gains; amplifications per se are uncommon [86]. The frequency of CIN correlates with tumor volume and disease stage, suggesting that genetic alterations accumulate during the natural history of a lesion [87]. Specifically, deletions within the 9p chromosomal region occur in ~30% and result in loss of *CDKN2A,* which encodes both the $p16^{INK4A}$ and $p14^{ARF}$ tumor suppressor proteins [88]. Loss at this locus therefore may promote tumorigenesis through dysregulation of the p53 and cyclin D1/RB activity [88]. Deletions in the p-arm of chromosome 16 occur in ~40% [89]. This region contains *TSC2,* loss of which leads to dysregulation of the PI_3K/AKT/mTOR pathway. A locus at 10q that contains the gene encoding PTEN, a phosphatase that dephosphorylates PIP_3 thereby attenuating AKT/mTOR signaling, is lost in ~30% [90, 91]. This is typically associated with malignancy. The clinical relevance of CIN is identified in sporadic insulinomas, where chromosomal loss rather than tumor size or proliferation rates are the most powerful predictors for the development of metastatic disease [92].

In small bowel tumors, losses at 18q22–qter occur in up to 90% of patients [93, 94], while losses in 11q22–23 (not related to regulation of the *MEN1* locus) occur in 33%. About 20% of tumors exhibit alterations in the distal part of 11q (which contains *SDHD*) [95]. Loss of chromosome 18 might be linked to alterations in the TGFβ/SMAD pathway [79] and is considered to represent a primary event in tumorigenesis. Alterations in the SDHD gene are related to hypoxia and VHL-mediated signaling pathways. Gain of copies of chromosome 14, which occurs in ~10%, has been identified as a marker of poor prognosis [96].

3.3.1 The Place of Epigenetics

The CpG island methylator phenotype (CIMP) is characterized by widespread promoter methylation. Methylation and histone modifications, i.e., chromatin remodeling, are the most prominent genetic alterations occurring in 20–40% of lung NET. None of these alterations, however, are currently clinically actionable. CpG island methylation is also well recognized in pancreatic and small bowel tumors although gene-specific hypermethylation or hypomethylation are less commonly observed in pancreatic than in gastrointestinal NET [97].

MGMT (6-*O*-methylguanine-DNA methyltransferase) is hypermethylated in ~25% of pancreatic tumors, and expression of this gene is decreased in 30–50% [98, 99]; these alterations have been show to correlate with responses to alkylating therapy. Progression-free survival is often longer when there is an MGMT protein loss or MGMT promoter methylation [98, 99]. Impairment of *VHL* gene expression via promoter methylation occurs in ~6% of pancreatic tumors and leads to activation of the HIF1α-signaling pathway and hypoxia responses which may be pro-angiogenic [100]. This mechanism, in particular, may be associated with an adverse outcome [100]. Interestingly, different types of pancreatic tumors have different methylation patterns. Insulinomas are hypermethylated at the *IGF2* locus, whereas gastrinomas exhibit hypomethylation of this gene locus [101].

In small bowel NET, pyrosequencing studies have revealed variation in promoter methylation at *WIF1* (WNT inhibitory factor 1), *RASSF1A*, (RAS association domain-containing protein 1), *CTNNB1* (β-catenin), *NKX2–3* (homeobox protein NKX-2.3), and *CDKN2A* (specifically, the promoter controlling p16^{INK4A} expression) [102]. By contrast, the promoter region of *CDKN2A* that drives p14^{ARF} expression and those of *SMAD*2 and *SMAD4* often exhibited low levels of methylation [102]. Global methylation of LINE1 repeats (which is indicative of chromatin remodeling) is also reduced and is associated with loss of chromosome 18 [102].

CIMP correlates with high Ki67 indices (>10%), and survival is directly related to the degree of CpG island methylation; low methylation is a better prognostic [103]. The clinical usefulness of chemical-based DNA modifications, e.g., methylation, has attracted much attention but as yet has failed to provide information that has clinical utility [104]. Further elucidation of this field may yield more insight.

3.3.2 The Promise of Molecular Transcriptomics

Gene expression data has been developed for lung, gastric pancreatic, and small bowel tumors. Transcriptome analysis of lung NET identifies expression of neuroendocrine-associated genes including insulinoma-associated gene 1, achaete-scute homologue 1, gastrin-releasing peptide, and chromogranin A [105]. Lung NET, as expected, was classified separately to other lung neoplasia confirming their different etiopathogenesis [105, 106]. In a second study, the genes associated with a poor prognosis were located at chromosome 11q [107]. Upregulated genes were associated with the mitotic spindle checkpoint, the chromosomal passenger complex (CPC), mitotic kinase CDC2 activity, and the BRCA-Fanconi anemia pathway. Interestingly, BIRC5 (survivin), BUB1, CD44, IL20RA, KLK12, and OTP were all prognostic in this dataset. More recently, GC (vitamin D-binding protein) and CEACAM1 (carcinoembryonic antigen family member) were identified as potential diagnostic markers as they differentiated typical from atypical NET [108]. miRNA profiles have been evaluated in these tumors. miR-21 expression is higher in lesions with lymph node metastasis [109]. A series of miRNAs is altered in lung neoplasia, some of which are dysregulated specifically in NET [110]. Overall, lung NET appears to have distinct miRNA expression profiles compared to other lung neoplasia [111].

In the stomach, DNA microarray studies have identified upregulation of CgA, with a lower expression of MTA1 and MAGE-D2 [112]; both markers are linked to a more aggressive phenotype. The miRNA profile of gastric NET is not known.

In pancreatic NET, two subtypes of pancreatic NENs: «benign» and «malignant» are readily evident based on gene expression patterns [113]. Malignant gene expression overlaps with the WHO category of a well-differentiated NEC and is characterized by overexpression of mRNAs encoding ADCY2, FEV, GADD45β, and NR4A2 [113]. Analyses of MEN1-associated pancreatic NET transcriptomes have revealed that expression of FGF-9, islet amyloid polypeptide (amylin), and SST, among other proteins, is altered by loss of menin function [114]. In insulinomas, somatostatin 2 receptor encoding mRNA is absent or expressed at low levels [91]. In a separate study, expression of *TSC2* and *PTEN* was decreased in ~80% and was associated with shorter disease-free and overall survival [91].

Hanahan et al. identified different genetic pNEN subtypes, which are associated with more aggressive behavior and metastasis [115]. It is noteworthy that these subtypes exhibited no correlation with the WHO classification. In this study, miRNA profiles were leveraged with gene expression patterns to identify three different classes of pNET, islet-like, intermediate (IT), and metastasis-like phenotype (MLP) that were characterized by distinct gene profiles [115]. Expression was associated with differences in genomic mutations, e.g., IT was not associated with DAXX/ATRX mutations but with MEN-1 alterations, while MLP did exhibit DAXX/ATRX mutations and was both more metabolically active as well as likely to have evolved from a less well-differentiated progenitor cell. This classification system has recently been confirmed [66].

Dysregulation of microRNA (miRNA) levels has also been noted including upregulation of miR-103 and miR-107 [116], whereas miR-21 overexpression was associated with both high proliferation and liver metastases [116]. In contrast, a separate study reported that expression of miR-642 correlated with proliferation while miR-210 was associated with metastatic disease [117]. Li et al. independently noted that downregulation of serum miR-1290 discriminated pancreatic NET from adenocarcinomas [118]. The precise role of miRNAs in pancreatic NEN tumorigenesis remains to be defined.

Two subtypes of small bowel NET have been identified through gene expression profiling: the first principally synthesize and secrete serotonin, and second subtype is characterized by expression of serotonin, substance P, and other tachykinins [119]. The former subtype is well-differentiated NENs, whereas the latter overlaps with NECs [119]. Overexpression of nucleosome assembly protein-like 1 (*NAP1L1*), melanoma-associated antigen D2 (*MAGED2*), and metastasis-associated protein MTA1 (*MTA1*) might identify metastatic tumors [120]. Other candidate genes with biomarker potential include paraneoplastic antigen Ma2 (*PNMA2*) [121, 122], expression of which has confirmed as an early biomarker of disease recurrence [122]. Small bowel tumors have a substantially different profile compared to pancreatic neoplasms [113], reinforcing other evidence that supports a different etiology and pathobiology. Global miRNA profiles do not overlap with pancreatic NET [116–118, 123]. In small bowel NET, five miRNAs including miR-96, miR-182, miR-183, miR-196, and miR-200 were upregulated during tumor progression, whereas four (miR-31, miR-129-5p, miR-133a, and miR-215) were significantly downregulated [123]. The cardiac-specific miRNA-133a has been confirmed to be downregulated in metastases [124], but the relevance of this observation remains to be determined. It is likely that network-based approaches may have more utility for identifying relevant miRNAs as well as determine biologically useful interactions that have potential clinical relevance. Alterations in miRNA have been identified in the circulation and levels may be decreased by SSA usage [125]. However, detection and quantification of miRNAs remain challenging since there is currently no standardization and normalization methodology has not been adequately characterized.

Table 3.2 Molecular abnormalities in bronchopulmonary, pancreatic, and GI NEN

Organ	Familial mutation(s)	Somatic	Methylation CIMP	Transcriptome	miRNA
Lung	*MEN1*	*ARID1*, *PSIP1*	Yes	Yes	Yes
Stomach	*MEN1*	No data	No data	Yes	No data
Duode-num	*MEN1*	No data	No data	No data	No data
Pancreas	*MEN1*, *VHL*, *NF-1*, *TSC*	*MEN1*, *ATRX*, *DAXX*, mTOR pathway, *YY1*, DNA repair pathway (*BRCA2*, *CHECK2*, *MUTYH*)	Yes	Yes	Yes
Small bowel	*IPMK*	*CDKN1B*	Yes	Yes	Yes
Appendix	No data	No data	No data	No data	No data
Colon	No data	No data	No	No data	No data
Rectum	No data	No data	No	No data	No data

ARID1 AT-rich interactive domain-containing protein 1, *ATRX* alpha thalassemia/mental retardation syndrome X-Linked, *BRCA2* breast cancer 2, CHEK2 = checkpoint kinase 2, *CIMP* CpG island methylator phenotype, *DAXX* death domain-associated protein, *CDKN1B* cyclin-dependent kinase inhibitor 1B (or $P27^{KIP1}$), *IPMK* inositol polyphosphate multikinase, *MEN1* multiple neoplasia type I, *MUTYH* mutYH DNA glycosylase, *NF-1* neurofibromatosis, *PSIP1* PC4- and SFRS1 interacting protein 1; *TSC* tuberous sclerosis, *VHL* von Hippel-Lindau, *YY1* yin-yang 1

Gene expression data can also be used to confirm different organs of origin of NENs and thus have been used to develop clinically relevant tests for detecting tumor origin in patients with CUPs [126]. Moreover, there is some utility at defining different lung neoplasia at a tissue level (miRview lung, Rosetta Genomics Ltd.) [127]. The most useful data from gene expression profiling, however, is the identification of circulating tumor RNA (NETest, Clifton Life Sciences) that has provided the basis for development of blood-based biomarker signatures (Table 3.2). Such multianalyte algorithmic analysis is significantly more accurate than monoanalyte determinations such as CgA [128]. Gene expression assays are clinically effective (~95% accurate) in the diagnosis of GEP-NENs [129]. In addition, circulating tumor RNA directly recapitulates tumor-based gene expression and is effective in predicting disease progression [130]. Similarly, after surgery, transcript analysis is decreased commensurate with the amount of tumor resected [131]. Transcript levels are effective in monitoring the efficacy of somatostatin analog therapy [132] and have also been shown to predict responsiveness to peptide radiotherapy (PRRT) [133, 134]. This is the first clinically useful application of transcriptomes in NET [134].

3.4 Conclusion

NENs represent a diverse group of neoplasia that exhibit a unique pathobiology and a neoplastic molecular profile that is substantially different to other epithelial cancers. Despite the apparent increase in NEN incidence in recent years, a commensurate increase in molecular and cellular biology of this disease has been lacking. Data derived from several clinical trials and traditional evaluation of tumor biology have, to date, yielded relatively little information about the underlying pathobiology of these lesions. The etiopathogenesis remains unclear as do the environmental factors responsible for a «second hit», except in the instance of gastric NETs.

While factors that regulate proliferation and angiogenesis have been identified (e.g., TGFβ, EGF, VEGF), the mechanisms underlying metastasis and target organ tropism remain to be defined. Traditional DNA sequencing approaches have revealed little regarding driver mutations but have played a role in confirming pancreatic NET is a tumor suppressor-driven disease with a limited mutational spectrum (MEN-1, ATRX, DAXX, mTOR, MUTYH). Individualized stratification of patients to specific treatments based on genetic or epigenetic profile still remains unattainable at this time for NENs, and a goal of precision medicine for these tumors, currently, is quixotic.

Gene expression arrays have provided further insights into tumor biology and have proven to be the most useful tool in diagnostics. A more accurate molecular delineation of NEN disease can be provided with the view to define the regulatory changes that occur as the primary tumor evolves into a metastatic phenotype and in so doing undergoes alteration in its spectrum of regulatory pathways and therefore druggable targets. Since tumors evolve as they progress (hence an individual therapeutic agent becomes ineffective), the need to identify real time molecular evolution and identify the advent of a new target is paramount. Repetitive biopsy of tumor tissue (either primary or metastases) is not a viable option given the need for repetitive invasive procedures. Thus, the development of blood-based strategies to measure and assess changes in the tumor by assessment of circulating molecular signatures is of critical relevance to both management strategy and outcome analysis for NENs.

Overall, our current knowledge of the molecular topography of NENs is extremely limited (for the most part descriptive and correlative rather than mechanistic) and represents a vast dark room illuminated by random lights – some of which are probably only reflections (◘ Fig. 3.3). Elucidation of the molecular machinery of NENs is indistinguishable from any possibility of rational or meaningful progress in the management of this disease.

3

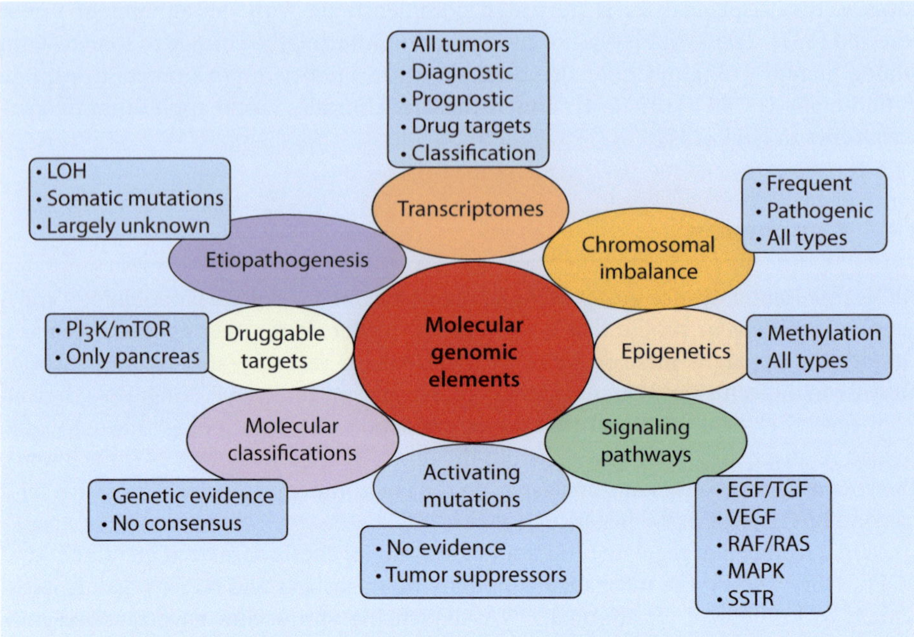

Fig. 3.3 Summary of the current understanding of molecular genomic events. Transcriptomic analysis has provided the most relevant and clinically applicable information. Information has allowed for the development of diagnostic and prognostic markers as well as identification of potential drug targets and information that could be used to better classify neuroendocrine neoplasia. Chromosomal imbalance is a consistent feature of NEN, occurring in all types. This it pathogenic and this information is potentially useful as a biomarker. Epigenetic modifications, especially methylation alterations, occur in all NEN evaluated. Signaling pathways linked to growth factors (proliferation, angiogenesis) have been defined in NEN; the somatostatin receptor (SSTR) pathway has provided the most clinical utility. Activating mutations are rare and NEN typically exhibit either germline or somatic mutations in tumor suppressor genes. Evidence for molecular classifications exists (gene expression arrays, specific mutational landscape) but while discussed [104] have, thus far, not been incorporated. Druggable targets, the PI3K/mTOR pathway, have been defined, particularly in pancreatic NEN, but this occurs in <5% of all tumors. The etiopathogenesis of these remains largely unclear. While loss of heterozygosity (LOH) and somatic mutations have been identified as factors, this information is only limited to lung and pancreatic NEN. The mechanisms and factors driving neoplasia at other sites remain to be defined

Bibliography

1. de Mestier L, Dromain C, d'Assignies G et al (2014) Evaluating digestive neuroendocrine tumor progression and therapeutic responses in the era of targeted therapies: state of the art. Endocr Relat Cancer 21:R105–R120. doi:10.1530/ERC-1513-0365. Print 2014
2. Bergsland EK (2013) The evolving landscape of neuroendocrine tumors. Semin Oncol 40:4–22. doi:10.1053/j.seminoncol.2012.1011.1013
3. Wang H, Chen Y, Fernandez-Del Castillo C, Yilmaz O, Deshpande V (2012) Heterogeneity in signaling pathways of gastroenteropancreatic neuroendocrine tumors: a critical look at notch signaling pathway. Mod Pathol 24:143
4. Sundin A, Rockall A (2012) Therapeutic monitoring of gastroenteropancreatic neuroendocrine tumors: the challenges ahead. Neuroendocrinology 96:261–271. doi:10.1159/000342270. Epub 000342012 Oct 000342212

5. Kidd M, Schimmack S, Lawrence B, Alaimo D, Modlin IM (2012) EGFR/TGFalpha and TGFbeta/CTGF signaling in neuroendocrine neoplasia: theoretical therapeutic targets. Neuroendocrinology 15:15
6. Chan JA, Kulke MH (2011) New treatment options for patients with advanced neuroendocrine tumors. Curr Treat Options in Oncol 12:136–148
7. Oberg K (2010) Pancreatic endocrine tumors. Semin Oncol 37:594–618
8. Garcia-Carbonero R, Capdevila J, Crespo-Herrero G et al (2010) Incidence, patterns of care and prognostic factors for outcome of gastroenteropancreatic neuroendocrine tumors (GEP-NETs): results from the National Cancer Registry of Spain (RGETNE). Ann Oncol 21:1794–1803. doi:10.1093/annonc/mdq1022. Epub 2010 Feb 1795
9. Strosberg J, Gardner N, Kvols L (2009) Survival and prognostic factor analysis of 146 metastatic neuroendocrine tumors of the mid-gut. Neuroendocrinology 89:471–476. Epub 2009 Jan 2028
10. Modlin IM, Oberg K, Chung DC et al (2008) Gastroenteropancreatic neuroendocrine tumours. Lancet Oncol 9:61–72
11. Frilling A, Modlin I, Kidd M et al (2014) Recommendations for management of patients with neuroendocrine liver metastases. Lancet Oncol 15:e8–21
12. Pusceddu S, Femia D, Lo Russo G et al (2016) Update on medical treatment of small intestinal neuroendocrine tumors. Expert Rev Anticancer Ther 16:969–976. doi:10.1080/14737140.14732016.11207534. Epub 14732016 Jul 14737113
13. Yao JC, Lagunes DR, Kulke MH (2013) Targeted therapies in neuroendocrine tumors (NET): clinical trial challenges and lessons learned. Oncologist 18:525–532. doi:10.1634/theoncologist. 2012-0434. Epub 2013 Apr 1624
14. Caplin ME, Pavel M, Cwikla JB et al (2014) Lanreotide in metastatic enteropancreatic neuroendocrine tumors. N Engl J Med 371:224–233. doi:10.1056/NEJMoa1316158
15. Rinke A, Muller HH, Schade-Brittinger C et al (2009) Placebo-controlled, double-blind, prospective, randomized study on the effect of octreotide LAR in the control of tumor growth in patients with metastatic neuroendocrine midgut tumors: a report from the PROMID Study Group. J Clin Oncol 27:4656–4663. Epub 2009 Aug 4624
16. Rankin EB, Giaccia AJ (2016) Hypoxic control of metastasis. Science 352:175–180. doi:10.1126/science.aaf4405. Epub 2016 Apr 1127
17. Yang Y (2015) Cancer immunotherapy: harnessing the immune system to battle cancer. J Clin Invest 125:3335–3337. doi:10.1172/JCI83871. Epub 82015 Sep 83871
18. Riihimaki M, Hemminki A, Sundquist K, Sundquist J, Hemminki K (2016) The epidemiology of metastases in neuroendocrine tumors. Int J Cancer 139:2679–2686. doi:10.1002/ijc.30400. Epub 32016 Sep 30409
19. Kidd M, Modlin I, Bodei L, Drozdov I (2015) Decoding the molecular and mutational ambiguities of gastroenteropancreatic neuroendocrine neoplasm pathobiology. Cellular and Molecular Gastroenterology and Hepatology 1:131–153
20. Leotlela PD, Jauch A, Holtgreve-Grez H, Thakker RV (2003) Genetics of neuroendocrine and carcinoid tumours. Endocr Relat Cancer 10:437–450
21. Elsasser SJ, Allis CD, Lewis PW (2011) Cancer. New epigenetic drivers of cancers. Science 331:1145–1146. doi:10.1126/science.1203280
22. Franklin DS, Godfrey VL, Lee H et al (1998) CDK inhibitors p18(INK4c) and p27(Kip1) mediate two separate pathways to collaboratively suppress pituitary tumorigenesis. Genes Dev 12:2899–2911
23. Metz DC, Jensen RT (2008) Gastrointestinal neuroendocrine tumors: pancreatic endocrine tumors. Gastroenterology 135:1469–1492
24. Modlin IM, Kidd M, Latich I, Zikusoka MN, Shapiro MD (2005) Current status of gastrointestinal carcinoids. Gastroenterology 128:1717–1751
25. Tomita H, Takaishi S, Menheniott TR et al (2011) Inhibition of gastric carcinogenesis by the hormone gastrin is mediated by suppression of TFF1 epigenetic silencing. Gastroenterology 140:879–891. doi:10.1053/j.gastro.2010.1011.1037. Epub 2010 Nov 1025
26. Selvik LK, Rao S, Steigedal TS et al (2014) Salt-inducible kinase 1 (SIK1) is induced by gastrin and inhibits migration of gastric adenocarcinoma cells. PLoS One 9:e112485. doi: 10.111371/journal.pone.0112485. eCollection 0112014
27. Porta C, Paglino C, Mosca A (2014) Targeting PI3K/Akt/mTOR signaling in cancer. Front Oncol 4:64

28. Svejda B, Kidd M, Kazberouk A, Lawrence B, Pfragner R, Modlin IM (2011) Limitations in small intestinal neuroendocrine tumor therapy by mTor kinase inhibition reflect growth factor-mediated PI3K feedback loop activation via ERK1/2 and AKT. Cancer 117:4141–4154
29. Li HJ, Kapoor A, Giel-Moloney M, Rindi G, Leiter AB (2012) Notch signaling differentially regulates the cell fate of early endocrine precursor cells and their maturing descendants in the mouse pancreas and intestine. Dev Biol 371:156–169
30. Rozengurt E, Walsh JH (2001) Gastrin, CCK, signaling, and cancer. Annu Rev Physiol 63:49–76
31. Treinies I, Paterson HF, Hooper S, Wilson R, Marshall CJ (1999) Activated MEK stimulates expression of AP-1 components independently of phosphatidylinositol 3-kinase (PI3-kinase) but requires a PI3-kinase signal To stimulate DNA synthesis. Mol Cell Biol 19:321–329
32. Kinoshita Y, Nakata H, Kishi K, Kawanami C, Sawada M, Chiba T (1998) Comparison of the signal transduction pathways activated by gastrin in enterochromaffin-like and parietal cells. Gastroenterology 115:93–100
33. Abraham NS (2012) Proton pump inhibitors: potential adverse effects. Curr Opin Gastroenterol 28:615–620
34. Kidd M, Modlin IM, Pfragner R et al (2007) Small bowel carcinoid (enterochromaffin cell) neoplasia exhibits transforming growth factor-beta1-mediated regulatory abnormalities including upregulation of C-Myc and MTA1. Cancer 109:2420–2431
35. Papouchado B, Erickson LA, Rohlinger AL et al (2005) Epidermal growth factor receptor and activated epidermal growth factor receptor expression in gastrointestinal carcinoids and pancreatic endocrine carcinomas. Mod Pathol 18:1329–1335
36. Gilbert JA, Adhikari LJ, Lloyd RV et al (2010) Molecular markers for novel therapies in neuroendocrine (carcinoid) tumors. Endocr Relat Cancer 17:623–636
37. Susini C, Buscail L (2006) Rationale for the use of somatostatin analogs as antitumor agents. Ann Oncol 17:1733–1742
38. Wolin EM (2012) The expanding role of somatostatin analogs in the management of neuroendocrine tumors. Gastrointestinal Cancer Res 5:161–168
39. Oberg K, Kvols L, Caplin M et al (2004) Consensus report on the use of somatostatin analogs for the management of neuroendocrine tumors of the gastroenteropancreatic system. Ann Oncol 15:966–973
40. Zhang J, Jia Z, Li Q et al (2007) Elevated expression of vascular endothelial growth factor correlates with increased angiogenesis and decreased progression-free survival among patients with low-grade neuroendocrine tumors. Cancer 109:1478–1486
41. Besig S, Voland P, Baur DM, Perren A, Prinz C (2009) Vascular endothelial growth factors, angiogenesis, and survival in human ileal enterochromaffin cell carcinoids. Neuroendocrinology 90:402–415. doi:10.1159/000245900. Epub 000242009 Oct 000245908
42. Olsson AK, Dimberg A, Kreuger J, Claesson-Welsh L (2006) VEGF receptor signalling - in control of vascular function. Nat Rev Mol Cell Biol 7:359–371
43. Bowen KA, Silva SR, Johnson JN et al (2009) An analysis of trends and growth factor receptor expression of GI carcinoid tumors. J Gastrointest Surg 13:1773–1780
44. Kidd M, Modlin IM, Shapiro MD et al (2007) CTGF, intestinal stellate cells and carcinoid fibrogenesis. World J Gastroenterol 13:5208–5216
45. Yao JC, Phan A, Hoff PM et al (2008) Targeting vascular endothelial growth factor in advanced carcinoid tumor: a random assignment phase II study of depot octreotide with bevacizumab and pegylated interferon alpha-2b. J Clin Oncol 26:1316–1323
46. Phan AT, Halperin DM, Chan JA et al (2015) Pazopanib and depot octreotide in advanced, well-differentiated neuroendocrine tumours: a multicentre, single-group, phase 2 study. Lancet Oncol 16:695–703
47. Raymond E, Dahan L, Raoul JL et al (2011) Sunitinib malate for the treatment of pancreatic neuroendocrine tumors. N Engl J Med 364:501–513
48. Walenkamp A, Crespo G, Fierro Maya F et al (2014) Hallmarks of gastrointestinal neuroendocrine tumours: implications for treatment. Endocr Relat Cancer 21:R445–R460. doi:10.1530/ERC-1514-0106
49. Jiang WG, Sanders AJ, Katoh M et al (2015) Tissue invasion and metastasis: Molecular, biological and clinical perspectives. Semin Cancer Biol 35:S244–S275. doi:10.1016/j.semcancer.2015.1003.1008. Epub 2015 Apr 1010

50. Boo YJ, Park SS, Kim JH, Mok YJ, Kim SJ, Kim CS (2007) Gastric neuroendocrine carcinoma: clinicopathologic review and immunohistochemical study of E-cadherin and Ki-67 as prognostic markers. J Surg Oncol 95:110–117
51. Fujimori M, Ikeda S, Shimizu Y, Okajima M, Asahara T (2001) Accumulation of beta-catenin protein and mutations in exon 3 of beta-catenin gene in gastrointestinal carcinoid tumor. Cancer Res 61:6656–6659
52. Galvan JA, Astudillo A, Vallina A et al (2013) Epithelial-mesenchymal transition markers in the differential diagnosis of gastroenteropancreatic neuroendocrine tumors. Am J Clin Pathol 140:61–72. doi:10.1309/AJCPIV1340ISTBXRAX
53. Jeffery N, McLean MH, El-Omar EM, Murray GI (2009) The matrix metalloproteinase/tissue inhibitor of matrix metalloproteinase profile in colorectal polyp cancers. Histopathology 54:820–828. doi:10.1111/j.1365-2559.2009.03301.x
54. Zhang Q, Yang M, Shen J, Gerhold LM, Hoffman RM, Xing HR (2010) The role of the intravascular microenvironment in spontaneous metastasis development. Int J Cancer 126:2534–2541. doi:10.1002/ijc.24979
55. Gurevich LE (2003) Role of matrix metalloproteinases 2 and 9 in determination of invasive potential of pancreatic tumors. Bull Exp Biol Med 136:494–498
56. Capurso G, Lattimore S, Crnogorac-Jurcevic T et al (2006) Gene expression profiles of progressive pancreatic endocrine tumours and their liver metastases reveal potential novel markers and therapeutic targets. Endocr Relat Cancer 13:541–558
57. Di Florio A, Adesso L, Pedrotti S et al (2011) Src kinase activity coordinates cell adhesion and spreading with activation of mammalian target of rapamycin in pancreatic endocrine tumour cells. Endocr Relat Cancer 18:541–554. doi:10.1530/ERC-1510-0153. Print 2011 Oct
58. Gaur P, Sceusi EL, Samuel S et al (2011) Identification of cancer stem cells in human gastrointestinal carcinoid and neuroendocrine tumors. Gastroenterology 141:1728–1737. doi:10.1053/j.gastro.2011.1707.1037. Epub 2011 Jul 1730
59. Scoazec JY (2013) Angiogenesis in neuroendocrine tumors: therapeutic applications. Neuroendocrinology 97:45–56. doi:10.1159/000338371. Epub 000332012 Jun 000338377
60. Sei Y, Zhao X, Forbes J et al (2015) A hereditary form of small intestinal carcinoid associated with a germline mutation in inositol polyphosphate multikinase. Gastroenterology 149:67–78. doi:10.1053/j.gastro.2015.1004.1008. Epub 2015 Apr 1059
61. Fernandez-Cuesta L, Peifer M, Lu X et al (2014) Frequent mutations in chromatin-remodelling genes in pulmonary carcinoids. Nat Commun 5:3518. doi:10.1038/ncomms4518
62. Simbolo M, Mafficini A, Sikora KO et al (2016) Lung neuroendocrine tumours: deep sequencing of the four World Health Organization histotypes reveals chromatin-remodelling genes as major players and a prognostic role for TERT, RB1, MEN1 and KMT2D. J Pathol 22
63. Zhang J, Francois R, Iyer R, Seshadri M, Zajac-Kaye M, Hochwald SN (2013) Current understanding of the molecular biology of pancreatic neuroendocrine tumors. J Natl Cancer Inst 105:1005–1017. doi:10.1093/jnci/djt1135. Epub 2013 Jul 1009
64. Agarwal SK, Jothi R (2012) Genome-wide characterization of menin-dependent H3K4me3 reveals a specific role for menin in the regulation of genes implicated in MEN1-like tumors. PLoS One 7:e37952. doi:10.31371/journal.pone.0037952. Epub 0032012 May 0037930
65. Marinoni I, Kurrer AS, Vassella E et al (2014) Loss of DAXX and ATRX are associated with chromosome instability and reduced survival of patients with pancreatic neuroendocrine tumors. Gastroenterology 146:453–460.e455. doi:10.1053/j.gastro.2013.1010.1020. Epub 2013 Oct 1019
66. Scarpa A, Chang DK, Nones K et al (2017) Whole-genome landscape of pancreatic neuroendocrine tumours. Nature 543:65–71. doi:10.1038/nature21063. Epub 22017 Feb 21015
67. Cao Y, Gao Z, Li L et al (2013) Whole exome sequencing of insulinoma reveals recurrent T372R mutations in YY1. Nat Commun 4:2810. doi:10.1038/ncomms3810
68. He Y, Sandoval J, Casaccia-Bonnefil P (2007) Events at the transition between cell cycle exit and oligodendrocyte progenitor differentiation: the role of HDAC and YY1. Neuron Glia Biol 3:221–231. doi:10.1017/S1740925X08000057
69. Zhuang Z, Vortmeyer AO, Pack S et al (1997) Somatic mutations of the MEN1 tumor suppressor gene in sporadic gastrinomas and insulinomas. Cancer Res 57:4682–4686

70. Zhou C, Dhall D, Nissen NN, Chen CR, Yu R (2009) Homozygous P86S mutation of the human glucagon receptor is associated with hyperglucagonemia, alpha cell hyperplasia, and islet cell tumor. Pancreas 38:941–946
71. Jiao Y, Shi C, Edil BH et al (2011) DAXX/ATRX, MEN1, and mTOR pathway genes are frequently altered in pancreatic neuroendocrine tumors. Science 331:1199–1203
72. Cromer MK, Choi M, Nelson-Williams C et al (2015) Neomorphic effects of recurrent somatic mutations in Yin Yang 1 in insulin-producing adenomas. Proc Natl Acad Sci U S A 112:4062–4067. doi:10.1073/pnas.1503696112. Epub 1503692015 Mar 1503696118
73. Francis JM, Kiezun A, Ramos AH et al (2013) Somatic mutation of CDKN1B in small intestine neuroendocrine tumors. Nat Genet 45:1483–1486. doi:10.1038/ng.2821. Epub 2013 Nov 1483
74. Lee M, Pellegata NS (2013) Multiple endocrine neoplasia syndromes associated with mutation of p27. J Endocrinol Investig 36:781–787. doi:10.3275/9021. Epub 2013 Jun 3226
75. Karnik SK, Hughes CM, Gu X et al (2005) Menin regulates pancreatic islet growth by promoting histone methylation and expression of genes encoding p27Kip1 and p18INK4c. Proc Natl Acad Sci U S A 102:14659–14664. Epub 12005 Sep 14629
76. Banck MS, Kanwar R, Kulkarni AA et al (2013) The genomic landscape of small intestine neuroendocrine tumors. J Clin Invest 15
77. Ghimenti C, Lonobile A, Campani D, Bevilacqua G, Caligo MA (1999) Microsatellite instability and allelic losses in neuroendocrine tumors of the gastro-entero-pancreatic system. Int J Oncol 15: 361–366
78. Arnold CN, Sosnowski A, Blum HE (2004) Analysis of molecular pathways in neuroendocrine cancers of the gastroenteropancreatic system. Ann N Y Acad Sci 1014:218–219
79. Banck MS, Kanwar R, Kulkarni AA et al (2013) The genomic landscape of small intestine neuroendocrine tumors. J Clin Investig 123:2502–2508
80. Kidd M, Eick G, Shapiro MD, Camp RL, Mane SM, Modlin IM (2005) Microsatellite instability and gene mutations in transforming growth factor-beta type II receptor are absent in small bowel carcinoid tumors. Cancer 103:229–236
81. House MG, Herman JG, Guo MZ et al (2003) Prognostic value of hMLH1 methylation and microsatellite instability in pancreatic endocrine neoplasms. Surgery 134:902–908. discussion 909
82. el-Naggar AK, Ballance W, Karim FW et al (1991) Typical and atypical bronchopulmonary carcinoids. A clinicopathologic and flow cytometric study. Am J Clin Pathol 95:828–834
83. Debelenko LV, Swalwell JI, Kelley MJ et al (2000) MEN1 gene mutation analysis of high-grade neuroendocrine lung carcinoma. Genes Chromosom Cancer 28:58–65
84. Swarts DR, Ramaekers FC, Speel EJ (2012) Molecular and cellular biology of neuroendocrine lung tumors: evidence for separate biological entities. Biochim Biophys Acta 1826:255–271. doi:10.1016/j.bbcan.2012.1005.1001. Epub 2012 May 1010
85. Padberg BC, Woenckhaus J, Hilger G et al (1996) DNA cytophotometry and prognosis in typical and atypical bronchopulmonary carcinoids. A clinicomorphologic study of 100 neuroendocrine lung tumors. Am J Surg Pathol 20:815–822
86. Speel EJ, Richter J, Moch H et al (1999) Genetic differences in endocrine pancreatic tumor subtypes detected by comparative genomic hybridization. Am J Pathol 155:1787–1794
87. Speel EJ, Scheidweiler AF, Zhao J et al (2001) Genetic evidence for early divergence of small functioning and nonfunctioning endocrine pancreatic tumors: gain of 9Q34 is an early event in insulinomas. Cancer Res 61:5186–5192
88. Simon B, Lubomierski N (2004) Implication of the INK4a/ARF locus in gastroenteropancreatic neuroendocrine tumorigenesis. Ann N Y Acad Sci 1014:284–299
89. Zikusoka MN, Kidd M, Eick G, Latich I, Modlin IM (2005) The molecular genetics of gastroenteropancreatic neuroendocrine tumors. Cancer 104:2292–2309
90. Perren A, Komminoth P, Saremaslani P et al (2000) Mutation and expression analyses reveal differential subcellular compartmentalization of PTEN in endocrine pancreatic tumors compared to normal islet cells. Am J Pathol 157:1097–1103
91. Missiaglia E, Dalai I, Barbi S et al (2010) Pancreatic endocrine tumors: expression profiling evidences a role for AKT-mTOR pathway. J Clin Oncol 28:245–255
92. Jonkers YM, Claessen SM, Perren A et al (2005) Chromosomal instability predicts metastatic disease in patients with insulinomas. Endocr Relat Cancer 12:435–447

93. Kytola S, Hoog A, Nord B et al (2001) Comparative genomic hybridization identifies loss of 18q22-qter as an early and specific event in tumorigenesis of midgut carcinoids. Am J Pathol 158:1803–1808
94. Lollgen RM, Hessman O, Szabo E, Westin G, Akerstrom G (2001) Chromosome 18 deletions are common events in classical midgut carcinoid tumors. Int J Cancer 92:812–815
95. Kytola S, Nord B, Elder EE et al (2002) Alterations of the SDHD gene locus in midgut carcinoids, Merkel cell carcinomas, pheochromocytomas, and abdominal paragangliomas. Genes Chromosom Cancer 34:325–332
96. Andersson E, Sward C, Stenman G, Ahlman H, Nilsson O (2009) High-resolution genomic profiling reveals gain of chromosome 14 as a predictor of poor outcome in ileal carcinoids. Endocr Relat Cancer 16:953–966
97. Chan AO, Kim SG, Bedeir A, Issa JP, Hamilton SR, Rashid A (2003) CpG island methylation in carcinoid and pancreatic endocrine tumors. Oncogene 22:924–934
98. Kulke MH, Hornick JL, Frauenhoffer C et al (2009) O6-methylguanine DNA methyltransferase deficiency and response to temozolomide-based therapy in patients with neuroendocrine tumors. Clin Cancer Res 15:338–345
99. Walter T, van Brakel B, Vercherat C et al (2015) O6-Methylguanine-DNA methyltransferase status in neuroendocrine tumours: prognostic relevance and association with response to alkylating agents. Br J Cancer 112:523–531
100. Schmitt AM, Schmid S, Rudolph T et al (2009) VHL inactivation is an important pathway for the development of malignant sporadic pancreatic endocrine tumors. Endocr Relat Cancer 16: 1219–1227
101. Dejeux E, Olaso R, Dousset B et al (2009) Hypermethylation of the IGF2 differentially methylated region 2 is a specific event in insulinomas leading to loss-of-imprinting and overexpression. Endocr Relat Cancer 16:939–952
102. Fotouhi O, Adel Fahmideh M, Kjellman M et al (2014) Global hypomethylation and promoter methylation in small intestinal neuroendocrine tumors: an in vivo and in vitro study. Epigenetics 9:987–997
103. Arnold CN, Sosnowski A, Schmitt-Graff A, Arnold R, Blum HE (2007) Analysis of molecular pathways in sporadic neuroendocrine tumors of the gastro-entero-pancreatic system. Int J Cancer 120:2157–2164
104. Kidd M, Modlin I, Oberg K (2016) Towards a new classification of gastroenteropancreatic neuroendocrine neoplasms. Nat Rev Clin Oncol 13:691–705. doi:10.1038/nrclinonc.2016.1085. Epub 2016 Jun 1037
105. Bhattacharjee A, Richards WG, Staunton J et al (2001) Classification of human lung carcinomas by mRNA expression profiling reveals distinct adenocarcinoma subclasses. Proc Natl Acad Sci U S A 98:13790–13795. Epub 12001 Nov 13713
106. Guo Y, Eichler GS, Feng Y, Ingber DE, Huang S (2006) Towards a holistic, yet gene-centered analysis of gene expression profiles: a case study of human lung cancers. J Biomed Biotechnol 2006:69141
107. Swarts DR, Van Neste L, Henfling ME et al (2013) An exploration of pathways involved in lung carcinoid progression using gene expression profiling. Carcinogenesis 34:2726–2737. doi:10.1093/carcin/bgt2271. Epub 2013 Aug 2728
108. Toffalorio F, Belloni E, Barberis M et al (2014) Gene expression profiling reveals GC and CEACAM1 as new tools in the diagnosis of lung carcinoids. Br J Cancer 110:1244–1249. doi:10.1038/bjc.2014.1241. Epub 2014 Feb 1211
109. Lee HW, Lee EH, Ha SY et al (2012) Altered expression of microRNA miR-21, miR-155, and let-7a and their roles in pulmonary neuroendocrine tumors. Pathol Int 62:583–591. doi:10.1111/j.1440-1827.2012.02845.x
110. Mairinger FD, Ting S, Werner R et al (2014) Different micro-RNA expression profiles distinguish subtypes of neuroendocrine tumors of the lung: results of a profiling study. Mod Pathol 27:1632–1640. doi:10.1038/modpathol.2014.1674. Epub 2014 May 1630
111. Rapa I, Votta A, Felice B et al (2015) Identification of MicroRNAs differentially expressed in lung carcinoid subtypes and progression. Neuroendocrinology 101:246–255. doi:10.1159/000381454. Epub 000382015 Mar 000381416
112. Kidd M, Modlin IM, Mane SM et al (2006) Utility of molecular genetic signatures in the delineation of gastric neoplasia. Cancer 106:1480–1488

3

113. Duerr EM, Mizukami Y, Ng A et al (2008) Defining molecular classifications and targets in gastroenteropancreatic neuroendocrine tumors through DNA microarray analysis. Endocr Relat Cancer 15:243–256
114. Dilley WG, Kalyanaraman S, Verma S, Cobb JP, Laramie JM, Lairmore TC (2005) Global gene expression in neuroendocrine tumors from patients with the MEN1 syndrome. Mol Cancer 4:9
115. Sadanandam A, Wullschleger S, Lyssiotis CA et al (2015) A cross-species analysis in pancreatic neuroendocrine tumors reveals molecular subtypes with distinctive clinical, metastatic, developmental, and metabolic characteristics. Cancer Discov 5:1296–1313
116. Roldo C, Missiaglia E, Hagan JP et al (2006) MicroRNA expression abnormalities in pancreatic endocrine and acinar tumors are associated with distinctive pathologic features and clinical behavior. J Clin Oncol 24:4677–4684. Epub 2006 Sep 4611
117. Thorns C, Schurmann C, Gebauer N et al (2014) Global MicroRNA profiling of pancreatic neuroendocrine neoplasias. Anticancer Res 34:2249–2254
118. Li A, Yu J, Kim H et al (2013) MicroRNA array analysis finds elevated serum miR-1290 accurately distinguishes patients with low-stage pancreatic cancer from healthy and disease controls. Clin Cancer Res 19:3600–3610. doi:10.1158/1078-0432.CCR-3612-3092. Epub 2013 May 3622
119. Kidd M, Modlin IM, Drozdov I (2014) Gene network-based analysis identifies two potential subtypes of small intestinal neuroendocrine tumors. BMC Genomics 15:595
120. Kidd M, Modlin IM, Mane SM, Camp RL, Eick G, Latich I (2006) The role of genetic markers--NAP1L1, MAGE-D2, and MTA1--in defining small-intestinal carcinoid neoplasia. Ann Surg Oncol 13: 253–262
121. Leja J, Essaghir A, Essand M et al (2009) Novel markers for enterochromaffin cells and gastrointestinal neuroendocrine carcinomas. Mod Pathol 22:261–272
122. Cui T, Hurtig M, Elgue G et al (2010) Paraneoplastic antigen Ma2 autoantibodies as specific blood biomarkers for detection of early recurrence of small intestine neuroendocrine tumors. PLoS One 5:e16010
123. Li SC, Essaghir A, Martijn C et al (2013) Global microRNA profiling of well-differentiated small intestinal neuroendocrine tumors. Mod Pathol 26:685–696. doi:10.1038/modpathol.2012.1216. Epub 2013 Jan 1018
124. Ruebel K, Leontovich AA, Stilling GA et al (2010) MicroRNA expression in ileal carcinoid tumors: downregulation of microRNA-133a with tumor progression. Mod Pathol 23:367–375
125. Li SC, Khan M, Caplin M, Meyer T, Oberg K, Giandomenico V (2015) Somatostatin analogs treated small intestinal neuroendocrine tumor patients circulating MicroRNAs. PLoS One 10:e0125553. doi: 10.0121371/journal.pone.0125553. eCollection 0122015
126. Kerr SE, Schnabel CA, Sullivan PS et al (2014) A 92-gene cancer classifier predicts the site of origin for neuroendocrine tumors. Mod Pathol 27:44–54. doi:10.1038/modpathol.2013.1105. Epub 2013 Jul 1012
127. Gilad S, Lithwick-Yanai G, Barshack I et al (2012) Classification of the four main types of lung cancer using a microRNA-based diagnostic assay. J Mol Diagn 14:510–517. doi:10.1016/j.jmoldx.2012.1003.1004. Epub 2012 Jun 1027
128. Modlin I, Drozdov I, Alaimo D et al (2014) A multianalyte PCR blood test outperforms single analyte ELISAs for neuroendocrine tumor detection. Endocr Relat Cancer 21:615–628
129. Modlin IM, Kidd M, Bodei L, Drozdov I, Aslanian H (2015) The clinical utility of a novel blood-based multi-transcriptome assay for the diagnosis of neuroendocrine tumors of the gastrointestinal tract. Am J Gastroenterol 110:1223–1232. doi:10.1038/ajg.2015.1160. Epub 2015 Jun 1222
130. Kidd M, Drozdov I, Modlin I (2015) Blood and tissue neuroendocrine tumor gene cluster analysis correlate, define hallmarks and predict disease status. Endocr Relat Cancer 22:561–575. doi:10.1530/ERC-1515-0092. Epub 2015 Jun 1532
131. Modlin IM, Frilling A, Salem RR et al (2016) Blood measurement of neuroendocrine gene transcripts defines the effectiveness of operative resection and ablation strategies. Surgery 159:336–347. doi:10.1016/j.surg.2015.1006.1056. Epub 2015 Oct 1019
132. Cwikla JB, Bodei L, Kolasinska-Cwikla A, Sankowski A, Modlin IM, Kidd M (2015) Circulating transcript analysis (NETest) in GEP-NETs treated with Somatostatin Analogs defines Therapy. J Clin Endocrinol Metab 100:E1437–E1445

133. Bodei L, Kidd M, Modlin IM et al (2016) Measurement of circulating transcripts and gene cluster analysis predicts and defines therapeutic efficacy of peptide receptor radionuclide therapy (PRRT) in neuroendocrine tumors. Eur J Nucl Med Mol Imaging 43:839–851. doi:10.1007/s00259-00015-03250-z. Epub 02015 Nov 00223
134. Kidd M, Modlin IM (2017) Therapy: The role of liquid biopsies to manage and predict PRRT for NETs. Nat Rev Gastroenterol Hepatol 15:26
135. Schimmack S, Svejda B, Lawrence B, Kidd M, Modlin IM (2011) The diversity and commonalities of gastroenteropancreatic neuroendocrine tumors. Langenbeck's Arch Surg 396:273–298
136. Spans L, Clinckemalie L, Helsen C et al (2013) The genomic landscape of prostate cancer. Int J Mol Sci 14:10822–10851. doi:10.13390/ijms140610822

Tumor Staging TNM

Laura A. Boos and Paul Komminoth

A. Colao et al. (eds.), *Neuroendocrine Tumors in Real Life*,
https://doi.org/10.1007/978-3-319-59024-0_4

4

Overview

Since the introduction of the TNM system for neuroendocrine neoplasms (NEN) 2010, several studies have shown that it is a significant prognostic parameter and that in general data are applicable and reproducible. It appears, however, that – at least for some locations – minor adjustments will be necessary and that a unified TNM classification incorporating the proposals of ENET and AJCC/UICC would be very useful.

In this book chapter, the most important facts and experiences concerning the prognostic significance of the TNM system NEN are summarized. This is done separately for the different tumor locations, and key points are tabulated at the end of each section.

4.1 Introduction

TNM classifications are used in order to assemble results of diagnostic procedures in a reproducible manner, which encodes information in a medically universally understandable encryption. They stratify patients, who are suffering from the same disease into categories according to prognosis, and therewith allow clinicians to choose the adequate course of treatment.

TNM classifications are used for nearly all malignant neoplasms in humans and serve as a connecting element between the diagnostic results obtained by pathologists and the clinical course of action. For neuroendocrine neoplasms (NEN), currently at least two TNM classifications exist simultaneously. Since the TNM for NEN has been implemented roughly 10 years ago, knowledge about the robustness of the proposed classifications is limited. Several studies have since been conducted in affected organs. They have shown that the parameters, which are stated in the TNM classifications, have an informative value regarding prognosis.

An assimilation of the different classification in the future is desirable, since the existence of differing systems leads to confusion in the daily practice. Furthermore, an alignment could provide a better comparability between different studies.

In this chapter the current knowledge about TNM and prognosis is summarized for different organ systems.

4.2 Neuroendocrine Tumors of the Pancreas (PNET)

A first approach for a unified classification of NET was made in 1980 [1]. 20 years later a new WHO classification was published [2], which advocated to categorize these tumors according to their malignant potential as (1) well-differentiated (neuro)endocrine tumors (with subdivision into «benign behavior» and «uncertain behavior»), (2) well-differentiated (neuro)endocrine carcinoma, and (3) poorly differentiated (neuro) endocrine carcinoma (of the small cell or large cell type). Unfortunately, this classification did not find universal acceptance.

Therefore in 2006 and 2007, a new TNM staging system, which included a grading classification, was proposed by the European Neuroendocrine Tumor Society (ENET) [3, 4].

In this TNM classification, the combined usage of a site-specific staging system as well as a grading classification was proposed.

Shortly afterward the American Joint Cancer Committee/International Union for Cancer Control/World Health Organization 2010 (AJCC/UICC/WHO 2010) *TNM* seventh edition was published and recommended a partly different categorization of NEN.

Alongside NEN of other locations, especially the classification of pancreatic NEN, shows major differences between the ENET and the AJCC/UICC/WHO 2010 system (◘ Tables 4.1 and 4.2).

Nevertheless, both systems, the novel AJCC/UICC/WHO 2010 classification as well as the ENET TNM classification, were reported to be highly prognostic for patients' survival [6]. However, although both systems were reported to provide prognostically relevant results, the parallel existence of two differing TNM systems leads to a confusion among clinicians and furthermore impaired the comparability of research results regarding prognostic factors and treatment stratification [5].

◘ Table 4.1 TNM classification of pancreatic NEN according to ENET and AJCC/UICC/WHO 2010

Definition	ENET TNM	AJCC/UICC/WHO 2010 TNM
T	*T-primary tumor*	
Tx	Primary tumor cannot be assessed	
T0	No evidence of primary tumor	
Tis		Carcinoma in situ
T1	Limited to pancreas, <2 cm	Limited to pancreas, ≤2 cm
T2	Limited to pancreas, 2–4 cm	Limited to pancreas, >2 cm
T3	Limited to pancreas, >4 cm or invading duodenum and/or bile duct	Invasion beyond pancreas without involvement of the superior mesenteric artery
T4	Invasion of adjacent organs or the wall of large vessels (celiac axis or superior mesenteric artery)	Invasion of major vessels (celiac axis or superior mesenteric artery)
N	*N-regional lymph node metastasis*	
Nx	Regional lymph nodes cannot be assessed	
N0	No regional lymph node metastasis	
N1	Regional lymph node metastasis	
M	*M-distant metastasis*	
Mx	Distant metastasis cannot be assessed	
M0	No distant metastasis	
M1	Distant metastasis	

Table 4.2 Tumor stage classification of pancreatic NEN according to ENET and the AJCC/UICC/WHO 2010

Stage definition	ENET TNM	AJCC/UICC/WHO 2010 TNM
Stage I	T1, N0, M0	
Stage IIa	T2, N0, M0	
Stage IIb	T3, N0, M0	
Stage IIIa	T4, N0, M0	
Stage IIIb	Any T, N1, M0	
Stage IV	Any T, any N, M1	
Stage 0		Tis, N0, M0
Stage IA		T1, N0, M0
Stage IB		T2, N0, M0
Stage IIA		T3, N0, M0
Stage IIB		T1-T3, N1, M0
Stage III		T4, any N, M0
Stage IV		Any T, any N, M1

Therefore, although several studies were conducted in the last years to provide information regarding the prognostic impact of factors included in TNM staging, only a comparatively small amount of data can be contrasted.

Several studies addressed the 5-year overall survival (OS) rate of patients with PNET according to their ENET TNM stage [6–9]. Taken together a total of 827 patients was evaluated regarding this parameter, and all included studies showed a significant correlation between ENET stage and 5-year OS (Table 4.3). Regarding the 5-year OS rate according to stratification by AJCC/UICC /WHO 2010 TNM stage, most of the included studies reported a significant correlation between stage and 5-year OS rate in a total of 2319 patients (Table 4.3) [6, 7, 9–12]. It should be noted, however, that due to a generally favorable prognosis of this entity, depending on the collective composition, 5 years might be a rather short follow-up time, which could be a possible limitation regarding the interpretation of the 5-year survival rate, as stated by Cho et al. [7].

A recent study conducted in a smaller collective reported an equal prognostic impact of both staging systems [7]. This is, however, in contrast to previous studies, which compared both staging systems and reported differing prognostic implications [9, 13].

Yang et al. stated a slight advantage of the ENET TNM staging system due to a statistically significant difference between survival stages III and IV, which could not be

Table 4.3 5-year overall survival rate of patients with pancreatic NEN according to AJCC/UICC/WHO 2010 seventh edition stage (grouped) and ENET stage (grouped)

Author	Patients (*n*)	AJCC stage I 5-year survival rate (%)	AJCC stage II 5-year survival rate (%)	AJCC stage III 5-year survival rate (%)	AJCC stage IV 5-year survival rate (%)	*p*-value
Cho et al. (2016)	153	100	100	100	11	<0.001
Qadan et al. (2014)	1202	84	72	65	55	0.36
Scarpa et al. (2010)	274	75	64	60	20	ND
Strosberg et al. (2011)	425	92	84	81	57	<0.001
Yang et al. (2015)	145	79,5	63,1	15	ND	<0.005
Yang et al. (2015)	120	84,6	70,7	ND	ND	<0.001
Author	**Patients (*n*)**	**ENET stage I 5-year survival rate (%)**	**ENET stage II 5-year survival rate (%)**	**ENET stage III 5-year survival rate (%)**	**ENET stage IV 5-year survival rate (%)**	***p*-value**
Cho et al. (2016)	153	100	100	100	11	<0.001
Han et al. (2014)	104	100	97	73	60	0.04
Strosberg et al. (2011)	425	100	88	85	57	0.001
Yang et al. (2015)	145	75.5	72.7	29	ND	<0.005

ND no data available

reported for the AJCC/UICC/WHO 2010 TNM classification [9]. Rindi et al. also conducted a comparison of both staging systems in a collective of 1072 patients and reported a higher sensitivity for ENET TNM staging regarding tumor-free survival [13].

Furthermore, they could show that a classification by complete TNM systems did not provide a consistently significant prognostic stratification in contrast to a grouped TNM stage system: ENET stages IIa and IIb as well as IIIa and IIIb were summarized as stage II and III, respectively, and AJCC/UICC/WHO 2010 stages IA and IB as well as IIA and IIB were summarized as stages I and II, respectively.

Having grouped the stages, the ENET system provided a statistically significant and progressive separation of patients into four risk groups, while there was an overlap in stages II and III using the AJCC/UICC/WHO 2010 system [13]. Therefore Rindi et al. proposed to simplify the ENET staging system into four single-stage classes [13]; this was supported by the results of Scarpa et al. [12].

A cross tabulation of the AJCC/UICC/WHO 2010 and the ENET classification in one study demonstrated that patients classified as stage III patients in the ENET staging system were split into AJCC/UICC/WHO 2010 stages II and III, while patients classified as stage I according to the AJCC/UICC/WHO 2010 staging system were distributed between stages I and II in the ENET classification [6].

The T-stage is defined differently in both staging systems. pT1 and pT2 are similar; however, ENET pT3 is either limited to the pancreas and exceeds a dimension of 4 cm or involves the duodenum or bile duct, while AJCC/UICC/WHO 2010 pT3 is defined as tumor growth beyond the pancreas but without involvement of the superior mesenteric artery, therewith comprising a larger portion of tumors. ENET pT4 on the other hand is defined as tumor invasion into adjacent organs or the wall of large vessels, while AJCC/UICC pT4 is used for NEN invading the celiac axis or the superior mesenteric artery (◘ Table 4.1).

ENET T-stage alone showed statistically different survival times [12, 14]. Brunner et al. reported a significant prognostic difference regarding the survival of patients with pT1 or pT2 or pT3 stages compared to pT4 stage [14]. In one study with a comparatively large collective, Kaplan-Meier analysis showed a significant difference between the survival rates of patients with combined pT1 and pT2 stage compared to pT3 or pT4, as well as between pT3 and pT4 but not between pT1 and pT2, suggesting that differences in tumor size in tumors <4 cm do not have a prognostic impact [12].

Lymph node (LN) metastases in patients with PNET were reported to be an impairing factor regarding prognosis [8, 11, 12, 14–16]; three studies reported a 5-year OS rate, which confirmed this result (◘ Table 4.4). These findings explain why ENET stage IIIb (tumors with LN metastases) shows significantly shorter survival times than stages I, IIa, IIb, IIIa, and IV [14] and underlines the reasonable demand for grouped TNM stages. Only in one study pN-status was not found to be a significant prognostic factor [17].

Regarding blood vessel invasion, two studies with a total of 186 patients reported 5-year OS rates of patients and found invasion of blood vessels to be a significant prognostic factor (◘ Table 4.4) [8, 17]. One other group published opposing results, reporting no prognostic impact of blood vessel invasion in 82 patients [16].

The role of perineural invasion as a prognostic factor remains unclear so far: one study reported a prognostic impact of perineural invasion [8], while another study with a comparable collective size reported no significant effect on survival [17].

Distant metastatic disease in patients with PNET was reported to impair the OS significantly according to 3 studies comprising a total of 460 patients (◘ Table 4.4) [8, 11, 12]. Two other studies, comprising a total of 194 patients, however, showed contrary results [16, 17].

Table 4.4 5-year overall survival rate of patients with pancreatic NEN according to pN/pV/pM-status

Author	Patients (*n*)	pN0 5-year survival rate (%)	pN1 5-year survival rate (%)	*p*-value
Han et al. (2014)	104	96	64	0.033
Demir et al. (2011)	82	42.7	73,3	0.04
Scarpa et al. (2010)	274	94	31	<0.001
Author	**Patients (*n*)**	**pV0 5-year survival rate (%)**	**pV1 5-year survival rate (%)**	***p*-value**
Han et al. (2014)	104	96	80	0.023
Demir et al. (2011)	82	62.2	35.9	0.1
Author	**Patients (*n*)**	**pM0 5-year survival rate (%)**	**pM1 5-year survival rate (%)**	***p*-value**
Han et al. (2014)	104	94	89	0.015
Demir et al. (2011)	82	59.6	53.3	0.83
Scarpa et al. (2010)	274	88	35	<0.001

Furthermore, R status was reported to have a significant impact on patient survival [17]. One study reported a significantly longer median survival in patients with R0 resection of the primary compared to patients with R1/R2 resection [16]. Another study supported these results; however, in this series with exclusion of R2 cases, R0 resections were not associated with a better survival, suggesting an important role of macroscopic tumor rests in the resection margin [18].

Key Points Pancreas

- ENET pT-stage has significant informative value regarding prognosis – significant difference exists especially between pT1/pT2/pT3 and pT4 [14].
- LN involvement is significantly associated with worse 5-year OS [8, 11, 12, 14–16].
- Vascular invasion is probably a significant prognostic factor; however, at this point conflicting results exist [8, 16, 17].
- The impact of perineural invasion is not clear [8, 17].
- Most studies report that distant metastatic disease is a significant prognostic factor [8, 11, 12, 16, 17].
- The majority of studies show that resection status is a significant prognostic factor [16–18].
- Both ENET TNM and AJCC/UICC/WHO 2010 staging classifications have significant informative value, with a slight superiority of the ENET TNM [6–12].
- Grouped TNM staging allows superior progressive stratification [12, 13].

4.3 Neuroendocrine Tumors of the Stomach

The ENET TNM system and the AJCC/UICC/WHO 2010 TNM system for gastric NEN differ slightly regarding the definition of the pT-stage (Tables 4.5 and 4.6). Both pT-stages incorporate tumor size and invasion; however, in the ENET TNM classification, pT3 is defined as invasion of the serosa [3], while in pT3 in the AJCC/UICC/WHO 2010 classification describes tumors that invade the subserosal tissue.

Both TNM systems are significantly correlated with survival and prognosis [19]; only the AJCC/UICC/WHO 2010 TNM system, however, was shown to be an independent prognostic factor in multivariate analysis [20].

Different series reported the size of the primary tumor to have significant impact on prognosis, although different cutoff values were used or the threshold was not clearly stated [19–22].

Table 4.5 TNM classifications of gastric NEN according to ENET and AJCC/UICC/WHO 2010

Definition	ENET TNM	AJCC/UICC/WHO 2010 TNM
T	*T-primary tumor*	
Tx	Primary tumor cannot be assessed	
T0	No evidence of primary tumor	
Tis	In situ tumor/dysplasia (<0,5 mm)	In situ tumor/dysplasia (<0,5 mm), confined to mucosa
T1	Tumor ≤1 cm and invasion of lamina propria or submucosa	Tumor 0,5 mm–1 cm and confined to mucosa or ≤1 cm and invasion of submucosa
T2	Tumor >1 cm or invasion of muscularis propria or subserosa	Tumor >1 cm or invasion of muscularis propria
T3	Penetrates serosa	Invasion of subserosa
T4	Invasion of other organs or adjacent structures	Invasion of visceral peritoneum or other organs or adjacent structures
(m)	*For any T, add (m) for multiple tumors*	
N	*N-regional lymph node metastasis*	
Nx	Regional lymph nodes cannot be assessed	
N0	No regional lymph node metastasis	
N1	Regional lymph node metastasis	
M	*M-distant metastasis*	
Mx	Distant metastasis cannot be assessed	
M0	No distant metastasis	
M1	Distant metastasis	

Table 4.6 Tumor stage classification for gastric NEN according to ENET and AJCC/UICC/WHO 2010

Stage definition	AJCC/UICC/WHO 2010	ENET
Stage 0		Tis N0 M0
Stage I	T1 N0 M0	
Stage IIA	T2 N0 M0	
Stage IIB	T3 N0 M0	
Stage IIIA	T4 N0 M0	
Stage IIIB	Any T N1 M0	
Stage IV	Any T any N M1	

The depth of invasion was shown to be an independent predictor of prognosis if invasion beyond the lamina muscularis propria was present [22].

Tumor size and degree of invasion were reported to be associated significantly with LN – and distant metastases [21].

Furthermore, LN metastases were significantly associated with prognosis [20, 22]. La Rosa et al. reported a difference in prognosis according to the amount of positive LN with a worse outcome in patients with >3 positive LN [21]. Accordingly, lymphangiosis carcinomatosa was also associated with a worse outcome [19, 20], while invasion of blood vessels did not correlate significantly [19].

Perineural invasion was reported to be a significant prognostic factor [20] as well as distant metastases, which were shown to affect the survival of 1752 patients in two series [21, 22]. Kubota et al., on the other hand, found no significant correlation between liver metastases and prognosis; this study, however, was conducted with a smaller collective of 27 patients and focused on hepatic metastases [19].

Key Points Stomach

- Size of primary tumor is a significant factor for prognosis [19–22].
- Depth of invasion is significant factor for prognosis [19–22] and an independent predictor when invasion occurs beyond the L. muscularis propria [22].
- Size of tumor and invasion level significantly predict LN and distant metastases [21].
- pN1 is a significant factor for prognosis [20, 22]; there is a prognostic difference between 1–3 and >3 positive LN [21].
- L0/L1 is a significant prognostic factor [19, 20].
- Pn0/Pn1 is a significant prognostic factor [20].
- Vascular invasion does not correlate significantly with survival [19].
- Most studies agree on the significance of distant metastases as a factor for prognosis; however, conflicting results exist [19, 21, 22].
- ENET TNM and AJCC TNM are different; nevertheless both significantly correlate with survival and prognosis [19]; however, only the AJCC staging system was reported as an independent prognostic factor [20].

4.4 Neuroendocrine Tumors of Duodenum, Jejunum, and Ileum

The ENET TNM system and the AJCC/UICC/WHO 2010 system for intestinal NEN are essentially identical (◘ Tables 4.7 and 4.8). The ENET pT1-stage is defined by size and «invasion of mucosa or submucosa» [4], while the AJCC/UICC/WHO 2010 uses a slightly different nomenclature by defining pT1-stage by size and «invasion of lamina propria or submucosa» [23]. Biologically these two descriptions can be viewed as identical.

According to the SEER registry, the incidence of intestinal NEN has risen about 35% in the last 35 years [24, 25]. Due to progressively earlier diagnosis, the 5-year OS rates have increased in the last decades [26]. Nowadays, nonfunctional NEN of the duodenum are mostly diagnosed in early, well treatable disease stages and at a size ≤10 mm [26]. In contrast, functional duodenal NEN were reported to present more frequently with metastatic disease at this point [26].

◘ **Table 4.7** TNM classification of intestinal NEN according to ENET and AJCC/UICC/WHO 2010

Definition	ENET TNM	AJCC/UICC/WHO 2010 TNM
T	*T-primary tumor*	
Tx	Primary tumor cannot be assessed	
T0	No evidence of primary tumor	
T1	Tumor ≤1 cm; invasion of mucosa/lamina propria or submucosa[a]	
T2	Tumor >1 cm or invasion of muscularis propria	
T3	Duodenum/ampulla/proximal jejunum: invasion of pancreas or retroperitoneum jejunum/ileum – invasion of subserosa	
T4	Invasion of visceral peritoneum/other organs/adjacent structures	
(m)	*For any T, add (m) for multiple tumors*	
N	*N-regional lymph node metastasis*	
Nx	Regional lymph nodes cannot be assessed	
N0	No regional lymph node metastasis	
N1	Regional lymph node metastasis	
M	*M-distant metastasis*	
Mx	Distant metastasis cannot be assessed	
M0	No distant metastasis	
M1	Distant metastasis	

[a]Tumor limited to ampulla of Vater for ampullary gangliocytic paraganglioma

Table 4.8 Tumor stage classification for intestinal NEN according ENET and AJCC/UICC/WHO 2010

Stage definition	ENET	AJCC/UICC/WHO 2010
Stage I	T1 N0 M0	
Stage IIA	T2 N0 M0	
Stage IIB	T3 N0 M0	
Stage IIIA	T4 N0 M0	
Stage IIIB	Any T N1 M0	
Stage IV	Any T any N M1	

The staging systems define subgroups (Table 4.8); nevertheless, most statistical analyses have been done on grouped collectives [27–30]. A significant prognostic impact of the grouped stages was demonstrated [27], especially when comparing local (stage I–IIIA) to regional (stage IIIB) and distant disease (stage IV) [28–30] and when comparing regional to distant disease [28, 29]. The worst survival was reported for stage IV [28–31]. In early-stage disease, however, an overlap was shown between some stage groups [31]; the TNM staging did not distinguish optimally between the early-stage tumors [30].

The 5-year survival rate was 100% for stage I and II and varied between 91% and 91.1% and between 72% and 84% for stage III and IV, respectively [27, 28, 30] . The 10-year survival rates showed similar results with a significant decrease in survival for distant disease: stage I and II had a 10-year survival rate of 100%, while the survival varied between 84.6% and 93% and between 39% and 59.1% for stage III and IV, respectively [27, 28]. However, a wide range of 35%–80% for the 5-year survival rates of patients with jejunal or ileal NEN with stage IV disease has been presented by Niederle et al., and in more recent data collections, even more favorable outcomes were reported [32].

A progressively worse disease-specific survival with advanced pT-stage was reported by Kim et al. [31]; another series observed significantly more frequent distant metastases, disease progression, and death in larger tumors [27].

LN involvement was also shown to be significantly associated with a lower 10-year OS rate compared to patients with pN0-stage [31]. The impact of pN1-stage on prognosis, however, varied according to the pT-stage; worse survival was observed in patients with pT1 and pT2 stage with LN involvement, but no adverse effect of LN metastases was detected in patients with more advanced disease [31].

Furthermore, a worse 5-year OS rate was observed for patients with non-resectable tumor-suspect LN in the mesenteric root compared to patients in whom resection was feasible [30].

Vascular invasion was reported to be more frequent in patients with higher TNM stage [27], which could be interpreted as an expression of the more aggressive nature of advanced disease.

A significantly worse 10-year OS rate was reported for patients whose tumors had metastasized [31]; more specifically a higher risk of disease progression, death in general, and death related to the intestinal NEN has been reported for patients with metastasized tumors [27].

Metastases to the bone were observed to occur rather late in disease progression; the 5-year survival rate of patients with jejunal or ileal NEN and skeletal metastases was 20% [33].

Liver tumor load, extra-abdominal metastases, and peritoneal carcinomatosis in tumors with jejunal or ileal primary have been reported to be independent prognostic factors by multivariate analysis [34].

A significant survival benefit was shown for patients that underwent resection of hepatic metastases compared to patients that did not undergo this intervention in presence of hepatic spread of disease [29]. Surgical resection of the jejunal or ileal primary tumor was not associated with a statistically significant improvement in survival in patients with metastatic disease [33].

Key Points Duodenum, Jejunum, and Ileum

- Progressively worse disease-specific survival with more advanced T-status [31].
- Significantly worse 10-year OS rate in pN1 compared to pN0 [31].
- Impact of pN1 disease varies according to T-status (impact observed in pT1 and pT2, none in higher pT-status) [31].
- Significantly worse 10-year OS rate in M1 compared to M0 [31].
- Significant survival benefit of patients that underwent liver resection if hepatic metastasis is present [29].
- Significant prognostic impact of TNM stages, especially when comparing local (I–IIIA) to regional (IIIB) and distant disease (IV) [27–31], but there is an overlap in some subgroups of patients with early-stage disease [31].

4.5 Neuroendocrine Tumors of the Appendix Vermiformis

The ENET TNM system and the AJCC/UICC/WHO 2010 TNM system for appendiceal NEN differ considerably from each other (◘ Tables 4.9 and 4.10). Both pT-stages include invasion and tumor size as defining factors; nevertheless, they propose different threshold values.

Volante et al. reported the pT-stage – ENET and AJCC/UICC/WHO 2010 – to be the most significant prognostic indicator [35]. In this series, however, the ENET pT-stage seemed to be less specific compared to the AJCC/UICC/WHO 2010 pT-stage; although all patients, who died from the disease, were staged as pT3 or pT4 according to ENET, a high pT-stage was also observed in up to 25% of patients, who were alive at the time of follow-up [35] .The AJCC/UICC/WHO 2010 pT-stage, on the other hand, was evaluated to be more accurate and specific in selecting the very few aggressive and fatal cases [35]. Furthermore, only AJCC/UICC/WHO 2010 pT-stage could be confirmed as an independent prognostic indicator on multivariate analysis [35].

Tumor invasion into the mesoappendix has been discussed controversially regarding its impact on survival and its part in the definition of pT-stage. One of the criteria of the ENET pT2-stage is an invasion of the subserosa or mesoappendix up to 3 mm; pT3-stage can be defined as an invasion of subserosa or mesoappendix >3 mm [4]. The AJCC/UICC/WHO 2010 definition of pT-stage does not include this parameter

Table 4.9 TNM classification of appendiceal NEN according to ENET and AJCC/UICC/WHO 2010

Definition	ENET TNM	AJCC/UICC/WHO 2010 TNM
T	*T-primary tumor*	
Tx	Primary tumor cannot be assessed	
T0	No evidence of primary tumor	
T1	Tumor ≤1 cm; invasion of submucosa or muscularis propria	T1a: tumor ≤1 cm
		T1b: tumor >1 but ≤2 cm
T2	Tumor ≤2 cm; invasion of submucosa, muscularis propria and/or ≤3 mm invasion of subserosa/mesoappendix	Tumor >2 cm but ≤4 cm or invasion of caecum
T3	Tumor >2 cm and/or >3 mm invasion of subserosa/mesoappendix	Tumor >4 cm or invasion of ileum
T4	Invasion of peritoneum/other organs/ adjacent structures	Invasion of peritoneum/other organs/adjacent structures
N	*N-regional lymph node metastasis*	
Nx	Regional lymph nodes cannot be assessed	
N0	No regional lymph node metastasis	
N1	Regional lymph node metastasis	
M	*M-distant metastasis*	
Mx	Distant metastasis cannot be assessed	
M0	No distant metastasis	
M1	Distant metastasis	

Table 4.10 Tumor stage classification in appendiceal NEN according to ENET and AJCC/UICC/WHO 2010

Stage definition	AJCC/UICC/ WHO 2010	ENET
Stage I	T1 N0 M0	T1 N0 M0
Stage II	T2–T3 N0 M0	Stage IIA: T2 N0 M0
		Stage IIB: T3 N0 M0
Stage III	T4 – any T N0 – N1 M0	Stage IIIA: T4 N0 M0
		Stage IIIB: any T N1 M0
Stage IV	Any T any N M1	Any T any N M1

(◘ Table 4.9). Mesoappendiceal invasion was observed in about 30–40% of appendiceal NEN in children and in about 10–20% of appendiceal NEN in adults [36]. In the past, the involvement of the mesoappendix has favored more radical surgery as reported by Moertel et al. [37]; nevertheless, the degree of invasion did not have an impact on outcome in a series of 40 children, as there were no metastases or recurrences although 85% of tumors invaded beyond the appendiceal submucosa [38]. Mesoappendiceal invasion in tumors <2 cm was reported to have no negative effect on survival [39, 40]; however, deep mesoappendiceal invasion has been observed to confer a relevant risk of disease recurrence [39]. Furthermore, tumors with an invasion into the mesoappendix were observed to show a higher rate of vascular and lymph vessel involvement than cases without [4, 36, 41].

Several series reported tumor size alone to have no impact on survival [35, 42]. MacGillivray et al. on the other hand reported a relation between tumor size and prognosis and mentioned a maximal diameter > 2 cm to be the most important parameter for prediction of survival [43].

Tumor size has, moreover, been reported to be a significant predictor of nodal involvement [44]. Deschamps et al. reported tumors <1 cm to have no LN or distant metastases [45], while Syracuse et al. observed 2 patients with tumors <1 cm and nodal spread in a series of 92 patients [46]. Anderson et al. reported 2 patients out of 147 with tumors <2 cm who had metastatic disease (1.3%) [47], while Deschamps et al. observed 10% of patients with tumors with a diameter 1–2 cm to have LN involvement [45]. In contrast, other series did not detect LN or distant metastases in tumors <2 cm [37, 48]. Dralle reported a higher risk of LN involvement in tumors <2 cm if mesoappendiceal invasion is present, (0.3% in tumors without invasion and 3.5% in tumors with invasion [36]).

Due to this controversial data, tumors >1 cm but <2 cm have been reported to be the most challenging, regarding the determination of the clinical approach [41].

Patients with appendiceal NEN exceeding a diameter of 2 cm have been observed to have an increased risk to develop metastatic lesions [49] or disease recurrence [39]. Moertel et al. published a series in 1987 that indicates this course of illness: of 150 patients with appendiceal NEN, 127 had tumors <2 cm, and none of those patients developed metastatic disease. 3 of 4 patients with tumors between 2 and 3 cm developed LN metastases (21%) and 4 of 9 patients with tumors >3 cm (44%) [37].

Localized (node negative), regional, and distant disease was reported to have a progressively worse 3-year/5-year/10-year survival rate [50]. LN involvement and distant metastatic disease were shown to be independent significant predictors of prognosis in multivariate analysis [51].

Only a trend to shorter survival was observed for tumors presenting with vascular invasion [35]; nevertheless, vascular invasion has been reported to favor more radical surgery in the past [37]. Rossi et al. stated the importance to examine areas of suspected vascular invasion immunohistochemically (CD31) due to potential accidental confusion with tissue artifacts [40].

The presence of perineural invasion did not have a significant impact on disease-related survival in univariate analysis [35].

Positive resection margins were associated with prognosis; this, however, could not be validated as independent prognostic marker in multivariate analysis [35].

Key Points Appendix

- Tumor size is a significant predictor of nodal involvement and distant metastases [44, 49]. Tumors <1 cm (< 2 cm) rarely have LN or distant metastases [37, 45, 48]; only 10% of tumors with LN metastases are between 1 and 2 cm [45].
- Tumor size ≥2 cm is an important prognostic factor [43] and is significantly associated with distant metastatic lesions [39, 47].
- Trend to significance is observed for V1 [35] and patients with metastases more frequently exhibit vascular invasion [37].
- Positive resection margin is associated with shorter survival [35].
- Prognostic impact of depth of invasion into mesoappendix is undisputable [4, 35] and is significantly correlated with lymph node involvement and vascular invasion [4, 36, 41].
- ENET pT-stage is less specific than AJCC pT-stage; only AJCC pT-stage was independent in multivariate analysis [35].

4.6 Neuroendocrine Tumors of the Rectum and Colon

The ENET TNM system and the AJCC/UICC/WHO 2010 TNM system are the same regarding NEN of the colon and rectum [52] (◘ Tables 4.11 and 4.12).

Regarding rectal NEN the TNM staging was reported to be a significant prognostic factor in several series [52, 53]. Comparable to the tumor staging for other NEN, stages I–IIIA represent local disease, while stage IIIB depicts LN involvement, and stage IV constitutes of patients with metastasized disease (◘ Table 4.12). Chi et al. observed a shorter survival in patients with stage IV tumors [53]; another series also reported significantly shorter survival time for patients with metastasized disease, although there was no clear statement whether metastases to the LN or distant metastases or both entities were addressed [52]. Patients, who suffered from tumors without LN involvement, were reported to survive without recurrence [54].

In several series the 5- and 10-year survival rate was examined according to localized, regional, or distant disease (◘ Table 4.13). «Localized» was defined as an invasive neoplasm confined to the organ of origin, «regional» was defined as either extending beyond the organ of origin or with regional LN involvement, and «distant» was defined as a tumor with spread to body parts remote of the primary tumor [25, 55, 56]. The survival rates show a clear and progressive decline when aligned with the extent of disease (◘ Table 4.13). This was verified additionally in a review by Scherübl et al., who reported a 5-year survival rate of 98.9–100% for localized disease (in patients with tumors ≤10 mm without vascular invasion and without invasion into the muscularis propria), 54–73% in regional disease, and 15–30% in distant disease [57]. Furthermore, another series showed similar results examining the 5- and 10-year OS rates. In this study slightly different terms were used, («locally confined,» «locally advanced,» and «distant» disease) without providing a detailed definition regarding the «locally advanced» stage in terms of local tumor extension and/or LN involvement and therefore affecting the comparability [58].

Tumor size was observed to have an impact on OS [53]; however, this could not be validated for every threshold value, since another series could only show a significant difference in prognosis comparing tumors <1 cm and tumors >1 cm but failed to show

Table 4.11 TNM classification of colorectal NEN according to ENET and AJCC/UICC/WHO 2010

Definition	ENET TNM	AJCC/UICC/WHO 2010 TNM
T	*T-primary tumor*	
Tx	Primary tumor cannot be assessed	
T0	No evidence of primary tumor	
T1	Invasion of lamina propria or submucosa T1a: ≤1 cm T1b: >1 but ≤2 cm	
T2	Invasion of muscularis propria or >2 cm	
T3	Invasion of subserosa/pericolic/perirectal fat	
T4	Invasion of peritoneum/other organs/adjacent structures	
(m)	*For any T, add (m) for multiple tumors*	
N	*N-regional lymph node metastasis*	
Nx	Regional lymph nodes cannot be assessed	
N0	No regional lymph node metastasis	
N1	Regional lymph node metastasis	
M	*M-distant metastasis*	
Mx	Distant metastasis cannot be assessed	
M0	No distant metastasis	
M1	Distant metastasis	

Table 4.12 Definition of tumor stage for colorectal NEN according to ENET and AJCC/UICC/WHO 2010

Stage definition	AJCC/UICC/WHO 2010	ENET
Stage I	T1 N0 M0	Stage IA: T1a N0 M0
		Stage IB: T1b N0 M0
Stage IIA	T2 N0 M0	T2 N0 M0
Stage IIB	T3 N0 M0	T3 N0 M0
Stage IIIA	T4 N0 M0	T4 N0 M0
Stage IIIB	Any T N1 M0	Any T N1 M0
Stage IV	Any T any N M1	Any T any N M1

Table 4.13 5-/10-year survival rate (%) according to extent of disease in colorectal NEN

Author	Localized 5-year survival rate (%)	Regional 5-year survival rate (%)	Distant 5-year survival rate (%)
Yao JC et al. (2008)	90	62	24
Modlin IM et al. (1997)	81	46.7	18.3
Modlin IM et al. 1973–1991 (2003)	84	36.4	32.2
Modlin IM et al. 1992–1999 (2003)	90.8	48.9	69.5
Author	**Localized 10-year survival rate (%)**	**Regional 10-year survival rate (%)**	**Distant 10-year survival rate (%)**
Yao JC et al. (2008)	80	47	3

Table 4.14 Lymph node metastases in rectal NEN (%) depending on tumor size in the US SEER and the Japanese Niigata registry

Tumor size (mm)	Lymph node metastasis in rectal NET (%) (SEER registry)	Lymph node metastases in rectal NET (%) (Niigata registry)
≤5 mm	ND	3.7
≤10 mm	3	9.7
10.1–20 mm	17–42	27.6
>20 mm	60–80	N.D.

ND: no data available

a difference between tumors with a diameter of 1–2 cm and >2 cm [52]. Furthermore, progressive tumor size was reported to predict increasing tumor progression [58] as well as LN metastases [57] and distant metastases [52].

The SEER registry documented nodal disease in about 3% of rectal NEN ≤ 10 mm, in about 17–42% of rectal NEN between 10.1 mm and 20 mm, and in about 60–80% in patients with rectal NEN ≥ 20 mm (Table 4.14) [57].

In a large Japanese series, patients with tumors ≤10 mm were reported to have LN metastases considerably more often. In detail, in the large series by Soga et al., comprising of 849 patients with rectal NEN (Japanese cancer registry Niigata), submucosal tumors ≤5 mm showed LN metastases in 3.7%, while tumors ≤10 mm led to LN metastases in 9.7% [59]. Interestingly, however, patients with tumors ≤10 mm without vascular invasion and without invasion of the L. muscularis propria did not develop LN metastases [59]. This patient group is reported to have an excellent 5-year survival rate of 98.9–100% as mentioned above (Table 4.4) [57].

Patients with tumors between 0.1 cm and 1 cm have been reported to have a 5-year OS rate of 81% and a distant metastases rate < 5%, while most patients with tumors ≥2 cm had metastases, and their 5-year survival rate was between 18% and 40% [53]. Nevertheless, also patients with rectal NEN < 1 cm were reported to be at a smaller but still present risk of developing metastases [52, 60, 61].

Although the same classifications are used for both tumor localizations, colonic NEN differ strongly from NEN located in the rectum.

Patients with rectal NEN are reported to have metastasized disease at diagnosis in 4–18% of cases [55, 62]; the tumors are usually between 1 and 2 cm [57].

Colonic NEN, however, have nodal or distant disease in about two-thirds of patients at the time of diagnosis; the average tumor diameter at presentation is 5 cm [63, 64].

The 5-year survival rate of colonic NEN has been reported to be 70.7% for localized disease compared to 46.7% for regional disease and 20.5% for distant disease [56].

Key Points Rectum and Colon

- At diagnosis rectal NEN are usually small and not advanced [55, 57, 62].
- In contrast, colonic NEN mostly exhibit a tumor diameter of about 5 cm, and there is metastatic disease in two-thirds of cases [63, 64].
- Tumor size has a significant impact on overall survival [53], although not for every defined increase in size a prognostic difference could be demonstrated [52].
- Progressive tumor size is associated with distant metastases [52]; patients with tumors between 0.1 and 1 cm have been reported to have a distant metastasis rate < 5% and a 5-year OS rate of 81%, while patients with tumors ≥2 cm had a 5-year OS rate of 18%–40% [53].
- Occurrence of LN metastases is dependent on tumor size [57]. Nevertheless, there is still a risk of metastasis in NEN <1 cm [52, 60, 61].
- Patients without LN metastases survive without recurrence [54].
- 5-year OS rate is dependent on localized/regional/systemic disease [25, 56–58].
- TNM staging is a significant prognostic factor [52, 53].

4.7 Neuroendocrine Tumors of the Lung

The AJCC/UICC/WHO 2010 classification for neoplasms of the lung is applicable for carcinomas of the lung including small cell carcinoma (SCLC) and large cell neuroendocrine carcinoma (LCNEC) as well as for well-differentiated pulmonary NEN also referred to as pulmonary carcinoids (PC): typical carcinoids (TC) and atypical carcinoids (AC) [23, 65].

The application of the AJCC/UICC/WHO 2010 seventh edition TNM staging for pulmonary NEN is recommended among others by the ENET [66].

For PCs a SEER database analysis reported survival outcomes to be consistently associated with stage of disease [65]. Another series observed N- and M-stage to have a significant prognostic impact in univariate analysis; this however could not be verified in a multivariate analysis [67]. Daddi et al. reported a significant association between progressive tumor size/TNM stage and worse survival for a collective of ACs in a univariate analysis. However, this could not be verified in a multivariate analysis [68].

The pT-stage is defined by size, degree of invasion, and relation to the main bronchus and carina (◘ Table 4.15 and 4.16). Travis et al. reported a significant overall effect

Table 4.15 TNM classification of malignant pulmonary neoplasms according to UICC/AJCC [23]

Definition	AJCC/UICC/WHO 2010 TNM
T	*T-primary tumor*
Tx	Primary tumor cannot be assessed or tumor proven by the presence of malignant cells in sputum or bronchial washings but not visualized by imaging or bronchoscopy
T0	No evidence of primary tumor
Tis	Carcinoma in situ
T1	Tumor ≤3 cm, surrounded by lung or visceral pleura, without bronchoscopic evidence of invasion more proximal than the lobar bronchus (i.e., not in the main bronchus)* T1a: tumor ≤2 cm T1b: tumor >2 cm – ≤3 cm
T2	Tumor >3 cm–≤ 7 cm or tumor with any of the following features* – involvement of main bronchus, ≥2 cm distal of carina – invasion of visceral pleura (Pl1 or Pl2) – association with atelectasis or obstructive pneumonitis that extends to the hilar region but does not involve the entire lung T2a: tumor >3 cm but ≤5 cm T2b: >5 cm but ≤7 cm
T3	Tumor >7 cm *or* direct invasion into any of the following structures: parietal pleura (Pl3), chest wall (including superior sulcus tumors), diaphragm, phrenic nerve, mediastinal pleura, parietal pericardium, *or* tumor in the main bronchus <2 cm distal to the carina but without involvement of carina *or* association with atelectasis or obstructive pneumonitis of the entire lung or separate tumor nodule(s) in the same lobe as the primary
T4	Tumor of any size with invasion into any of the following structures: mediastinum, heart, great vessels, trachea, recurrent laryngeal nerve, esophagus, vertebral body, and carina. Separate tumor nodule(s) in a different ipsilateral lobe
N	*N-regional lymph node metastasis*
Nx	Regional lymph nodes cannot be assessed
N0	No regional lymph node metastasis
N1	Metastasis in ipsilateral peribronchial and/or ipsilateral hilar lymph nodes or intrapulmonary nodes (including involvement by direct extension)
N2	Metastasis in ipsilateral mediastinal and/or subcarinal lymph node(s)
N3	Metastasis in contralateral mediastinal, contralateral hilar, ipsilateral or contralateral scalene or supraclavicular lymph node(s)
M	*M-distant metastasis*
Mx	Distant metastasis cannot be assessed
M0	No distant metastasis
M1	Distant metastasis M1a: separate tumor nodule(s) in a contralateral lobe, tumor with pleural nodules, or malignant pleural (or pericardial) effusion⁺ M1b: distant metastasis (in extrathoracic organs)

4

Table 4.16 Tumor stage classification for malignant tumors of the lung according to AJCC/UICC/WHO 2010

Stage Definition	AJCC/UICC/WHO 2010
Occult carcinoma	Tx N0 M0
Stage 0	Tis N0 M0
Stage IA	T1a–T1b N0 M0
Stage IB	T2a N0 M0
Stage IIA	T2b N0 M0
	T1a–T2a N1 M0
Stage IIB	T2b N1 M0
	T3 N0 M0
Stage IIIA	T1a–T2b N2 M0
	T3 N1–N2 M0
	T4 N0–N1 M0
Stage IIIB	T1a–T3 N3 M0
	T4 N2–N3 M0
Stage IV	Any T any N M1a–M1b

of pT-stage on survival. Furthermore, in that series a significantly worse survival for patients with T1 N0 PCs with a diameter of >2–3 cm compared to patients with T1 N0 PCs with a primary tumor ≤2 cm was observed [69].

In contrast to the definition of N-stage in other NEN, the N-stage for malignant neoplasms of the lung incorporates the location of positive LN separating the N-stages according to vicinity (Table 4.15).

A significant impact of LN involvement on survival in patients with PCs has been reported [69]. This result could be reproduced in a multivariate analysis in a collective of ACs [68].

Well-differentiated pulmonary NEN were reported to have progressively worse survival rates in «localized,» «regional,» and «distant» disease [65]. «Localized» was defined as a tumor confined to the organ of origin, and these tumors showed a 5- and 10-year survival rate of 84% and 56%, respectively; «regional» spread of disease was defined as extent beyond the limits of the organ of origin and/or as spread to regional LN, and these tumors showed a 5- and 10-year survival rate of 72% and 56%, respectively. The worst 5- and 10-year survival rates with 27% and 15%, respectively, were observed for tumors with spread to distant body parts remote from the primary tumor, which was defined as «distant» [70].

Nevertheless, it must be stated that pulmonary NEN are classified according to their mitotic activity, their ki-67 index, their cell morphology, as well as the presence of necrosis [70], and it should be noted that their prognosis varies according to their degree of malignancy, with a progressively worse outcome from TCs via ACs to LCNEC and SCLC [71]. The diagnostic criteria are said to still rely primarily on histology [66].

Battafarano et al. reported no significant association between prognosis and TNM stage regarding LCNEC in a multivariate analysis [72]. Furthermore, patients with LCNEC were reported to have a significantly worse outcome after resection compared to patients with large cell carcinomas, even in TNM tumor stage I [72].

Planchard et al. observed a 5-year survival rate of 25% for SLCL without metastases and a survival rate of around 10% after 2 years in patients with metastatic disease [73]. Tumor staging was reported to have prognostic ramification in SCLC, and a further collection of data in future studies and databases was called for [74].

Since the submission of the manuscript a new and updated version of the TNM classification system (version 8) has been published by the UICC in which the differences between the ENETS and the UICC system for neuroendocrine neoplasms of the pancreas and the appendix have mostly been eliminated.

Key Points Lung

- Pulmonary NEN are mainly classified according to their cell morphology, mitotic activity, ki-67 index, and necrosis [70].
- Prognosis is associated with tumor type with a progressively worse outcome for typical CD (TC) - > atypical CD (AC) - > LCLC and - > SCLC [71].
- Survival outcomes for carcinoids are consistently associated with histological grade and stage of disease in the SEER registry [65].
- Overall effect of pT-status on survival is significant in carcinoids [69].
- For T1 N0 carcinoids, there is significant worse outcome for those with tumor >2–3 cm compared with tumors ≤2 cm [69].
- Effect of pN-status on survival is significant in TC and AC [68].
- 5- and 10-year survival rates decrease progressively for localized – regional – distant disease in carcinoids.
- N status and M status are statistically significant regarding carcinoids in univariate analysis, however, not in multivariate analysis [67].
- TNM stage and tumor size are significantly associated with worse outcome in patients with AC in univariate analysis but not in multivariate analysis [68].
- TNM stage is not significantly associated with outcome in LCNEC in a multivariate analysis [72].

Bibliography

1. Williams ED, Siebenmann RE, Sobin LH (1980) Histological typing of endocrine tumours. World Health Organization, Geneve
2. Solcia E, Klöppel G, Sobin LH (2000) Histological typing of endocrine tumours. Springer, New York
3. Rindi G, Kloppel G, Alhman H, Caplin M, Couvelard A, de Herder WW, Erikssson B, Falchetti A, Falconi M, Komminoth P, Korner M, Lopes JM, McNicol AM, Nilsson O, Perren A, Scarpa A, Scoazec JY, Wiedenmann B (2006) TNM staging of foregut (neuro)endocrine tumors: a consensus proposal including a grading system. Virchows Arch 449:395–401
4. Rindi G, Kloppel G, Couvelard A, Komminoth P, Korner M, Lopes JM, McNicol AM, Nilsson O, Perren A, Scarpa A, Scoazec JY, Wiedenmann B (2007) TNM staging of midgut and hindgut (neuro) endocrine tumors: a consensus proposal including a grading system. Virchows Arch 451:757–762

4

5. Klöppel G, Rindi G, Perren A, Komminoth P, Klimstra DS (2010) The ENET and AJCC/UICC TNM classifications of the neuroendocrine tumors of the gastrointestinal tract and the pancreas: a statement. Virchows Arch 456:595–597
6. Strosberg JR, Cheema A, Weber J, Han G, Coppola D, Kvols LK (2011) Prognostic validity of a novel American joint committee on cancer staging classification for pancreatic neuroendocrine tumors. J Clin Oncol 29(22):3044–3049
7. Cho JH, Ryu JK, Song SY, Hwang JH, Lee DK, Woo SM, Joo YE, Jeong S, Lee SO, Park BK, Cheon YK, Han J, Kim TN, Lee JK, Moon SH, Kim H, Park ET, Hwang JC, Kim TH, Jeon TJ, Cho CM, Choi HS, Lee WJ (2016) Prognostic validity of the American joint committee on cancer and the European neuroendocrine Tumors staging classifications for pancreatic neuroendocrine Tumors: a retrospective Nationwide Multicenter study in South Korea. Pancreas 45(7):941–946. doi: 10.97/MPA.0000000000000586
8. Han X, Xu X, Jin D, Wang D, Ji Y, Lou W (2014) Clinicopathological characteristics and prognosis-related factors of Resectable pancreatic neuroendocrine Tumors: a retrospective study of 104 cases in a single Chinese center. Pancreas 43(4):526–531
9. Yang M, Zeng L, Zhang Y, Wang WG, Wang L, Ke NW, Liu XB, Tian BL (2015) TNM staging of pancreatic neuroendocrine tumors: an observational analysis and comparison by both AJCC and ENET systems from 1 singe institution. Medecine (Baltimore) 94(12):e660
10. Yang M, Ke NW, Zeng L, Zhang Y, Tan CL, Zhang H, Mai G, Tian BL, Liu XB (2015) Survival analyses for patients with surgically resected pancreatic neuroendocrine tumors by World Health Organization 2010 grading Classifications and American joint committee on cancer 2010 staging systems. Medecine (Baltimore) 94(48):e2156
11. Qadan M, Ma Y, Visser BC, Kunz PL, Fisher GA, Norton JA, Poultsides GA (2014) Reassessment of the current American joint Committee on cancer staging system for pancreatic neuroendocrine tumors. J Am Coll Surg 218(2):188–195
12. Scarpa A, Mantovani W, Capelli P, Beghelli S, Boninsegna L, Bettini R, Panzuto F, Pederzoli P, delle Fave G, Falconi M (2010) Pancreatic endocrine tumors: improved TNM staging and histopathological grading permit a clinically efficient prognostic stratification of patients. Mod Pathol 23(6): 824–833
13. Rindi G, Falconi M, Klersy C, Albarello L, Boninsegna L, Buchler MW, Capella C, Caplin M, Couvelard A, Doglioni C, Delle Fave G, Fischer L, Fusai G, de Herder WW, Jann H, Komminoth P, de Krijger RR, La Rosa S, Luong TV, Pape U, Perren A, Ruszniewski P, Scarpa A, Schmitt A, Solcia E, Wiedenmann B (2012) TNM staging of neoplasms of the endocrine pancreas: results form a large international cohort study. J Natl Cancer Inst 104(10):764–777
14. Brunner SM, Weber F, Werner JM, Agha A, Farkas SA, Schlitt HJ, Hornung M (2015) Neuroendocrine tumors of the pancreas: a retrospective single-center analysis using the ENET TNM-classification and immunohistochemical markers for risk stratification. BMC Surg 15:49. doi:10.1186/s12893-015-0033-1
15. Boninsegna L, Panzuto F, Partelli S, Capelli P, Delle Fave G, Bettini R, Pederzoli P, Scarpa A, Falconi M (2012) Malignant pancreatic neuroendocrine tumour: lymph node ratio and Ki67 are predictors of recurrence after curative resections. Eur J Cancer 48(11):1608–1615
16. Demir R, Pohl J, Agaimy A, Peros G, Perrakis A, Merkel S, Hohenberger W, Klein P (2011) Necrosis and angioinvasion predict adverse outcome in pancreatic neuroendocrine tumors after curative surgical resection: results of a single-center series. World J Surg 35(12):2764–2772
17. Gao C, Fu X, Pan Y, Li Q (2010) Surgical treatment of pancreatic neuroendocrine Tumors: report of 112 cases. Dig Surg 27(3):197–204
18. Pomianowska E, Gladhaug IP, Grzyb K, Røsok BI, Edwin B, Bergestuen DS, Mathisen O (2010) Survival following resection of pancreatic endocrine tumors: importance of R-status and the WHO and TNM classification systems. Scand J Gastroenterol 45(7–8):971–979
19. Kubota T, Ohyama S, Hiki N, Nunobe S, Yamamoto N, Yamaguchi T (2012) Endocrine carcinoma of the stomach: clinicopathological analysis of 27 surgically treated cases in a single institute. Gastric Cancer 15(3):323–330. doi:10.1007/s10120-011-0122-5
20. Kim BS, Park YS, Yook JH, Kim BS (2016) Comparison of the prognostic values of the 2010 WHO classification, AJCC 7th edition, and ENET classification of gastric neuroendocrine tumors. Medicine (Baltimore) 95(30):e3977. doi:10.1097/MD.0000000000003977

21. La Rosa S, Inzani F, Vanoli A, Klersy C, Dainese L, Rindi G, Capella C, Bordi C, Solcia E (2011) Histologic characterization and improved prognostic evaluation of 209 gastric neuroendocrine neoplasms. Hum Pathol 42(10):1373–1384. doi:10.1016/j.humpath.2011.01.018
22. CS FL, Brock G, Scoggins CR, McMasters KM, Martin RC 2nd (2009) A proposed staging system for gastric carcinoid tumors based on an analysis of 1,543 patients. Ann Surg Oncol 16(1):51–60. doi:10.1245/s10434-008-0192-8
23. Sobin LH, Gospodarowicz MK, Wittekind CH (2010) TNM classification of malignant tumours, 7th edn. John Wiley & Sons
24. Modlin IM, Oberg K, Chung DC, Jensen RT, de Herder WW, Thakker RV, Caplin M, Delle Fave G, Kaltsas GA, Krenning EP, Moss SF, Nilsson O, Rindi G, Salazar R, Ruszniewski P, Sundin A (2008) Gastroenteropancreatic neuroendocrine tumours. Lancet Oncol 9(1):61–72
25. Yao JC, Hassan M, Phan A, Dagohoy C, Leary C, Mares JE, Abdalla EK, Fleming JB, Vauthey JN, Rashid A, Evans DB (2008) One hundred years after "carcinoid": epidemiology of and prognostic factors for neuroendocrine tumors in 35,825 cases in the United States. J Clin Oncol 26(18):3063–3072
26. Scherübl H, Schwertner C, Steinberg J, Stölzel U, Pohl J, Dralle H, Klöppel G (2010) Neuroendocrine tumors of the small bowels are on the rise: early tumors and their management. Z Gastroenterol 48(3):406–413
27. Araujo PB, Cheng S, Mete O, Serra S, Morin E, Asa SL, Ezzat S (2013) Evaluation of the WHO 2010 grading and AJCC/UICC staging systems in prognostic behavior of intestinal neuroendocrine tumors. PLoS One 8(4):e61538. doi:10.1371/journal.pone.0061538
28. Jann H, Roll S, Couvelard A, Hentic O, Pavel M, Müller-Nordhorn J, Koch M, Röcken C, Rindi G, Ruszniewski P, Wiedenmann B, Pape UF (2011) Neuroendocrine tumors of midgut and hindgut origin: tumor-node-metastasis classification determines clinical outcome. Cancer 117(15):3332–3341. doi:10.1002/cncr.25855
29. Srirajaskanthan R, Ahmed A, Prachialias A, Srinivasan P, Heaton N, Jervis N, Quaglia A, Vivian G, Ramage JK (2013) ENET TNM staging predicts prognosis in small bowel neuroendocrine tumours. ISRN Oncol 2013:420795. doi:10.1155/2013/420795
30. Strosberg JR, Weber JM, Feldman M, Coppola D, Meredith K, Kvols LK (2013) Prognostic validity of the American joint committee on cancer staging classification for midgut neuroendocrine tumors. J Clin Oncol 31(4):420–425. doi:10.1200/JCO.2012.44.5924
31. Kim MK, Warner RR, Roayaie S, Harpaz N, Ward SC, Itzkowitz S, Wisnivesky JP (2013) Revised staging classification improves outcome prediction for small intestinal neuroendocrine tumors. J Clin Oncol 31(30):3776–3781. doi:10.1200/JCO.2013.51.1477
32. Niederle B, Pape UF, Costa F, Gross D, Kelestimur F, Knigge U, Öberg K, Pavel M, Perren A, Toumpanakis C, O'Connor J, O'Toole D, Krenning E, Reed N, Kianmanesh R, all other Vienna Consensus Conference participants (2016) ENET consensus guidelines update for neuroendocrine neoplasms oft he jejunum and ileum. Neuroendocrinology 103:125–138
33. Strosberg J, Gardner N, Kvols L (2009) Survival and Prognostic factor analysis of 146 metastatic neuroendocrine Tumors of the mid-gut. Neuroendocrinology 89:471–476
34. Norlén O, Stålberg P, Öberg K, Eriksson J, Hedberg J, Hessman O, Janson ET, Hellman P, Åkerström G (2012) Long-term results of surgery for small intestinal neuroendocrine tumors at a tertiary referral center. World J Surg 36(6):1419–1431
35. Volante M, Daniele L, Asioli S, Cassoni P, Comino A, Coverlizza S, De Giuli P, Fava C, Manini C, Berruti A, Papotti M (2013) Tumor staging but not grading is associated with adverse clinical outcome in neuroendocrine Tumors of the appendix. A retrospective clinical pathologic analysis of 138 cases. Am J Surg Pathol 37(4):606–612. doi:10.1097/PAS.0b013e318275d1d7
36. Dralle H (2011) Surgical strategies for accidental detection of appendix carcinoids. Chirurg 82(7):598–606
37. Moertel CH, Weiland LH, Nagorney DM, Dockerty MB (1987) Carcinoid tumor of the appendix: treatment and prognosis. N Engl J Med 317(27):1699–1701
38. Parkes SE, Muir KR, Sheyyab MA, Cameron AH, Pincott JR, Raafat F, Mann JR (1993) Carcinoid tumours of the appendix in children 1957-1986: incidence, treatment and outcome. Br J Surg 80:502–504
39. Plöckinger U, Couvelard A, Falconie M, Sundin A, Salazar R, Christ E, de Herder WW, Gross D, Knapp WH, Knigge UP, Kulke MH, Pape UF, all other Frascati Consensus Conference participants (2008)

Consensus guidelines for the Management of Patients with digestive neuroendocrine tumours: well-differentiated tumour/carcinoma of the appendix and goblet cell carcinoma. Neuroendocrinolgy 87:20–30
40. Rossi G, Valli R, Bertolini F, Sighinolfi P, Losi L, Cavazza A, Rivasi F, Luppi G (2003) Does mesoappendix infiltration predict a worse prognosis in incidental neuroendocrine tumors of the appendix? A clinicopathologic and immunohistochemical study of 15 cases. Am J Clin Pathol 120(5): 706–711
41. Pape UF, Niederle B, Costa F, Gross D, Kelestimur F, Kianmanesh F, Knigge U, Öberg K, Pavel M, Perren A, Toumpanakis C, O'Connor J, Krenning E, Reed E, O'Toole D, all other Vienna Consensus Conference participants (2016) ENET consensus guidelines for neuroendocrine neoplasms of the appendix (excluding goblet cell carcinomas). Neuroendocrinology 103:144–152
42. Alexandraki KI, Griniatsos J, Bramis KI, Ballian N, Dimitriou N, Giannakakis T, Tsigris C, Felekouras E, Kaltsas GA (2011) Clinical value of right hemicolectomy for appendiceal carcinoids using pathologic criteria. J Endocrinol Investig 34:255–259. doi:10.3275/7286
43. MacGillivray DC, Heaton RB, Rushin JM, Cruess DF (1992) Distant metastasis from a carcinoid tumor of the appendix less than one centimeter in size. Surgery. Apr;111(4):466–71
44. Mullen JT, Savarese DM (2011) Carcinoid tumors of the appendix: a population-based study. J Surg Oncol 104(1):41–44. doi:10.1002/jso.21888
45. Deschamps L, Couvelard A (2010) Endocrine tumors of the appendix: a pathologic review. Arch Pathol Lab Med 134(6):871–875. doi:10.1043/1543-2165-134.6.871
46. Syracuse DC, Perzin KH, Price JB, Wiedel PD, Mesa-Tejada R (1979) Carcinoid tumors of the appendix. Mesoappendiceal extension and nodal metastases. Ann Surg 190(1):58–63
47. Anderson JR, Wilson BG (1985) Carcinoid tumours of the appendix. Br J Surg 72(7):545–546
48. Bamboat ZM, Berger DL (2006) Is right hemicolectomy for 2.0-cm appendiceal carcinoids justified? Arch Surg 141(4):349–352
49. Pape UF, Perren A, Niederle B, Gross D, Gress T, Costa F, Arnold R, Denecke T, Plöckinger U, Salazar R, Grossman S et al (2012) ENET Consensus guidelines for the Management of Patients with neuroendocrine neoplasms from the Jejuno-ileum und the appendix Including goblet cell carcinomas. Neuroendocrinology 95:135–156
50. Boudreaux JP, Klimstra DS, Hassan MM, Woltering EA, Jensen RT, Goldsmith SJ, Nutting C, Bushnell DL, Caplin ME, Yao JC, North American Neuroendocrine Tumor Society (NANET) (2010) The NANET consensus guideline for the diagnosis and management of neuroendocrine tumors: well-differentiated neuroendocrine tumors of the jejunum, ileum, appendix, and cecum. Pancreas 39(6):753–766. doi:10.1097/MPA.0b013e3181ebb2a5
51. Landry CS, Woodall C, Scoggins CR, McMasters K, Martin RCG II (2008) Analysis of 900 Appendiceal carcinoid Tumors for a proposed predictive staging system. Arch Surg 143(7):664–670
52. Weinstock B, Ward SC, Harpaz N, Warner RR, Itzkowitz S, Kim MK (2013) Clinical and prognostic features of rectal neuroendocrine tumors. Neuroendocrinology 98(3):180–187. doi:10.1159/000355612. Epub 2013 Nov 5
53. Chi Y, Du F, Zhao H, Wang JW, Cai JQ (2014) Characteristics and long-term prognosis of patients with rectal neuroendocrine tumors. World J Gastroenterol 20(43):16252–16257. doi:10.3748/wjg.v20.i43.16252
54. Tsukamoto S, Fujita S, Yamaguchi T, Yamamoto S, Akasu T, Moriya Y, Taniguchi H, Shimoda T (2008) Clinicopathological characteristics and prognosis of rectal well-differentiated neuroendocrine tumors. Int J Color Dis 23(11):1109–1113. doi:10.1007/s00384-008-0505-1
55. Modlin IM, Lye KD, Kidd M (2003) A 5-decade analysis of 13,715 carcinoid tumors. Cancer 97(4): 934–959
56. Modlin IM, Sandor A (1997) An analysis of 8305 cases of carcinoid tumors. Cancer 79(4):813–829
57. Scherübl H, Klöppel G (2009) Rectal carcinoids on the rise – update. Z Gastroenterol 47(4):365–371. doi:10.1055/s-2008-1027930. Epub 2009 Apr 8
58. Gleeson FC, Levy MJ, Dozois EJ, Larson DW, Wong Kee Song LM, Boardman LA (2014) Endoscopically identified well-differentiated rectal carcinoid tumors: impact of tumor size on the natural history and outcomes. Gastrointest Endosc 80(1):144–151. doi:10.1016/j.gie.2013.11.031
59. Soga J (2005) Early-stage carcinoids of the gastrointestinal tract: an analysis of 1914 reported cases. Cancer 103(8):1587–1595

60. Kulke MH, Mayer RJ (1999) Carcinoid tumors. N Engl J Med 340(11):858–868
61. Landry CS, Brock G, Scoggins CR, McMasters KM, Martin RC 2nd (2008) A proposed staging system for rectal carcinoid tumors based on an analysis of 4701 patients. Surgery 144(3):460–466. doi:10.1016/j.surg.2008.05.005. Epub 2008 Jul 25
62. Modlin I Drozdov I, Gustafsson B (2007) Rectal neuroendocrine tumors – Diagnosis and treatment. In: Modlin I, Oberg K A (eds) century of advances in neuroendocrine tumor biology and treatment (ISBN 978-3-00-023 638-9) Felsenstein C.C.C.P, 124–133
63. Rosenberg JM, Welch JP (1985) Carcinoid tumors of the colon: a study of 72 patients. Am J Surg 149:775–779
64. Ballantyne GH, Savoca PE, Flannery JT, Ahlmann MH, Modlin IM (1992) Incidence and mortality of carcinoids of the colon: data from the Connecticut tumor registry. Cancer 69:2400–2405
65. Phan AT, Oberg K, Choi J, Harrison LH Jr, Hassan MM, Strosberg JR, Krenning EP, Kocha W, Woltering EA, Maples WJ, North American Neuroendocrine Tumor Society (NANET) (2010) NANET consensus guideline for the diagnosis and management of neuroendocrine tumors: well-differentiated neuroendocrine tumors of the thorax (includes lung and thymus). Pancreas 39(6):784–798. doi:10.1097/MPA.0b013e3181ec1380
66. Caplin ME, Baudin E, Ferolla P, Filosso P, Garcia-Yuste M, Lim E, Oberg K, Pelosi G, Perren A, Rossi RE, Travis WD (2015) ENET consensus conference participants. Pulmonary neuroendocrine (carcinoid) tumors: European neuroendocrine tumor society expert consensus and recommendations for best practice for typical and atypical pulmonary carcinoids. Ann Oncol 26(8):1604–1620. doi:10.1093/annonc/mdv041
67. Cao C, Yan TD, Kennedy C, Hendel N, Bannon PG, McCaughan BC (2011) Bronchopulmonary carcinoid tumors: long-term outcomes after resection. Ann Thorac Surg 91(2):339–343. doi:10.1016/j.athoracsur.2010.08.062
68. Daddi N, Schiavon M, Filosso PL, Cardillo G, Ambrogi MC, De Palma A, Luzzi L, Bandiera A, Casali C, Ruffato A, De Angelis V, Andriolo LG, Guerrera F, Carleo F, Davini F, Urbani M, Mattioli S, Morandi U, Zannini P, Gotti G, Loizzi M, Puma F, Mussi A, Ricci A, Oliaro A, Rea F (2014) Multi-institutional Italian pathology group. Prognostic factors in a multicentre study of 247 atypical pulmonary carcinoids. Eur J Cardiothorac Surg 45(4):677–686
69. Travis WD, Giroux DJ, Chansky K, Crowley J, Asamura H, Brambilla E, Jett J, Kennedy C, Rami-Porta R, Rusch VW, Goldstraw P (2008) International staging committee and participating institutions. The IASLC lung cancer staging project: proposals for the inclusion of broncho-pulmonary carcinoid tumors in the forthcoming (seventh) edition of the TNM classification for lung Cancer. J Thorac Oncol 3(11):1213–1223
70. Schnabel PA, Junker K (2015) Pulmonary neuroendocrine tumors in the new WHO 2015 classification: start of breaking new grounds? Pathologe 36(3):283–292. doi:10.1007/s00292-015-0030-2
71. Skuladottir H, Hirsch FR, Hansen HH, Olsen JH (2002) Pulmonary neuroendocrine tumors: incidence and prognosis of histological subtypes. A population-based study in Denmark. Lung Cancer 37(2):127–135
72. Battafarano RJ, Fernandez FG, Ritter J, Meyers BF, Guthrie TJ, Cooper JD, Patterson GA (2005) Large cell neuroendocrine carcinoma: an aggressive form of non-small cell lung cancer. J Thorac Cardiovasc Surg 130(1):166–172
73. Planchard D, Le Péchoux C (2011) Small cell lung cancer: new clinical recommendations and current status of biomarker assessment. Eur J Cancer 47(Suppl 3):S272–S283. doi:10.1016/S0959-8049(11)70173-3
74. Gaspar LE, McNamara EJ, Gay EG, Putnam JB, Crawford J, Herbst RS, Bonner JA (2012) Small-cell lung cancer: prognostic factors and changing treatment over 15 years. Clin Lung Cancer 13(2):115–122. doi:10.1016/j.cllc.2011.05.008

Clinical Cases and Their Implications (From Clinical Practice to Guidelines)

Contents

Prognostic Factors: Grading (Ki-67 Index)

Marco Volante, Caterina Marchiò, Luisella Righi, Eleonora Duregon, Alessandro Piovesan, and Mauro Papotti

A. Colao et al. (eds.), *Neuroendocrine Tumors in Real Life*,
https://doi.org/10.1007/978-3-319-59024-0_5

Overview

While Ki-67 index is crucial for the diagnosis and grading and for prognostic and predictive purposes in digestive neuroendocrine tumors (NET), it does not play the same established role in lung NET. In fact, gastroenteropancreatic NE neoplasms are classified into two groups of NET and NE carcinomas, both of them further graded into G1, G2, and G3. The assumption that all G3 neoplasms are NE carcinomas by definition has been recently challenged by the identification of a new category of well-differentiated G3 tumors, named NET G3, based on the organoid architecture but a high proliferative activity (Ki-67 ranging 20–40%). Conversely, tumor grading in lung NET is defined by the histological classification based on mitotic count and necrosis, identifying typical carcinoids (low-grade), atypical carcinoids (intermediate-grade), large cell NE carcinomas, and small cell lung carcinomas (high-grade malignancies). Although Ki-67 index is not a diagnostic parameter, proposals were made to combine mitoses, necrosis, and Ki-67 index to grade lung NET in a system significantly correlated with survival. The presently reported patient exemplifies a rare case classified as atypical carcinoid of the lung with a relatively high Ki-67 index (16%). The patient refused any further treatment after surgery despite the mitotic count at the upper limit of the category, foci of necrosis, and the intermediate Ki-67 count. Additional data are needed on well-differentiated lung NET displaying a relatively high proliferative activity that parallel the novel category of NET G3 of the digestive tract and that might require a therapeutic strategy different from the current postsurgical «wait and see» approach.

Clinical Case

A female patient, aged 59, medical doctor, sought medical advice complaining shortness of breathing and cough. A chest X ray and CT scan confirmed the presence of a pulmonary nodule, located in the upper left lobe in paramediastinal position, close to the main bronchus, and measuring 3 cm in its largest diameter. The tumor was resected together with regional lymph node dissection and had a smooth border with a partial fibrous capsule. On cut surface, it was grayish in color, had a subpleural location, and was 29 mm in size.

Histologically, the tumor displayed an organoid architecture and was partially encapsulated and focally extended into the alveolar spaces (◘ Fig. 5.1). Cells were mostly round and uniform in size with very limited atypia (◘ Fig. 5.1). Occasional foci of necrosis were observed. The mitotic count was 8/10 high-power fields (hpf), corresponding to two square mm. Surgical margins were free. Regional mediastinal lymph nodes were affected by metastases (two peribronchial and six subcarinal nodes) (◘ Fig. 5.2).

The immunoprofile confirmed the neuroendocrine nature of the tumor with strong reactivity for both chromogranin A and synaptophysin. The proliferative activity assessed by Ki-67 immunostaining was 16% in hot spots of the primary tumor and slightly higher (20%) in the metastatic deposits (◘ Fig. 5.2).

A diagnosis of atypical carcinoid of the lung was reported, based on the current WHO classification of lung tumors [1], and the tumor was staged as pT2-N2.

A multidisciplinary discussion followed on the appropriate subsequent treatments, if any. No clear indication on the efficacy of adjuvant medical (somatostatin analogues, traditional chemotherapy, or targeted therapy) or peptide receptor radionuclide therapy (PRRT) after radical surgery is available for this type of tumors [2, 3]. Despite the lack of evidence of disease at postoperative imaging study, the opportunity of adjuvant medical treatment was considered, based on the metastatic lymph nodes and a value of mitotic count borderline with large cell neuroendocrine carcinoma/LCNEC (eight mitoses in this patient with a cutoff set at nine, also supported by a Ki-67 index up to 16%). The patient refused any treatments and strongly supported the decision of «watchful waiting» with a close follow-up program. This decision stemmed from a large series of consultations the patient autonomously decided to take in Italy and abroad.

The patient remained free of disease and asymptomatic for 15 months when an increase in circulating chromogranin A leads to perform a ^{68}Ga-Dotatate CT-PET, which revealed multiple skeletal uptakes (cranial theca, dorsal and lumbar vertebrae, ribs, iliac crest, and sacrum). Although no biopsy was performed on the suspected metastases, they were assumed to be secondary lesions of neuroendocrine origin, and a treatment with a somatostatin analogue (lanreotide autogel 120 mg/28 days) was started. After 5 months on lanreotide, another ^{68}Ga-Dotatate CT-PET showed progression of disease (PD) in all the skeletal sites, and therefore, the patient was offered PRRT with ^{177}Lu-Dotatate. She then underwent four consecutive administrations (1 every 8–10 weeks) of ^{177}Lu-Dotatate for a cumulative activity of 20 GBq from May 2015 to Jan 2016 and four infusions of zoledronate 4 mg (1 every 2 months). PPRT was poorly tolerated by the patient, who complained of profound asthenia and was accompanied by grade 1–2 hematological toxicity.

Imaging studies confirmed stable skeletal disease and no other metastatic sites, 10 months after the start of PRRT and 41 months after the original diagnosis.

According to the current WHO classification of lung tumors [1], the presently reported case was classified as an atypical lung carcinoid. In addition, it was associated to a high proliferative index (Ki-67, 16%) and followed an aggressive behavior with distant metastases to the bone in a 15-month period.

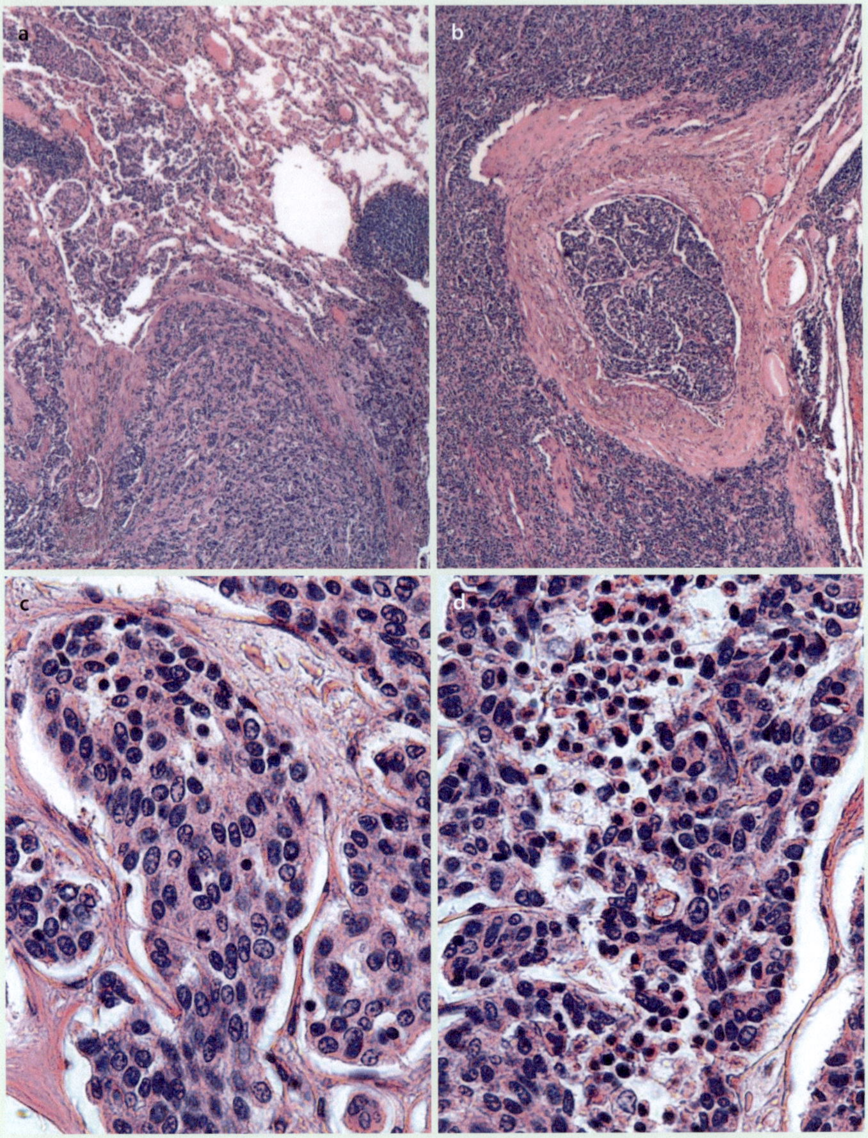

Fig. 5.1 The neoplasm had an organoid architecture, was partially encapsulated, was focally extended into the alveolar spaces **a**, and showed vascular invasion **b**. The cells were mostly round and had a uniform size with focal atypia **c** and limited foci of necrosis **d** (hematoxylin and eosin, **a** and **b** original magnification 40×; **c**, **d** original magnification 400×)

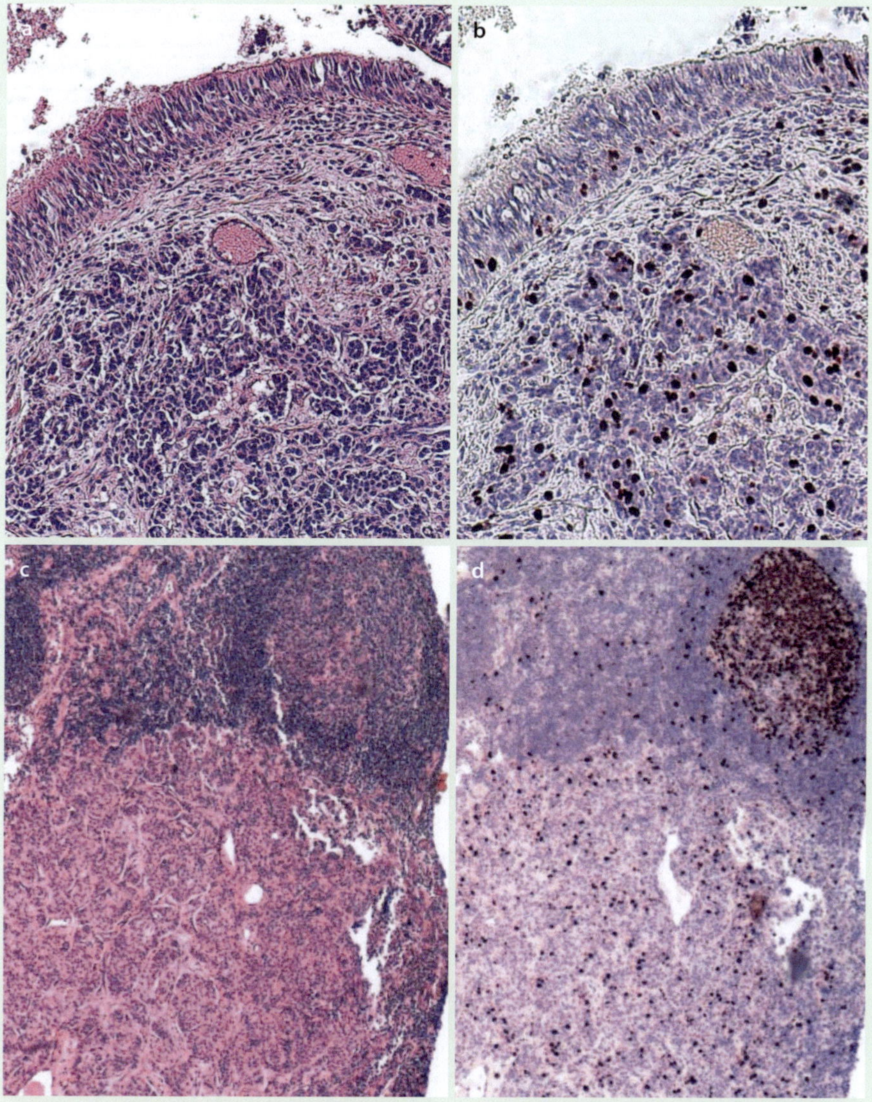

Fig. 5.2 The proliferative activity assessed by Ki-67 immunostaining was 16% in hot spots of the primary tumor **a**, **b** and slightly higher (20%) in metastatic regional lymph nodes **c**, **d**. (hematoxylin and eosin, **a** original magnification 200×, **c** original magnification 40×; immunoperoxidase, **b** original magnification 200×, **d** original magnification 40×)

5.1 Comments to the Case

This case offers several points of debate. The least debated is the classification, since the morphological parameters currently accepted by the WHO classification of neuroendocrine lung (and thymic) tumors clearly indicate the cutoffs to be applied, and in this particular case, the mitotic index of eight mitoses per ten high-power fields definitely supports a diagnosis of atypical carcinoid. Nevertheless, a nonmandatory parameter, i.e., the Ki-67 proliferation index, was particularly high in these cases, both in the primary tumor and the lymph node metastasis, in line with the mitotic count at the upper limit of the atypical carcinoid category. This suggests a potential biological aggressiveness of the tumor itself. A more debated issue is the therapeutic strategy for such a case. Adjuvant medical or radionuclide therapy after radical surgery has been suggested, but there are no proofs of a definite efficacy. This option was proposed (considering lymph node metastases and a relatively high Ki-67 index and mitotic count), but the patient refused further treatments. A final controversy is related to the therapeutic options at the time of possible disease progression, which indeed occurred some 15 months after surgery with bone spread. Somatostatin analogues and radionuclide therapy were administrated, but other regimens including chemotherapy might also be considered.

Questions

1. Is the diagnosis correct?
2. Is the current classification of NE tumors adequate and exhaustive to encompass such cases, or would a further intermediate category be needed to best classify lesions in between atypical carcinoid and LCNEC (that would ideally include «high-grade atypical carcinoids» and/or «less aggressive LCNEC»)? Or should this type of tumors be labeled LCNEC in any case?
3. Do any other parameters of relevance exist in this gray area?

Answers

1. It seems that the diagnosis was correct, when the criteria proposed by the current WHO classification of lung tumors are applied [1]. Based on mitotic count and presence of necrosis, both parameters were consistent in addressing the diagnosis to the category of atypical carcinoid, which is the rarest subtype, requiring a mitotic count ranging from 2 to 9/10 hpf and/or spotty necrosis.
2. Within this rare group of NET, there is an even rarer subgroup of tumors with an apparently high proliferative potential, as better recognized by the Ki-67 index. From a classification standpoint, since no other parameters, neither morphological (e.g., invasion, metastases, etc.) nor immunophenotypic (e.g., proliferation markers, oncogenes, genetic alterations, etc.), are currently accepted, no further stratification is expected for these tumors. The only alternative diagnostic option is the category of high-grade neuroendocrine carcinomas of the large (or small) cell type. Despite this latter category is by definition encompassing malignant NET having a mitotic count higher than 10/10 hpf, carcinomas in this category generally have an extremely high mitotic count exceeding 40 or 50/10 hpf (i.e., figures corresponding to a Ki-67 index

higher than 50%), thus leaving those rare cases with intermediate features in an area that is poorly represented but also poorly understood. The current treatment for such cases is debated, and if chemotherapy does not seem appropriate for atypical carcinoids after radical surgery, no other treatment is at present recommended, despite a proliferative activity ranging between 10 and 25% of Ki-67-positive cells may envisage something more than a close follow-up after surgery.

3. To address question 3, an answer or the answer is at present heavily related to the proliferative activity as measured by the Ki-67 immunodetection. Although the current WHO classification scheme for lung NET does *not* require the Ki-67 index, as opposed to gastroenteropancreatic NET, still its measurement is often solicited by clinicians, being considered a useful complementary tool for treatment decision making. It turns out then that a relevant issue is to establish its real role and—if so—how to measure Ki-67 index. With regard to the first point, there are over 2000 lung NET cases published having Ki-67 investigated as part of their morphological and phenotypic description [4]. Most of these studies recognize a usefulness of Ki-67 index reporting, and a multicentric study on almost 400 NET cases of lung origin proposed a novel grading system for lung NET that combined the Ki-67 index with the two conventional morphological parameters (mitoses and necrosis) ([2]; see also below). As for the methods to measure Ki-67 index, a more articulated discussion is needed, as detailed here below.

Up to Date of the Topic

Role of Grading and Ki-67 Index for Clinical Decision: Differences in GEP vs *Thoracic Areas*

Before entering the specific field of GEP and pulmonary NET grading by Ki-67 measurement, it is of relevance to spend a word on the different approaches to Ki-67 counting. A marked variability of measurement is detected among different observers, especially in low proliferating tumors [5]. This is in part related to the various methods in use for Ki-67 determination, which include random manual counts, counts in areas of higher labeling density as assessed at low power (so-called hot spots), Ki-67 index determination by automated count on digitalized slides, manual count on printed tumor areas from previously digitalized and selected tumor fields, and still other procedures. In general, the count in hot spots, either manually or as a result of an automated count in preselected hot spot regions, provided the most reliable results [2, 6]. This option best fits also for those rare cases featuring mixed patterns, both architectural and phenotypic, with organoid areas admixed with solid less differentiated fields and showing a markedly different proliferative activity. The question is about which Ki-67 value is to be accepted and which grade is to be assigned. As a general rule, the highest values and the highest grades rather than the most represented are those to be preferred [6].

Gastroenteropancreatic (GEP) NET are now clearly including a heterogeneous G3 category that needs to be split into two subgroups based on different proliferative activity and generally associated to a different architecture. As for Ki-67, no official cutoff is proposed, but an early study [7], subsequently confirmed [8], showed that cases with a Ki-67 < 55% had a better prognosis than highly proliferating neuroendocrine carcinomas (NEC). In general, a tumor displaying a Ki-67 index ranging between 20 and 50% has a different malignant potential compared to highly proliferating NECs that usually exceed 80% of proliferating cells. This difference is paralleled by a different tumor architecture, being the latter poorly differentiated tumors associated to a solid growth of small or large cells, while the former usually maintain some degree of organoid structure, as seen in carcinoid tumors. This stratification into well-differentiated and poorly differentiated grade 3 neuroendocrine neoplasms (i.e., NET-G3 and NEC-G3) will be probably incorporated in the upcoming new WHO classification of endocrine tumors (announced March 2017). The proposed stratification heavily impacts on the therapeutic decisions with regard to the administration of chemotherapy versus alternative treatments.

In pulmonary NET, no grading system has been developed to date, being tumor grade intrinsic to the histological classification [1, 9], which includes typical carcinoids (TC, low-grade malignant), atypical carcinoids (AC, intermediate-grade malignant), and large and small cell neuroendocrine carcinomas (LCNEC/SCLC) and high-grade malignant neoplasms. Some years ago, other authors proposed to label «carcinoma» in all types of lung NET and then introduced a grading that directly translated TC into G1 carcinomas, AC into G2 carcinomas, and LCNEC and SCLC into G3 carcinomas [10, 11]. Therefore, the stratification in grades proposed for GEP NET does not apply to thoracic NET (lung and thymus), nor is Ki-67 a relevant parameter for tumor classification or grading. Apparently, well-differentiated carcinoid tumors (typical and atypical) have accurately been distinguished from high-grade neuroendocrine carcinomas by the definition of the entity «large cell neuroendocrine carcinoma/LCNEC» [12]. Indeed, the vast majority of LCNECs shares the clinical behavior and some biological features (including its proliferative potential) with small cell lung cancer, and only rare cases labeled LCNEC show both morphological and clinical features more similar to carcinoids. This small subgroup has a well-differentiated organoid structure, resembling carcinoids, but a higher proliferative activity and invasive capacity (including distant spread). In our opinion, the currently reported case represents an example of this intermediate category between AC and LCNEC, which most likely parallels the novel «NET-G3» category of the GEP area. Whether these are carcinoids with a higher malignant potential or poorly differentiated neuroendocrine carcinomas «of intermediate grade» is yet to be understood. Only future studies unraveling the genetic background of such cases may provide a more accurate interpretation, in light of recent evidence of different genetic profiles between carcinoid tumors on the one side and high-grade small and large cell neuroendocrine carcinomas on the other [13].

Regardless of the real nature of such thoracic carcinoids with a relatively high Ki-67 index, indeed the use of Ki-67 is not officially required for the classification of thoracic NET, although the recent WHO classification [1] mentions that Ki-67 index might have a role in stratifying neuroendocrine lung tumors. A recent study of almost 400 pulmonary NET proposed a grading system that combined morphological parameters (mitotic count and necrosis) with the Ki-67 index [2]. The abovementioned grading proposal by Rindi turned out superior not only to the morphological WHO 2015 classification of lung tumors but also to WHO 2010 of digestive NET by jointly assembling this tripartite combination according to lung-specific cutoff thresholds [2]. By combining mitoses, necrosis, and Ki-67 index thresholds, a grading system (G1 to G3) was generated based on the occurrence of at least two of three parameters meeting the required cutoff levels. At the histological level, all typical carcinoids resulted to be G1, while among 75 atypical carcinoids, 45 were attributed to G2 (the remaining 29 being downgraded to G1 and 1 upgraded to G3). In the poorly differentiated group, 78 of 86 LCNEC and 76 of 82 small cell carcinomas were confirmed G3; however, 8 and 6, respectively, were downgraded to G2. Of note, this multiparametric grading system approach turned out to be an accurate predictor of lung NET behavior.

This piece of evidence might lead to a diagnostic/grading approach similar to that of GEP NET, although it seems that cutoff values may be different between the two sites (despite the similar embryological origin of all these foregut-derived thoracic, gastroduodenal, and pancreatic tumors). At the same time, it has to be acknowledged that this parameter still represents a challenge for clinicians, since no universal recommendations are available at present. Tentatively, a Ki-67 index ranging from 8 to 30% (very approximate figures), which most often should correspond to a mitotic count in the range of the entity currently called «atypical carcinoid» (i.e., 2–9 mitoses/10 hpf or rarely higher), identifies a subgroup of thoracic NET with an unpredictable behavior and a currently poorly defined therapeutic strategy. The partial overlapping of carcinoid tumors with LCNECs is also confirmed by recent genetic studies of a series of pulmonary NET (including carcinoids, large LCNECs, and «borderline tumors») that confirmed specific genetic signatures for these tumor entities, but also identified rare outlier cases, having gene alterations more closely related to other histotypes [14, 15]. In our laboratory, a study is in progress on a series of NET having a high proliferative index but well-differentiated, carcinoid-like, architecture that followed a clinical course intermediate between carcinoid tumors and high-grade small/large cell carcinomas. Preliminary results seem to suggest that specific cutoff values of Ki-67 may help stratify subgroups with different malignant potential and possibly therapeutic requirements (*Marchiò, Volante, Papotti, unpublished observation*).

Additional criteria are to be combined with morphology and Ki-67 index determination to best predict prognosis in this gray area and select those NET associated to a higher metastatic potential. The relevance of the problem is well represented by the currently reported case in which adjuvant therapeutic options, medical or PRRT, were discussed with the patient (incidentally a medical doctor) who, following several second opinions, refused any kind of therapy, most likely perceived as overtreatment. The lack of strong evidence on the efficacy of adjuvant treatment also for more aggressive pulmonary carcinoids enforced the patient's preference for the «watchful waiting.» The rapid progression of disease following this decision and the need to use more aggressive treatments (PRRT) after a relatively short span of time may confirm the need of additional criteria to properly select patients eligible for adjuvant therapy [16] or other biological drugs [17].

5.2 Concluding Remarks

In GEP NET, tumor grading is well established and performs well with some exceptions. The recent stratification of G3 tumors into G3a and G3b to separate lower-grade tumors from poorly differentiated neuroendocrine carcinomas (also introducing again the old morphological distinction between well and poorly differentiated tumors) may heavily impact on the therapeutic decisions in pancreatic and gastric NE neoplasms. An open issue remains the cutoff value to separate G1 from G2 tumors, which is currently set at 3% of Ki-67, but some evidence suggest that it should more appropriately fall at 5%, at least for pancreatic locations. Another possible exception is represented by appendiceal NET, which are extremely low-grade tumors in the vast majority of cases (virtually all are graded G1). This location contains tumors that are stratified with difficulty in significant prognostic groups when the current grading system is employed, as opposed to the old WHO classification dated 2000 [18].

In lung and thymic NET, the grading still largely corresponds to histological classification, according to the current WHO criteria [1]. The behavioral heterogeneity of some lung AC and LCNEC and the proven clinical utility of tumor grading in other NE neoplasms support the generation of such a grading also in the lung. To this regard, no single parameter is sufficient to predict behavior (neither the sole morphology nor Ki-67 index alone); however, a combination of the two may derive an accurate grading system of potential prognostic stratification and therapeutic usefulness.

Bibliography

1. Travis WD, Brambilla E, Muller-Hermelink KM (2015) WHO classification of tumours of the lung, pleura. Thymus and Heart, Lyon
2. Rindi G, Klersy C, Inzani F, Fellegara G, Ampollini L, Ardizzoni A, Campanini N, Carbognani P, De Pas TM, Galetta D, Granone PL, Righi L, Rusca M, Spaggiari L, Tiseo M, Viale G, Volante M, Papotti M, Pelosi G (2014) Grading the neuroendocrine tumors of the lung: an evidence-based proposal. Endocr Relat Cancer 21(1):1–16. doi:10.1530/ERC-13-024621/1/1. [pii]
3. Caplin ME, Baudin E, Ferolla P, Filosso P, Garcia-Yuste M, Lim E, Oberg K, Pelosi G, Perren A, Rossi RE, Travis WD, Participants Ecc (2015) Pulmonary neuroendocrine (carcinoid) tumors: European Neuroendocrine Tumor Society expert consensus and recommendations for best practice for typical and atypical pulmonary carcinoids. Ann Oncol 26(8):1604–1620. doi:10.1093/annonc/mdv041mdv041. [pii]
4. Pelosi G, Rindi G, Travis WD, Papotti M (2014) Ki-67 antigen in lung neuroendocrine tumors: unraveling a role in clinical practice. J Thorac Oncol 9(3):273–284. doi:10.1097/JTO.0000000000000092S1556-0864(15)30209-4. [pii]
5. Blank A, Wehweck L, Marinoni I, Boos LA, Bergmann F, Schmitt AM, Perren A (2015) Interlaboratory variability of MIB1 staining in well-differentiated pancreatic neuroendocrine tumors. Virchows Arch 467(5):543–550. doi:10.1007/s00428-015-1843-310.1007/s00428-015-1843-3. [pii]
6. Tang LH, Untch BR, Reidy DL, O'Reilly E, Dhall D, Jih L, Basturk O, Allen PJ, Klimstra DS (2016) Well-differentiated neuroendocrine Tumors with a morphologically apparent high-grade component: a pathway distinct from poorly differentiated neuroendocrine carcinomas. Clin Cancer Res 22(4):1011–1017. doi:10.1158/1078-0432.CCR-15-05481078-0432.CCR-15-0548. [pii]
7. Sorbye H, Welin S, Langer SW, Vestermark LW, Holt N, Osterlund P, Dueland S, Hofsli E, Guren MG, Ohrling K, Birkemeyer E, Thiis-Evensen E, Biagini M, Gronbaek H, Soveri LM, Olsen IH, Federspiel B, Assmus J, Janson ET, Knigge U (2013) Predictive and prognostic factors for treatment and survival in 305 patients with advanced gastrointestinal neuroendocrine carcinoma (WHO G3): the NORDIC NEC study. Ann Oncol 24(1):152–160. doi:10.1093/annonc/mds276mds276. [pii]

8. Milione M, Maisonneuve P, Spada F, Pellegrinelli A, Spaggiari P, Albarello L, Pisa E, Barberis M, Vanoli A, Buzzoni R, Pusceddu S, Concas L, Sessa F, Solcia E, Capella C, Fazio N, La Rosa S (2016) The Clinicopathologic heterogeneity of grade 3 Gastroenteropancreatic neuroendocrine neoplasms: morphological differentiation and proliferation identify different prognostic categories. Neuroendocrinology. doi:000445165 [pii]10.1159/000445165
9. Blank A, Schmitt A, Perren A (2015) Pathology: classification and immunoprofile. Front Horm Res. 44:104–114. doi: 10.1159/000382135
10. Huang Q, Muzitansky A, Mark EJ (2002) Pulmonary neuroendocrine carcinomas. A review of 234 cases and a statistical analysis of 50 cases treated at one institution using a simple clinicopathologic classification. Arch Pathol Lab Med 126(5):545–553. doi:10.1043/0003-9985(2002)126<0545:PNC>2.0.CO;2
11. Moran CA, Suster S, Coppola D, Wick MR (2009) Neuroendocrine carcinomas of the lung: a critical analysis. Am J Clin Pathol 131(2):206–221. doi:10.1309/AJCP9H1OTMUCSKQWJ17112PG86V536G2. [pii]
12. Travis WD, Linnoila RI, Tsokos MG, Hitchcock CL, Cutler GB Jr, Nieman L, Chrousos G, Pass H, Doppman J (1991) Neuroendocrine tumors of the lung with proposed criteria for large-cell neuroendocrine carcinoma. An ultrastructural, immunohistochemical, and flow cytometric study of 35 cases. Am J Surg Pathol 15(6):529–553
13. Swarts DR, Ramaekers FC, Speel EJ (2012) Molecular and cellular biology of neuroendocrine lung tumors: evidence for separate biological entities. Biochim Biophys Acta 1826(2):255–271. doi:10.1016/j.bbcan.2012.05.001S0304-419X(12)00035-2. [pii]
14. Rekhtman N, Pietanza MC, Hellmann MD, Naidoo J, Arora A, Won H, Halpenny DF, Wang H, Tian SK, Litvak AM, Paik PK, Drilon AE, Socci N, Poirier JT, Shen R, Berger MF, Moreira AL, Travis WD, Rudin CM, Ladanyi M (2016) Next-generation sequencing of pulmonary large cell neuroendocrine carcinoma reveals small cell carcinoma-like and non-small cell carcinoma-like subsets. Clin Cancer Res. doi: 1078-0432.CCR-15-2946 [pii]10.1158/1078-0432.CCR-15-2946
15. Vivero M, Sholl LM (2016) "Borderline" neuroendocrine carcinomas of the lung are clinically and genomically distinct from large cell neuroendocrine carcinoma. Mod Pathol 29(S1)
16. Cives M, Strosberg J (2015) The expanding role of somatostatin analogs in gastroenteropancreatic and lung neuroendocrine tumors. Drugs 75(8):847–858. doi:10.1007/s40265-015-0397-7
17. Cives M, Soares HP, Strosberg J (2016) Will clinical heterogeneity of neuroendocrine tumors impact their management in the future? Lessons from recent trials. Curr Opin Oncol 28(4):359–366. doi:10.1097/CCO.0000000000000299
18. Volante M, Daniele L, Asioli S, Cassoni P, Comino A, Coverlizza S, De Giuli P, Fava C, Manini C, Berruti A, Papotti M (2013) Tumor staging but not grading is associated with adverse clinical outcome in neuroendocrine tumors of the appendix: a retrospective clinical pathologic analysis of 138 cases. Am J Surg Pathol 37(4):606–612. doi:10.1097/PAS.0b013e318275d1d7

Prognostic Factors: Molecular Pathway – Somatostatin Receptors

Giovanni Vitale, Massimo Milione, and Natalie Prinzi

A. Colao et al. (eds.), *Neuroendocrine Tumors in Real Life*,
https://doi.org/10.1007/978-3-319-59024-0_6

Overview

Somatostatin receptors (SSTRs) are commonly expressed by neuroendocrine tumours (NET), providing the molecular basis for diagnostic and therapeutic interventions in these tumours.

We reported a case of a woman with liver metastases from an ileal NET G1, showing a very high expression of SSTR-2a at the level of tumour cells. After 1 year of treatment with long-acting octreotide acetate, a complete remission of the disease has been observed.

Several reports suggested that the expression of SSTRs represents a positive prognostic factor for survival in NET and predicts the responses to somatostatin analogues and peptide receptor radionuclide treatment.

6

Clinical Case

In January 2007, a 51-year-old woman was referred to the emergency department due to abdominal pain accompanied by nausea and vomiting. Imaging and laboratory tests were suggestive of bowel obstruction due to a tumour-like mass. She underwent surgery with resection of distal ileum, right colon and loco regional lymph nodes. Histology revealed a well-differentiated neuroendocrine tumour (NET) of the ileum (G1 according to WHO 2010; Ki67, 0.5%; TNM staging pT4 pN1 M0; Stage III – AJCC/ENET) (Fig. 6.1).

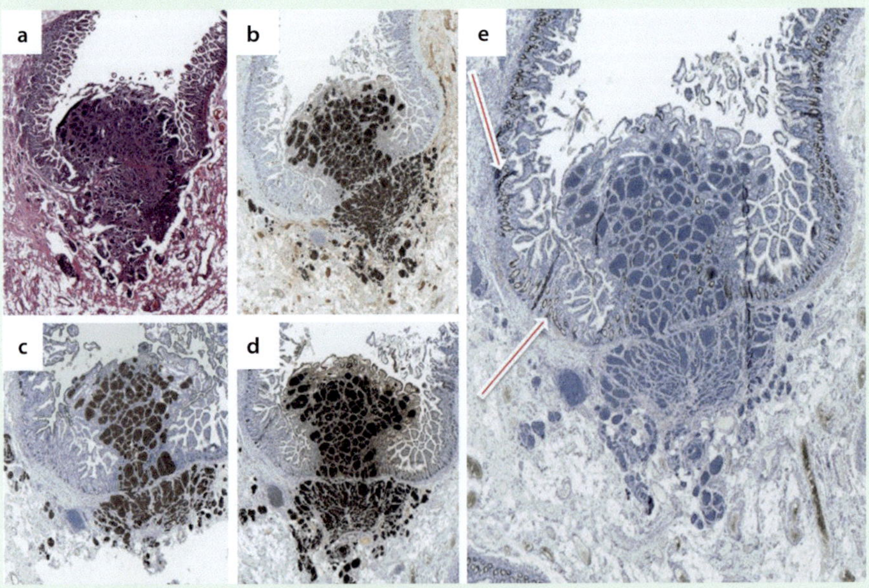

Fig. 6.1 Ileal NET histology. Neuroendocrine tumour of the ileum (haematoxylin-eosin, original magnification ×10) **a** showed intense dot-like staining for chromogranin-A (original magnification ×10) **b**, CDX2 (original magnification ×10) **c** and serotonin (original magnification ×10) **d**. Mib-1/Ki-67 proliferative index (original magnification ×40), counted on a minimum of 2000 tumour cells (WHO 2010), resulted 0.5% **e**; basal crypt cells were used as positive internal control (*arrows*)

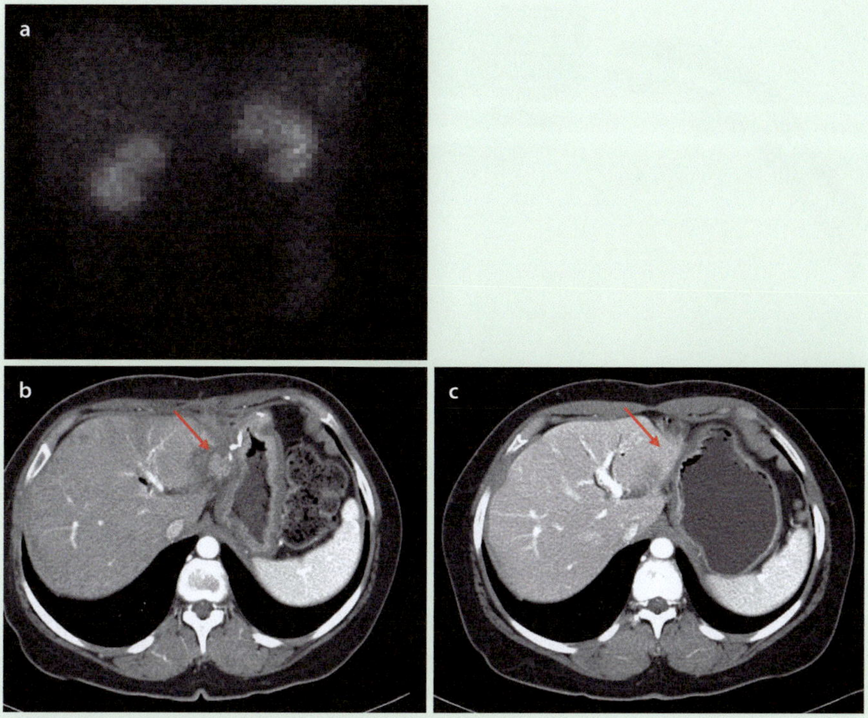

Fig. 6.2 Ileal NET imaging: **a** OctreoScan, performed before treatment with octreotide LAR, did not reveal any pathologic uptake. **b** Computed tomography scan, performed in November 2009 (before starting treatment), showed liver secondary lesion in the III segment (*arrow*). **c** Computed tomography scan, performed 1 year after treatment with octreotide, showed a complete response

During follow-up, she had no symptoms of flushing, diarrhoea or local discomfort; in addition blood values of chromogranin-A and neuron-specific enolase and urinary levels of 5-hydroxyindoleacetic acid were normal. The patient was disease-free until November 2009, when abdominal computed tomography detected multiple liver metastases sited at III and VII liver segments (Fig. 6.2). Liver metastases were negative at somatostatin receptor scintigraphy using ^{111}In-DTPA-D-Phe 1-Octreotide (OctreoScan) (Fig. 6.2). In order to obtain a better histological disease characterization, patient underwent liver biopsy, and the diagnosis of metastases from a well-differentiated NET was confirmed (Fig. 6.3). Even if liver metastases were negative at OctreoScan, immunohistochemistry revealed a positive and strong somatostatin receptor type 2a (SSTR-2a) staining (Fig. 6.3f).

Treatment with long-acting octreotide acetate 30 mg every 28 days by intramuscular injection was initiated. This therapy was well tolerated, and 6 months later, abdominal computed tomography revealed a partial remission according to the RECIST criteria of the largest liver nodule. One year later, computed tomography showed a complete regression of all liver metastases (Fig. 6.2c).

The patient is currently alive without any evidence of recurrence.

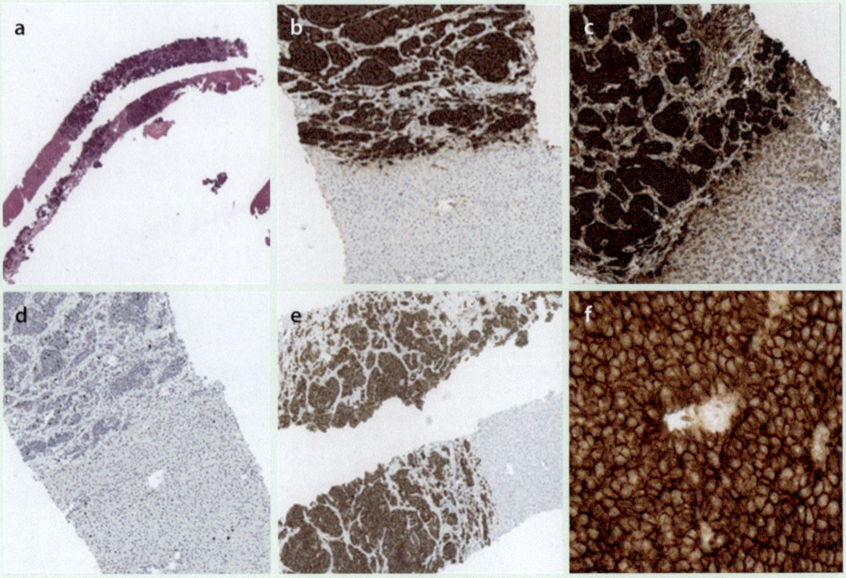

Fig. 6.3 Neuroendocrine tumour liver metastasis. Biopsy specimens from liver metastasis (haematoxylin-eosin, original magnification ×4) **a**. The positive intense cytoplasm staining for synaptophysin (data not shown), chromogranin-A (original magnification ×10) **b** and serotonin (original magnification ×10) **c** confirmed the neuroendocrine nature of this metastasis. Mib-1/Ki67 staining (original magnification ×10), depicted in rare nuclei of tumour cells, showed the low grade of this tumour (NET G1) **d**. CDX-2 intense and diffuse nuclear staining suggested the bowel origin (original magnification ×10) **e**. Intense continuous membranous staining for SSTR-2a in most tumour cells, classified as score 3 according to the method proposed by Volante M et al. Modern Pathology 2007 (original magnification ×40) **f**

6.1 Comments to the Case

Somatostatin receptors (SSTRs) are commonly expressed by NET. This provides the molecular basis for diagnostic and therapeutic interventions in these tumours.

In this chapter we described a case report of a patient with liver metastasis from an ileal NET G1, showing a very high expression of SSTR-2a at the level of tumour cells detected by immunohistochemistry. Surprisingly, OctreoScan resulted negative in this patient. After 1 year of monotherapy with octreotide, a complete remission of the disease has been observed, confirming in this case the validity of the immunohistochemistry for the detection of SSTR-2a. This case draws attention on (1) the importance of treatment with somatostatin analogues not only in the control of hormonal symptoms but also in the inhibition of tumour growth and (2) the potential role of SSTR expression as a predictive marker of response to somatostatin analogues in NET.

Questions

1. Which is the role of SSTR expression in NET as a prognostic marker useful in therapy decision-making?
2. Which are the procedures to detect SSTR expression in NET?

Tentative Answers

1. The expression of SSTRs represents a positive prognostic factor for survival in NET and appears to predict the responses to somatostatin analogues and peptide receptor radionuclide treatment.
2. SSTR expression in NET can be performed by SSTR scintigraphy/PET or directly on tumour tissue through immunohistochemical staining or real-time RT-PCR method.

Up to Date of the Topic

Somatostatin analogues and peptide receptor radionuclide treatment (PRRT) represent targeted therapies SSTR-oriented widely used in NET.

Somatostatin analogues (octreotide and lanreotide) have been demonstrated in numerous studies to be a milestone for the management of NET and the control of NET-related syndromes [1–3]. In addition, recent investigations (PROMID and CLARINET studies) have pointed out the ability of long-acting somatostatin analogues to control also tumour growth in NET, showing a better time to tumour progression [4] and progression-free survival [5] in the treatment group compared to placebo control. Biological response to somatostatin analogues depends on distribution and level of expression of SSTR subtypes in tumours and the expression of selective SSTR signalling pathway molecules. Unlike natural somatostatin, octreotide and lanreotide bind with high affinity only to SSTR-2 and with lower affinity to SSTR-5 subtype. Interestingly, patients with low-grade tumours and preserved SSTR-2 and SSTR-5 expressions have better survival times while are treated with somatostatin analogues [6]. Therefore, most clinicians agree that the presence of SSTRs should be verified before treatment with a somatostatin analogue is initiated [7]. Usually this is done in vivo by SSTR scintigraphy or PET, but immunohistochemical staining of tumour tissue specimens with specific antibodies against the receptors can also be used. According to a recent ENET Consensus [8], immunohistochemical staining for SSTR-2a has been considered optional, since methodological variations and current data do not show a completely conclusive pattern. Thus, treatment with somatostatin analogues may be initiated although SSTR-2 staining may be weak or even absent on immunohistochemistry. However, data on correlations between tumour SSTR profile evaluated by immunohistochemistry and response to somatostatin analogues are scanty, and most of these studies adopted polyclonal anti-SSTR antibodies.

One of the most clinically relevant therapeutic innovations in NET has been the development of PRRT through the use of somatostatin analogues labelled with β-emitting radionuclides, such as yttrium-90 or lutetium-177. Current guidelines support the use of PRRT in patients with unresectable grade 1 or 2 NET and high SSTR expression at known tumour sites [9]. In these cases, SSTR scintigraphy, which depends on the expression of SSTR (especially SSTR-2), has some predictive ability in determining functional response in these tumours. A recent paper showed that tumour SSTR-2a expression was an independent predictor of survival but had no greater value than OctreoScan in predicting the in vivo NET response to PRRT [10].

Several studies suggested a favourable prognostic value of SSTR expression in patients with NET, even if it is difficult to exclude the effects of treatment with somatostatin analogues from this analysis. In patients with pancreatic NET, an immunohistochemical SSTR-2a score <1 was an independent predictor of poor outcomes [11, 12], and it resulted stronger compared to Ki-67 labelling index [12]. In gastroenteropancreatic NET multivariate analysis confirmed that SSTR-2 expression was an independent factor impacting positively on survival [13, 14]. Corleto et al. [6] reported that neither SSTR-2 and SSTR-5 expression nor Ki-67 level alone correlated with survival. However, a significantly better 5-year survival rate was observed in patients with NET expressing SSTR-2, SSTR-5 and Ki-67 < 2% (91%), compared to those with SSTR-2- and SSTR-5-negative tumours and Ki-67>2% (43%). In pulmonary NET, SSTR-1 expression levels, evaluated both by immunohistochemistry and quantitative RT-PCR, were positively correlated with patient survival [15].

6

On the other hand, few studies reported contradictory results. In 114 gastrointestinal and bronchopulmonary NET, SSTR-2 expression did not correlate with the proliferative rate assessed through using MIB-1 immunohistochemistry [16]. Righi et al. [17] reported a SSTR-2a overexpression in metastatic typical carcinoids as compared with atypical carcinoids and clinically benign typical carcinoids.

In conclusion, SSTR expression appeared to be a prognostic marker in NET that can be used for patient stratification and to optimize treatment decisions. The next efforts of research should be devoted to improve the detection and complete characterization of SSTR expression in this tumour, also in view of clinical use of new SSTR panligands.

Bibliography

1. Pusceddu S, De Braud F, Festinese F, Bregant C, Lorenzoni A, Maccauro M, Milione M, Concas L, Formisano B, Leuzzi L, Mazzaferro V, Buzzoni R (2015) Evolution in the treatment of gastroenteropancreatic-neuroendocrine neoplasms, focus on systemic therapeutic options: a systematic review. Future Oncol 11(13):1947–1959
2. Lupoli G, Cascone E, Arlotta F, Vitale G, Celentano L, Salvatore M, Lombardi G (1996) Treatment of advanced medullary thyroid carcinoma with a combination of recombinant interferon alpha-2b and octreotide. Cancer 78(5):1114–1118
3. Vitale G, Tagliaferri P, Caraglia M, Rampone E, Ciccarelli A, Bianco AR, Abbruzzese A, Lupoli G (2000) Slow release lanreotide in combination with interferon-alpha2b in the treatment of symptomatic advanced medullary thyroid carcinoma. J Clin Endocrinol Metab 85(3):983–988
4. Rinke A, Müller HH, Schade-Brittinger C, Klose KJ, Barth P, Wied M, Mayer C, Aminossadati B, Pape UF, Bläker M, Harder J, Arnold C, Gress T, Arnold R, PROMID Study Group (2009) Placebo-controlled, double-blind, prospective, randomized study on the effect of octreotide LAR in the control of tumor growth in patients with metastatic neuroendocrine midgut tumors: a report from the PROMID Study Group. J Clin Oncol 27(28):4656–4663
5. Caplin ME, Pavel M, Ćwikła JB, Phan AT, Raderer M, Sedláčková E, Cadiot G, Wolin EM, Capdevila J, Wall L, Rindi G, Langley A, Martinez S, Blumberg J, Ruszniewski P, CLARINET Investigators (2014) Lanreotide in metastatic enteropancreatic neuroendocrine tumors. N Engl J Med 371(3):224–233. doi:10.1056/NEJMoa1316158

6. Corleto VD, Falconi M, Panzuto F, Milione M, De Luca O, Perri P, Cannizzaro R, Bordi C, Pederzoli P, Scarpa A, Delle FG (2009) Somatostatin receptor subtypes 2 and 5 are associated with better survival in well-differentiated endocrine carcinomas. Neuroendocrinology 89(2):223–230. doi:10.1159/000167796
7. Janson ET (2006) Treatment of neuroendocrine tumors with somatostatin analogs. Pituitary 9:249–256. doi:10.1007/s11102-006-0271-4
8. Niederle B, Pape UF, Costa F, Gross D, Kelestimur F, Knigge U, Öberg K, Pavel M, Perren A, Toumpanakis C, O'Connor J, O'Toole D, Krenning E, Reed N, Kianmanesh R, Vienna Consensus Conference participants (2016) ENET consensus guidelines update for neuroendocrine neoplasms of the jejunum and ileum. Neuroendocrinology 103(2):125–138
9. Bodei L, Mueller-Brand J, Baum RP, Pavel ME, Hörsch D, O'Dorisio MS, O'Dorisio TM, Howe JR, Cremonesi M, Kwekkeboom DJ, Zaknun JJ (2013) The joint IAEA, EANM, and SNMMI practical guidance on peptide receptor radionuclide therapy (PRRNT) in neuroendocrine tumours. Eur J Nucl Med Mol Imaging 40(5):800–816. doi:10.1007/s00259-012-2330-6
10. van Adrichem RC, Kamp K, van Deurzen CH, Biermann K, Feelders RA, Franssen GJ, Kwekkeboom DJ, Hofland LJ, de Herder WW (2016) Is there an additional value of using somatostatin receptor subtype 2a immunohistochemistry compared to somatostatin receptor Scintigraphy uptake in predicting Gastroenteropancreatic neuroendocrine tumor response? Neuroendocrinology 103(5):560–566
11. Okuwaki K, Kida M, Mikami T, Yamauchi H, Imaizumi H, Miyazawa S, Iwai T, Takezawa M, Saegusa M, Watanabe M, Koizumi W (2013) Clinicopathologic characteristics of pancreatic neuroendocrine tumors and relation of somatostatin receptor type 2A to outcomes. Cancer 119(23):4094–4102. doi:10.1002/cncr.28341
12. Mehta S, de Reuver PR, Gill P, Andrici J, D'Urso L, Mittal A, Pavlakis N, Clarke S, Samra JS, Gill AJ (2015) Somatostatin receptor SSTR-2a expression is a stronger predictor for survival than Ki-67 in pancreatic neuroendocrine tumors. Medicine (Baltimore) 94(40):e1281. doi:10.1097/MD.0000000000001281
13. Pinato DJ, Tan TM, Toussi ST, Ramachandran R, Martin N, Meeran K, Ngo N, Dina R, Sharma R (2014) An expression signature of the angiogenic response in gastrointestinal neuroendocrine tumours: correlation with tumour phenotype and survival outcomes. Br J Cancer 110(1):115–122. doi:10.1038/bjc.2013.682
14. Kim HS, Lee HS, Kim WH (2011) Clinical significance of protein expression of cyclooxygenase-2 and somatostatin receptors in gastroenteropancreatic neuroendocrine tumors. Cancer Res Treat 43(3):181–188. doi:10.4143/crt.2011.43.3.181
15. Kaemmerer D, Specht E, Sänger J, Wirtz RM, Sayeg M, Schulz S, Lupp A (2015) Somatostatin receptors in bronchopulmonary neuroendocrine neoplasms: new diagnostic, prognostic, and therapeutic markers. J Clin Endocrinol Metab 100(3):831–840. doi:10.1210/jc.2014-2699
16. Körner M, Waser B, Reubi JC (2015) Does somatostatin or gastric inhibitory peptide receptor expression correlate with tumor grade and stage in gut neuroendocrine tumors? Neuroendocrinology 101(1):45–57. doi:10.1159/000371804
17. Righi L, Volante M, Tavaglione V, Billè A, Daniele L, Angusti T, Inzani F, Pelosi G, Rindi G, Papotti M (2010) Somatostatin receptor tissue distribution in lung neuroendocrine tumours: a clinicopathologic and immunohistochemical study of 218 'clinically aggressive' cases. Ann Oncol 21(3):548–555. doi:10.1093/annonc/mdp334

Prognostic Factors: Molecular Pathway – Oncogene (mTOR)

Maria Chiara Zatelli

A. Colao et al. (eds.), *Neuroendocrine Tumors in Real Life*,
https://doi.org/10.1007/978-3-319-59024-0_7

Overview

The factors that can be used to estimate the chance of recovery from or recurrence of neuroendocrine neoplasms (NEN) are yet to be fully clarified. Molecular pathways have been investigated in order to find prognostic markers that could predict the survival of NEN patients and that could help in planning the best therapeutic approach. Recently, the mammalian target of rapamycin (mTOR) pathway has emerged as an important therapeutic target for the medical treatment of NEN. We here review the available information on the prognostic value of mTOR pathway derangements in patients with NET.

Clinical Case

7

A 76-year-old man was referred to the NEN clinic for the incidental detection of a 23 mm solid lesion in the body of the pancreas at an abdominal computerized tomography (CT) scan performed after an abdominal ultrasound (as a follow-up of previously diagnosed gallbladder stones). The patient was asymptomatic and hormonal screening was negative for any hypersecretion. Octreoscan was positive for a neuroendocrine lesion of the pancreas, with no further uptake in any other site. Endoscopic ultrasound-guided biopsy was indicative of a G1 NEN of the pancreas with a Ki-67 = 2%. The patient was followed up and after 6 months the control abdominal CT scan showed an increase in tumour diameter (28 mm, +21%); therefore the patient started medical therapy with a somatostatin analogue (SSA, lanreotide autogel 90 mg every 4 weeks) and ursodeoxycholic acid. After 6 months (12 months after diagnosis), the abdominal CT scan found the pancreatic lesion further increased in diameter, measuring 35 mm (+25%), in the absence of metastatic sites. ^{68}Ga-DOTATOC positron emission tomography (PET) did not show further sites of tracer uptake except for the pancreatic lesion. Due to disease progression and lack of extra-pancreatic localization, a surgical approach was undertaken, and the histological diagnosis was consistent with a G1 pancreatic NET (pNET, Ki67 ≥ 2%, T1 N0 M0, stage I). The patient was in good conditions and the postsurgical recovery was uneventful. SSA and ursodeoxycholic acid therapy was discontinued.

At the time of surgery, after patient informed consent was obtained, a primary culture of the surgical specimen was performed, as previously described [1]. Cells were treated in vitro with the mTOR inhibitor everolimus that caused a significant reduction in primary culture cell viability as compared to vehicle-treated cells after 48 h (−15%; $p < 0.05$). The tissue was also evaluated by AlphaScreen [2] for the expression levels of three mTOR pathway components, i.e. the phosphorylated forms of AKT, mTOR and 4EBP1, and compared to those recorded in the BON1 cell line (◘ Fig. 7.1). BON1 cells were used as reference for an everolimus-sensitive in vitro model, since it has been previously shown that everolimus is capable of reducing BON1 cell viability in vitro [3]. As shown in ◘ Fig. 7.1, the patient's primary culture displayed phosphorylated levels of AKT, mTOR and 4EBP1 similar or greater than those observed in the everolimus-sensitive human pancreatic NET cell line, BON1.

Six months after surgery (18 months after diagnosis), liver metastases to the VII (8 mm) and VIII (1 cm) liver segment were detected at CT and then confirmed at biopsy. Therefore, everolimus treatment was started, with stabilization of the disease and a progression-free survival of >20 months. These data are in line with previous reports showing an increased mTOR pathway activation in pNET [4, 5] and support the hypothesis that the expression levels of mTOR pathway components may represent a prognostic marker in pNET as well as a predictive marker of responsiveness to mTOR inhibitors [6–8].

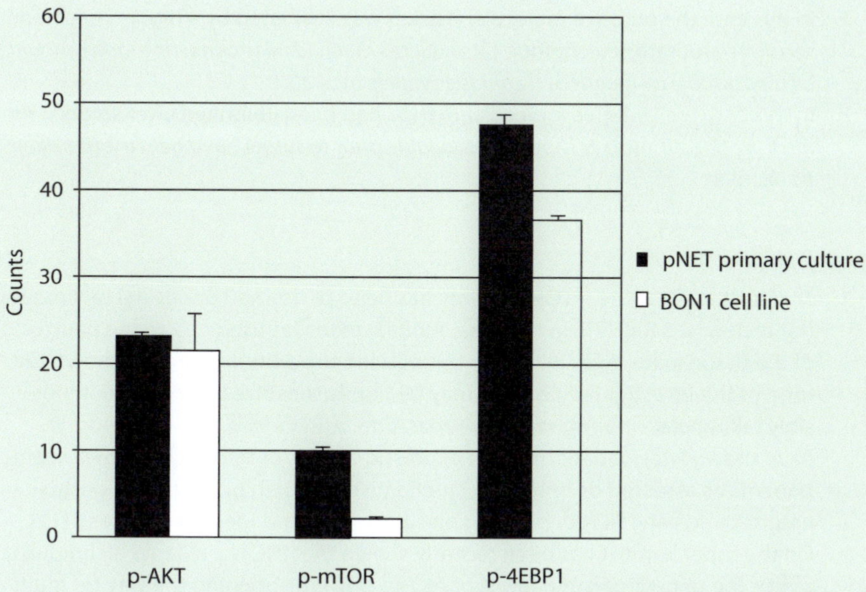

Fig. 7.1 mTOR signalling pathway expression in the primary culture of the patient. Total proteins were isolated and AlphaScreen analysis for phosphorylated AKT (*p-AKT*), mTOR (*p-mTOR*) and 4EBP1 (*p-4EBP1*) expression levels was performed. Values are expressed after normalization against glyceraldehyde-3-phosphate dehydrogenase (GAPDH) as AlphaScreen signal (counts)

7.1 Comments to the Case

The ENET guidelines on the management of pNET indicate as negative prognostic factors age (>40 years), Ki-67 labelling index (>2%), positive surgical margins, calcifications on CT scan, number of metastatic lymph nodes, the presence of symptoms, a rapid progression of liver metastases (>25% volume increase within 6–12 months) and the development of bone metastases [9, 10]. The reported case displayed only one of the clinical negative prognostic factors (i.e. age >40 years), but showed progression after treatment with SSA. At the same time, the molecular findings of this pNET patient are in keeping with the evidence that baseline AKT activation characterizes an aggressive clinical course and that it may predict an increased progression-free survival (PFS) under treatment with everolimus [6]. Moreover, AKT activation has been recently indicated as a putative predictive marker of response to everolimus [8]. These findings underline the relevant clinical potential of molecular markers that have been intensively investigated in the last years, since the «classical» clinical markers have shown their limited value, as underlined by the presented case. Indeed, a conservative management was chosen on the basis of the low likelihood of progression, as indicated by the clinical characteristics. On the contrary, the pNET turned out to be much more aggressive, requiring surgery and displaying metastatic spread after surgery. The availability of improved prognostic markers is therefore necessary in order to plan the appropriate treatment and follow-up in NEN patients.

Questions

1. In this case the putative molecular marker was evaluated by a highly specific and sensitive laboratory technique (AlphaScreen). *An ideal prognostic marker should be measurable by means of techniques widely available.*
2. In this case the putative molecular marker had been identified after surgery. *An ideal prognostic marker should be available prior to surgery and help the therapeutic decision.*

Answers

1. The evaluation of the mTOR pathway has been performed by several techniques (for review, see Ref. [7]). In this case, AlphaScreen was used due to the paucity of the tissue material available for this patient. In addition, the phosphorylated form of the investigated proteins may be highly sensitive to degradation possibly taking place during sample preparation. And indeed, previous reports have shown wide variations in the expression levels of the mTOR pathway components as assessed by immunohistochemistry (IHC) in patients with gastro-entero-pancreatic NEN depending on tumour site and metastatic spread [11]. On the other hand, it has been recently shown that IHC is a reliable technique to assess the phosphorylated levels of AKT in pNET [8], opening the way for multicentre validation studies. The availability of markers that can be assessed by IHC (i.e. in any Pathology Department) might importantly improve the possibility to provide prognostic information.
2. The prognostic value of circulating markers that could be assessed more easily, in multiple occasions, and independently of the availability of a tissue sample is a matter of great discussion. Single markers, the «mono-analyte biomarkers», such as chromogranin A and other circulating proteins, display poor sensitivity and specificity for diagnosis and have limited prognostic value. In addition, the routine use of miRNA or circulating tumour cells as useful prognostic markers in NEN still needs to be confirmed in clinical validation studies. Indeed, the value of each mono-analyte remains uncertain, since their involvement in the mechanistic processes of NEN disease is still unclear. On the other hand, multi-analyte biomarkers have the potential for higher diagnostic sensitivity and specificity as well as prognostic value, since they may better reflect the molecular events that cause NEN development, deeply influencing prognosis and response to treatment [12]. Along the line of multi-analyte strategies, multigene signatures have been considered as potentially useful on clinical grounds in order to provide real-time information about tumour activity and response to treatment. In these settings, transcript analysis provides copious information that has been employed to implement multi-analyte assays with algorithm analyses (MAAA) [13]. The NET MAAA biomarker panel has already been employed displaying high sensitivity and specificity, not depending on age, gender, ethnicity, fasting, or medications [14, 15]. However, this method requires a dedicated laboratory and the necessary technical hardware, software and skilled personnel that are not widely available.

Up to Date of the Topic

The issue of prognostic markers in the NET field is highly debated and generates more reviews that original research articles. A recent Delphic consensus assessment concluded that current mono-analyte biomarkers have a limited diagnostic and prognostic value [16]. Nevertheless, there is evidence supporting a prognostic role for the components of the mTOR pathway. Mutations of genes encoding for proteins included in the mTOR pathway were found in 14% of pNET in a study from the United States [17] and in 54% of pNET in a study from China [18]. Next-generation sequencing revealed that components of the PI3K/AKT/mTOR pathway are more frequently mutated in large-cell and small-cell lung carcinomas of the lung (11.7%) as compared to typical and atypical bronchial carcinoids (2.3%), possibly suggesting that mTOR pathway mutations associate with a more aggressive biological and clinical behaviour [19]. Besides genetic alterations, mTOR pathway deranged activity may also be assessed by IHC in lung NEN. Indeed, it has been shown that in lung carcinoids, low p-mTOR expression correlated with lymph node metastases, recurrent disease and survival. IHC scores for p-mTOR were found to be significantly higher in G1/G2 as compared to G3 also in GEP NEN [20]. These results confirm previous findings showing a significant association between the expression levels of the mTOR pathway components and tumour invasion, proliferation and advanced stage in pNET [21] or with Ki67 index in GEP NEN [22], supporting the hypothesis that an activated mTOR pathway may represent a negative prognostic factor. In addition, phosphatase and tensin homologue (PTEN), a negative regulator of the mTOR pathway, was found to be a potential prognostic marker, since low PTEN IHC scores, together with negative progesterone receptor staining, associated with the shortest median overall survival among 160 resected pNET [23]. Taken together, these data suggest that mTOR pathway profiling might have a prognostic role in lung and pNET. However, validation studies are still lacking, both from the technical and the clinical point of view.

Bibliography

1. Molè D, Gagliano T, Gentilin E, Tagliati F, Pasquali C, Ambrosio MR, Pansini G, Degli Uberti EC, Zatelli MC (2011) Targeting protein kinase C by Enzastaurin restrains proliferation and secretion in human pancreatic endocrine tumors. Endocr Relat Cancer 18:439–450. doi:10.1530/ERC-11-0055
2. Gagliano T, Bellio M, Gentilin E, Molè D, Tagliati F, Schiavon M, Cavallesco NG, Andriolo LG, Ambrosio MR, Rea F et al (2013) mTOR, p70S6K, AKT, and ERK1/2 levels predict sensitivity to mTOR and PI3K/mTOR inhibitors in human bronchial carcinoids. Endocr Relat Cancer 20:463–475. doi:10.1530/ERC-13-0042
3. Zitzmann K, De Toni EN, Brand S, Göke B, Meinecke J, Spöttl G, Meyer HH, Auernhammer CJ (2007) The novel mTOR inhibitor RAD001 (everolimus) induces antiproliferative effects in human pancreatic neuroendocrine tumor cells. Neuroendocrinology 85(1):54–60. Erratum in: Neuroendocrinology. 2009;90(3):250. Dosage error in article text. PubMed PMID: 17310129
4. Shida T, Kishimoto T, Furuya M, Nikaido T, Koda K, Takano S, Kimura F, Shimizu H, Yoshidome H, Ohtsuka M et al (2010) Expression of an activated mammalian target of rapamycin (mTOR) in gastroenteropancreatic neuroendocrine tumors. Cancer Chemother Pharmacol 65:889–893. doi:10.1007/s00280-009-1094-6

5. Righi L, Volante M, Rapa I, Tavaglione V, Inzani F, Pelosi G, Papotti M (2010) Mammalian target of rapamycin signaling activation patterns in neuroendocrinetumors of the lung. Endocr Relat Cancer 17:977–987. doi:10.1677/ERC-10-0157
6. Ghayouri M, Boulware D, Nasir A, Strosberg J, Kvols L, Coppola D (2010) Activation of the serine/threonine protein kinase Akt in enteropancreatic neuroendocrine tumors. Anticancer Res 30:5063–5067
7. Zatelli MC, Fanciulli G, Malandrino P, Ramundo V, Faggiano A, Colao A, NIKE Group (2016) Predictive factors of response to mTOR inhibitors in neuroendocrine tumours. Endocr Relat Cancer 23(3):R173–R183. doi:10.1530/ERC-15-0413. Review. PubMed PMID: 26666705
8. Falletta S, Partelli S, Rubini C, Nann D, Doria A, Marinoni I, Polenta V, Di Pasquale C, Degli Uberti E, Perren A, Falconi M, Zatelli MC (2016) mTOR inhibitors response and mTOR pathway in pancreatic neuroendocrine tumors. Endocr Relat Cancer 23(11):883–891. PubMed PMID: 27697900
9. Falconi M, Bartsch DK, Eriksson B, Klöppel G, Lopes JM, O'Connor JM, Salazar R, Taal BG, Vullierme MP, O'Toole D, Barcelona Consensus Conference participants (2012) ENETS consensus guidelines for the management of patients with digestive neuroendocrine neoplasms of the digestive system: well-differentiated pancreatic non-functioning tumors. Neuroendocrinology 95(2):120–134. doi:10.1159/000335587. PubMed PMID: 22261872
10. Falconi M, Eriksson B, Kaltsas G, Bartsch DK, Capdevila J, Caplin M, Kos-Kudla B, Kwekkeboom D, Rindi G, Klöppel G, Reed N, Kianmanesh R, Jensen RT, Vienna Consensus Conference participants (2016) ENETS consensus guidelines update for the Management of Patients with functional pancreatic neuroendocrine tumors and non-functional pancreatic neuroendocrine tumors. Neuroendocrinology 103(2):153–171. doi:10.1159/000443171. PubMed PMID: 26742109; PubMed Central PMCID: PMC4849884
11. Kasajima A, Pavel M, Darb-Esfahani S, Noske A, Stenzinger A, Sasano H, Dietel M, Denkert C, Röcken C, Wiedenmann B et al (2011) mTOR expression and activity patterns in gastroenteropancreatic neuroendocrine tumours. Endocr Relat Cancer 18:181–192. doi:10.1677/ERC-10-0126
12. Oberg K, Modlin IM, De Herder W, Pavel M, Klimstra D, Frilling A, Metz DC, Heaney A, Kwekkeboom D, Strosberg J, Meyer T, Moss SF, Washington K, Wolin E, Liu E, Goldenring J (2015) Consensus on biomarkers for neuroendocrine tumour disease. Lancet Oncol 16(9):e435–e446. doi:10.1016/S1470-2045(15)00186-2. Review. PubMed PMID: 26370353; PubMed Central PMCID: PMC5023063
13. Modlin IM, Bodei L, Kidd M (2016) Neuroendocrine tumor biomarkers: from monoanalytes to transcripts and algorithms. Best Pract Res Clin Endocrinol Metab 30(1):59–77. doi:10.1016/j.beem.2016.01.002. Review. PubMed PMID: 26971844
14. Modlin I, Drozdov I, Kidd M (2014) Gut neuroendocrine tumor blood qpcr fingerprint assay: characteristics and reproducibility. Clin Chem 52:419e29
15. Modlin IM, Kidd M, Bodei L et al (2015) The clinical utility of a novel blood-based multi-transcriptome assay for the diagnosis of neuroendocrine tumors of the gastrointestinal tract. Am J Gastroenterol 110:1223e32–1210.1038/ajg.2015.1160. Epub 2015 Jun 1222
16. Oberg K, Krenning E, Sundin A, Bodei L, Kidd M, Tesselaar M, Ambrosini V, Baum RP, Kulke M, Pavel M, Cwikla J, Drozdov I, Falconi M, Fazio N, Frilling A, Jensen R, Koopmans K, Korse T, Kwekkeboom D, Maecke H, Paganelli G, Salazar R, Severi S, Strosberg J, Prasad V, Scarpa A, Grossman A, Walenkamp A, Cives M, Virgolini I, Kjaer A, Modlin IM (2016) A Delphic consensus assessment: imaging and biomarkers in gastroenteropancreatic neuroendocrine tumor disease management. Endocr Connect 5(5):174–187. doi:10.1530/EC-16-0043. PubMed PMID: 27582247; PubMed Central PMCID: PMC5045519
17. Jiao Y, Shi C, Edil BH, de Wilde RF, Klimstra DS, Maitra A, Schulick RD, Tang LH, Wolfgang CL, Choti MA, Velculescu VE, Diaz LA Jr, Vogelstein B, Kinzler KW, Hruban RH, Papadopoulos N (2011) DAXX/ATRX, MEN1, and mTOR pathway genes are frequently altered in pancreatic neuroendocrine tumors. Science 331(6021):1199–1203. doi:10.1126/science.1200609. PubMed PMID: 21252315; PubMed Central PMCID: PMC3144496
18. Yuan F, Shi M, Ji J, Shi H, Zhou C, Yu Y, Liu B, Zhu Z, Zhang J (2014) KRAS and DAXX/ATRX gene mutations are correlated with the clinicopathological features, advanced diseases, and poor prognosis in Chinese patients with pancreatic neuroendocrine tumors. Int J Biol Sci 10(9):957–965. doi:10.7150/ijbs.9773. PubMed PMID: 25210493; PubMed Central PMCID: PMC4159686

19. Simbolo M, Mafficini A, Sikora KO, Fassan M, Barbi S, Corbo V, Mastracci L, Rusev B, Grillo F, Vicentini C, Ferrara R, Pilotto S, Davini F, Pelosi G, Lawlor RT, Chilosi M, Tortora G, Bria E, Fontanini G, Volante M, Scarpa A (2016) Lung neuroendocrine tumours: deep sequencing of the four World Health Organization histotypes reveals chromatin-remodelling genes as major players and a prognostic role for TERT, RB1, MEN1 and KMT2D. J Pathol 241(4):488–500. doi:10.1002/path.4853. [Epub ahead of print] PubMed PMID: 27873319
20. Circelli L, Sciammarella C, Guadagno E, Tafuto S, del Basso de Caro M, Botti G, Pezzullo L, Aria M, Ramundo V, Tatangelo F, Losito NS, Ieranò C, D'Alterio C, Izzo F, Ciliberto G, Colao A, Faggiano A, Scala S (2016) CXCR4/CXCL12/CXCR7 axis is functional in neuroendocrine tumors and signals on mTOR. Oncotarget 7(14):18865–18875. doi:10.18632/oncotarget.7738. PubMed PMID: 26934559; PubMed Central PMCID: PMC4951335
21. Komori Y, Yada K, Ohta M, Uchida H, Iwashita Y, Fukuzawa K, Kashima K, Yokoyama S, Inomata M, Kitano S (2014) Mammalian target of rapamycin signalling activation patterns in pancreatic neuroendocrine tumors. J Hepatobiliary Pancreat Sci 21(4):288–295. doi:10.1002/jhbp.26. PubMed PMID: 24002888
22. Qian ZR, Ter-Minassian M, Chan JA, Imamura Y, Hooshmand SM, Kuchiba A, Morikawa T, Brais LK, Daskalova A, Heafield R, Lin X, Christiani DC, Fuchs CS, Ogino S, Kulke MH (2013) Prognostic significance of MTOR pathway component expression in neuroendocrine tumors. J Clin Oncol 31(27):3418–3425. doi:10.1200/JCO.2012.46.6946. PubMed PMID: 23980085; PubMed Central PMCID: PMC3770868
23. Estrella JS, Broaddus RR, Mathews A, Milton DR, Yao JC, Wang H, Rashid A (2014) Progesterone receptor and PTEN expression predict survival in patients with low- and intermediate-grade pancreatic neuroendocrine tumors. Arch Pathol Lab Med 138(8):1027–1036. doi:10.5858/arpa.2013-0195-OA. PubMed PMID: 25076292

Prognostic Factors: Molecular Pathway – Tumour Suppressor Gene (MEN1)

Marie-Lise Jaffrain-Rea, Liliya Rostomyan, and Albert Beckers

A. Colao et al. (eds.), *Neuroendocrine Tumors in Real Life*,
https://doi.org/10.1007/978-3-319-59024-0_8

Overview

Multiple endocrine neoplasia type 1 (MEN1) is the most prevalent inherited cause of neuroendocrine tumours (NETs) of foregut origin, and gastroenteropancreatic (GEP) NETs are part of the characteristic MEN1 triad in association with primary hyperparathyroidism and pituitary adenomas. Lung and thymic NETs may also be present. MEN1 is an autosomal dominant disorder with a nearly complete penetrance, characterized by germline inactivating mutations in the *MEN1* gene encoding the nuclear protein menin, which somatic inactivation may also play a role in sporadic NETs. Compared with their sporadic counterpart, MEN1-NETs are typically characterized by an earlier onset and frequent multiplicity of tumours developing synchronously or metachronously within and across different neuroendocrine tissues/organs. Some phenotypes are also more aggressive or even malignant, representing a major cause of death in MEN1 patients. Due to the complexity of MEN1, prognostic factors identified in sporadic NETs may not correctly apply in this setting and surgical indications may differ. Expert clinical guidelines have been developed in order to identify a MEN1 condition and achieve an early diagnosis of MEN1 neoplasia in mutation carriers, with proven benefits for affected patients. However, this represents a heavy psychological and economic burden and open issues remain. Optimizing early tumour detection with acceptable diagnostic modalities is still challenging in real life, especially in young patients (<20 year) in whom there is increasing evidence of asymptomatic NETs.

Clinical Case

The proband: A 44-year-old woman came to our observation at the Neuromed Institute in May 2004 for a recurrent invasive macroprolactinoma. The disease presented at the age of 25 year as an apparently sporadic macroprolactinoma, which was successfully removed by transsphenoidal surgery (TS) and recurred 14 years later as an invasive recurrent macroprolactinoma with increasing dopamine-agonist resistance, requiring repeated TS (2002, 2004, 2008) and radiotherapy (2004). Due to uncontrolled tumour growth, she also received temozolomide (TMZ) (2011–2013) with PRL normalization lasting for 3 years after treatment withdrawal. She had type 2 diabetes mellitus and hypertension in a familial context. In 1995 she underwent a left hemithyroidectomy for a benign nodular disease, and thyroidectomy was totalized in 2005 during parathyroid surgery. Indeed, despite symptomatic bilateral urinary microlithiasis since the age of 37 years, hypercalcaemia was noticed in 2004, and primary HPT was diagnosed with rapid worsening (calcemia and PTH up to 13.4 mg/dl and 483 pg/ml ($N < 72$), respectively). Pathological examination confirmed the presence of a 1.8 cm right superior parathyroid adenoma in the setting of bilateral parathyroid hyperplasia and recurrent multinodular goitre, and a c.202_206dupGCCCC germline *MEN1* mutation was found [1]. She also had cutaneous lipomas and angiofibromas. A pancreatic mass was found and subsequently ascribed to the sequelae of an acute pancreatitis due to biliary lithiasis, leading to cholecystectomy in 2006, with subsequent spontaneous regression. Before starting TMZ, a whole-body PET-CT showed an isolated area of ^{18}F-DOPA uptake in the sellar region, which was no more evident in 2012. The patient is currently on replacement therapy for hypothyroidism/hypoparathyroidism, cabergoline being recently restarted (1.0 mg weekly) for a modest recurrent hyperprolactinemia without change on pituitary MRI.

Genetic familial screening revealed that the proband (II.a, ◘ Fig. 8.1) had inherited the *MEN1* mutation from her father, while two other mutation carriers were identified.

The proband's father (I.b) was 71 years old at the time of screening. He also had hypertension, type 2 diabetes mellitus and a previous thyroidectomy for a compressive multinodular goitre with post-operative hypoparathyroidism. A 1.5 cm right pulmonary nodule was found in 1999 following an episode of bronchitis, and a poorly conclusive fine-needle biopsy was performed in 2001 after a 0.5 cm increase in size. The patient refused surgery until symptomatic growth occurred in 2010. In January 2011, a whole-body PET-CT showed increased ^{18}F-FDG uptake by the bronchial lesion and revealed a focal hepatic uptake, with no uptake by a few thoracic lymph nodes and two nodules in the pancreatic tail (15 and 7 mm). In contrast, increased ^{18}F-DOPA uptake was present at the bronchial, hepatic and pancreatic sites, strongly suggesting associated NETs (◘ Fig. 8.2). Plasma NE markers were normal, including NSE. An inferior right bi-lobectomy was performed, and a well-delimited bronchial nodule (4.0 × 3.1 × 2.5 cm) was removed, with a final diagnosis of a lung neuroendocrine tumour (L-NET) with peribronchial invasion and lymphatic metastasis (pT2 N1). The proliferative activity was intermediate (mitosis 5HPF/10HPF, Ki67 7%), all tumour cells were positive for CrgA and synaptophysin, and a minority of proximal lymph nodes were metastatic. The patient was started on lanreotide 90 mg monthly. In 2012 a residual ^{18}F-DOPA uptake was limited to the dominant pancreatic nodule. Treatment with somatostatin analogues (SSA) was maintained through the years with regular CT imaging (the last one on April 2016) showing the stability of the dominant pancreatic nodule, a cystic evolution of the hepatic nodule and no additional lesion. Pituitary screening was repeatedly negative. Yet, the patient is asymptomatic on octreotide LAR 20 mg monthly and replacement therapy for hypothyroidism/hypoparathyroidism.

The proband's sister (II.b) was 40 years old at the time of screening. She was suffering from renal lithiasis, intermittent menstrual irregularities and unexplained episodes of

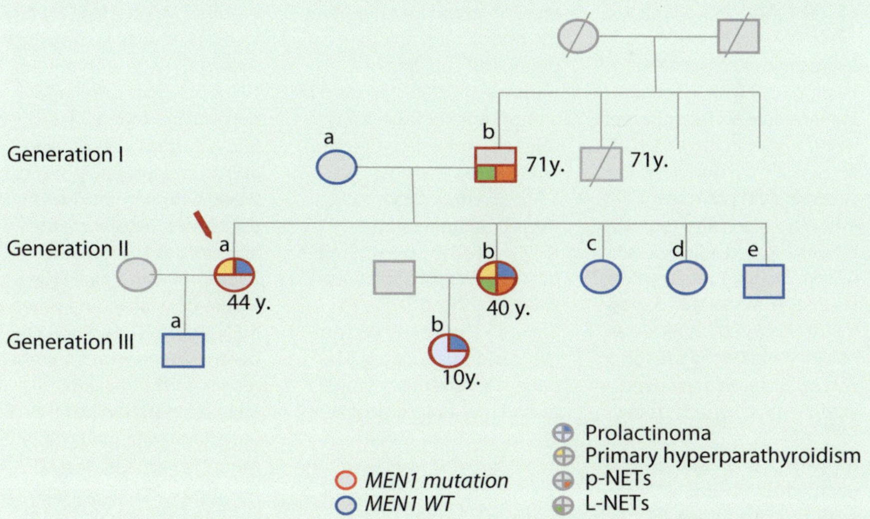

◘ **Fig. 8.1** An Italian MEN1 kindred with NETS – genealogical tree – the proband is indicated by an *arrow* (II.a)

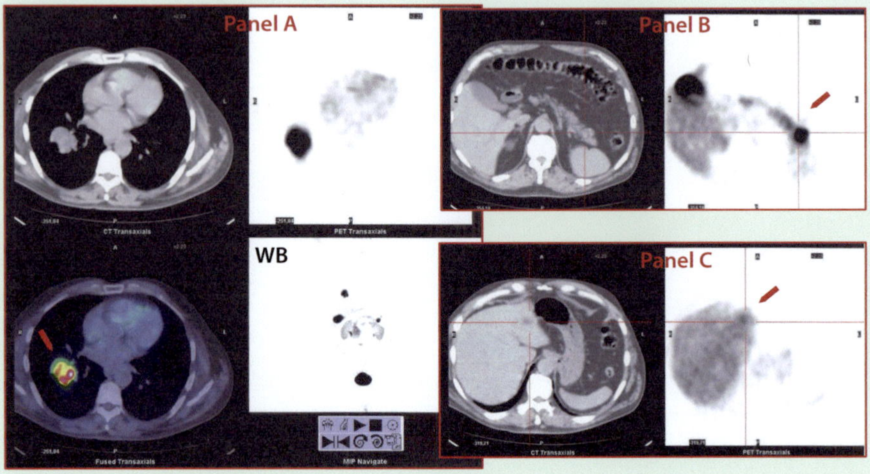

Fig. 8.2 ^{18}F-DOPA PET/TC in the proband's father – the right bronchial tumour (Panel **a**), the NF-P-NETs (Panel **b**) and to a lesser extent a small hepatic nodule (Panel **c**) showed a pathological uptake. The whole-body PET scan is also shown (Panel **a**, *WB*)

«dizziness» suggestive for hypoglycaemia. She was diagnosed with primary HPT and incipient hypercalcaemia (calcemia 10.3–11.0 mg/dl, PTH up to 273 pg/ml, *N* < 72), a microprolactinoma (PRL 35–50 ng/ml, *N* < 25 with a 3 mm PA on MRI) and hyperinsulinaemic hypoglycaemia (fasting test) with a 2 cm dominant nodule and an adjacent micronodule in the pancreatic tail, and a 1 cm nodule in the superior right pulmonary lobe. Pancreatic and thoracic lesions showed a significant uptake on octreoscan-111-In. Plasma NE markers were normal. In April 2007, a retrosternal left parathyroid adenoma (2.0 × 1.5 cm) was removed along with a thyroidectomy for incipient multinodular goitre, with post-operative hypoparathyroidism and no evidence of parathyroid hyperplasia. Six months later she underwent a left pancreatectomy, and multifocal insulinomas (2.0 and 0.7 cm) were confirmed by pathological examination. The dominant nodule had a low proliferative activity (mitosis <2/10 HPF, Ki 67 < 2%) and no vascular or lymphatic invasion were found. A bronchial carcinoid was confirmed by a fine-needle biopsy, and radiofrequency (RF) ablation was performed (2008), followed by a right superior lobectomy due to tumour growth (2015). Tumour size at surgery was 1.8 × 1.5 cm, with some necrotic changes and a Ki67 < 1%. The poorly symptomatic microprolactinoma was left untreated due to patient's choice and PRL normalized at menopause. The patient is currently asymptomatic on replacement therapy for post-operative hypothyroidism/hypoparathyroidism and no evidence of additional lesion.

The proband's niece (III.b) was 10 years old at first screening. A microprolactinoma was diagnosed on the basis of hyperprolactinemia (66.8 ng/ml, *N* < 23.5) with a 7 × 5 mm PA at MRI. Her height at first visit was at the 75° percentile with advanced bone age, and menarche occurred 6 months after cabergoline was started (1.0 mg/week). IGF1 was in the upper pubertal range with normal GH suppression after a 75 g oral glucose tolerance test. She is currently asymptomatic on cabergoline (0.5 mg/week) with normal PRL/GH/IGF1 levels, regular menses and a residual 4 × 3 mm microprolactinoma. Plasma NE are normal and no other MEN1-related condition has been recognized yet, except a recent normocalcaemic increase in PTH to be re-evaluated after vitamin D replacement therapy. Cervical US revealed a 1 cm hypoechoic/vascularized thyroid nodule (THY1 with haemorrhagic changes at cytology) and no evidence of enlarged parathyroid gland.

8.1 Comments to the Case

The *MEN1* c.20_206dupGCCCC mutation (previously indicated as c.317insGCCC) was already reported in MEN1 patients [2], including two apparently unrelated Italian kindreds [3]. It generates a stop codon in exon 2, expected to encode a short protein (p. P69fsX51) unable to interact with almost all its molecular partners. In this kindred, disease penetrance in mutation carriers was 100%. Prolactinomas and NETs were the most prevalent features, HPT being possibly masked by previous surgical complications of thyroidectomy in one case. The «top of the iceberg» was an aggressive prolactinoma associated with severe HPT and was partially reported previously [4]. Albeit isolated resistant prolactinomas are not a recognized indication for *MEN1* sequencing yet [5], a genetic background may be more frequently found [4, 6], suggesting that personal and familial anamnesis as well as minimal biological screening is advisable in such patients [4]. Instead, NETs have caused a significant morbidity in two proband's relatives.

Questions

1. How should we approach multiple simultaneous MEN1 lesions revealed by systematic screening in a single patient?
2. How can we effectively plan surveillance in paediatric MEN1 carriers in real life?
3. May a single drug target multiple NETs in a single MEN1 patient?

Answers

1. The proband's sister was diagnosed with four relatively small and moderately symptomatic endocrine tumours within a short period of time, generating anxiety and raising the issue of therapeutic priorities. Because she was mostly symptomatic for renal lithiasis with incipient hypercalcaemia, parathyroid surgery was proposed first. Of note, treating HPT may significantly improve hypergastrinemia and related symptoms in the presence of ZES if present [7]. Our patient had normal plasma gastrin and a dominant insulinoma was likely, though the possibility of an associated NF-P-NET was also considered due to frequent multiple P-NETs in MEN1 [5, 8]. In either case pancreatic surgery was indicated [5, 9] revealing two benign insulinomas. A hormonally silent small L-NET was also found. Since no surgical size threshold has been established for such tumours [5], follow-up of small lesions may be an option [10]. In this case RF ablation was proposed after a fine-needle biopsy had confirmed the diagnosis. The tumour was stable for 7 years before asymptomatic growth leads to thoracic surgery. Longitudinal observation of MEN1 L-NETs showed a mean annual increase in size of 17%, with a faster progression in men (doubling time 2.5 years vs 5.5 years in women) [10]. This family illustrates the more aggressive course of L-NETs in males [10, 11] and their metastatic potential, further supporting surgical indications adapted to the clinical context.
2. Clinical screening in paediatric *MEN1* mutation carriers is a heavy burden for the patients and for their family. Early genetic screening reassures the parents if the child does not carry mutation and allows to start an early surveillance programme where needed, as illustrated herein. Based on the earliest age of onset of MEN1 tumours in the literature, the last expert consensus [5] confirmed previous recommendations [12] to start screening for PA and insulinomas since

the age of 5 years and HPT since the age of 8 years, anticipating the age of screening for other P-NETs and thoracic NETs from 20 years to <10 years and 15 years, respectively. Screening for adrenal lesions before the age of 10 years is also recommended [5]. Early-onset P-NETs have been increasingly recognized [13–15], and the occurrence of NF-P-NETs detected by endoscopic US (EUS) was found to increase from <10% to 54% between the age of 16 and 20 years [14]. This is an important issue since plasma markers have a low diagnostic accuracy [16, 17] and the early detection of NETs mainly relies on radiological imaging [5]. Repeated exposure to ionizing radiations is of special concern in young patients, repeated MRI may not be well accepted and EUS is rather invasive. EUS was not performed in our patients, possibly missing small lesions. The issue is that small NF-P-NETS (<1 cm) have no surgical indications so that enhanced diagnostic sensitivity encourages surveillance while increasing patient's anxiety and management controversies [18]. Thus, applying the recommendations for CT/MRI/EUS every 1–2 years for the early detection of P-NETs is a challenge in real life, especially when starting from infancy. Further studies would be useful to delineate more personalized guidelines according to patient's age, gender and the presence of suspect MEN1 neoplasia at first screening.

3. No specific target therapy for MEN1 neoplasia is available yet. The common expression of somatostatin receptors (SSRs) by NETs and PA may be used for diagnostic and therapeutic purposes [19, 20], including peptide radiolabelled receptor therapy (PPRT) in selected cases [21]. First-generation somatostatin analogues (SSA) – octreotide and lanreotide – have been successfully used in MEN1 GEP-NETs [22] and unexpectedly in MEN1 HPT [23]. We used long-term SSA in the proband's father with a good tolerance, no recurrence of his metastatic L-NET and an improvement of pancreatic and hepatic lesions over time. Another example of potential double target treatment is the successful addition of cabergoline to other drugs in a MEN1 insulinoma [24]. In advanced NETs, chemotherapy (including TMZ) and/or molecular target therapies may be indicated [25]. When our family's proband started TMZ for an aggressive prolactinoma, no evidence of P-NET was present, so we were unable to analyse its potential effect on a concomitant tumour. However, everolimus was successfully used in a MEN1 patient with P-NET and multifactorial hypercalcaemia [26].

Up to Date of the Topic

1. Screening for MEN1 in NET patients

Although the majority of NETs are sporadic, genetic forms should be thought due to their impact on patient management and familial counselling. MEN1 is the main inherited cause of NETs deriving from the foregut [5], which is not surprising due to the role of *MEN1*/menin alterations in sporadic forms [27, 28]. Besides hyperparathyroidism (HPT) and pituitary adenomas (PA), NETs are the most common feature of MEN1 and are part of the MEN1 triad (HPT/PA/NETs) [5, 12]. Germline *MEN1* mutations are found in approximately 80% of patients developing a clinical MEN1 syndrome and more frequently in unselected NETs than in unselected HPT (1%) or PA (3%) [5, 12], with a high risk in GEP- and Thy-NETs [29]. Up to 33% of gastrinomas, 20% of Th-NETs but a minority of insulinomas and bronchial carcinoids (<5%) have been associated with MEN1 [28, 30]. *MEN1* sequencing is recommended in GEP-NETs occurring in a familial context or in the presence of another element of the MEN1 triad as well as in gastrinomas, early-onset insulinomas or multiple P-NETs at any age [5, 12, 30] and should be undertaken in a certified molecular diagnostic laboratory keeping in mind that: (1) though a large majority of genetically proven MEN1 patients turn out to have an inherited mutation, *de novo* mutations occur in 10% of the cases and are also transmissible to the offspring, (2) the difference between mutations and benign polymorphisms is not always clear-cut and this may complicate genetic counselling and follow-up and (3) if no pathogenic mutation is detected by direct sequencing, additional techniques should be used to detect deletions (e.g. multiplex ligation-dependent probe amplification, MLPA) and if still negative, mutations in cyclin-dependent kinase inhibitor genes, which may rarely induce MEN1-like syndromes (e.g. MEN4 due to *CDKN1B*/p27^{Kip1}mutations), should be thought [31, 32]. Once a causative *MEN1* mutation has been identified, familial screening starting from the closest relatives should be soon proposed to detect and treat MEN1 neoplasia in non-index cases [5, 33]. *MEN1* mutations have been listed in the literature and in publicly available web-based databases [34, 35]. Due to the lack of consistent genotype-phenotype correlations [5], all *MEN1* mutation carriers should enter a similar consensus-based surveillance programme.

2. Characteristics of MEN1-associated NETs (MEN1-NETs)

Several peculiarities distinguish MEN1-NETs from unselected cases. Typically, MEN1-NETs occur earlier than their sporadic counterpart, multiple tumours may develop in a synchronous or metachronous way in different NE tissues or in the same organ and additional MEN1 conditions may complicate the clinical picture at any time. Associations between multiple NETs, e.g. functioning and NF-P-NETs, may complicate their diagnosis and staging [8], and malignant NETs represent the leading cause of death in MEN1 [36, 37].

GEP-NETs: MEN1 gastrinomas are the most frequent (20–60%) and typically localize to the duodenum with multicentric small nodules (≤1 cm) in the setting of gastrin-producing cell hyperplasia. As in sporadic cases, their small size frequently contrasts with their ability to metastasize to lymph nodes (up to 60–80% at diagnosis) or to the liver (10–20%), with metastatic lesions exceeding in size the primary tumours [30]. Pancreatic gastrinomas are rare but generally larger and more aggressive than their duodenal counterpart and both may coexist [30, 38]. Overall, the prognosis of MEN1 gastrinomas is better than in sporadic cases, possibly due to an earlier diagnosis [8]. Since medical treatment for gastric hyperacidity has dramatically reduced the morbidity and mortality of ZES, acute gastrointestinal complications are no more a cause of death, and malignancy remains the major concern [36, 37]. Insulinomas develop at any age in 10–30% of MEN1 patients with a modest female predominance [5, 12, 14, 15], but most patients are young and up to 24% may occur before the age of 20 years [39]. Most of them localize to the body or tail of the pancreas; they are variable in size (<1 to >4 cm) and may be multiple, explaining recurrent hypoglycaemia after successful surgery. A large majority are benign but malignancy is more frequent than in sporadic cases [8]. Recently, insulinomas were found in 86/741 MEN1 patients (11.6%), 7 of them were metastatic at diagnosis, 19% were associated with other functional GEP-NETs (mostly gastrinomas) and 64% were with multiple P-NETs at pathological examination (64.4%), including insulin-immunostaining NETs (37.1%) [40]. Other functional P-NETs are too rare to be compared with sporadic cases (<5%). Instead, NF-P-NETs can now be recognized in >80% of MEN1 patients. Though a minority (0–13%) become large or symptomatic [38], they represent a significant cause of death [36–38]. If small NF-P-NETs are slowly growing with doubling times around 5–10 years [41, 42], the risk of metastasis increases with size, from ≤10% to >40% for tumours ≤2 cm and ≥3 cm, respectively [43], and distant metastases are major determinants of mortality [8, 43].

Thoracic NETs: L-NETs are typically diagnosed in middle-aged MEN1 patients [8] and not before the age of 21 years [8–11]. Female predominance has been mitigated by recent series [10, 11]. Systematic CT screening has revealed a higher prevalence of L-NETs than previously reported, with pulmonary nodules observed in 51/188 MEN1 patients, though not all were primary L-NETs [10]. Indeed, MEN1 L-NETs may be multiple and should not be confounded with metastasis of other NETs, so that fine-needle biopsy may be required [10]. Paraneoplastic endocrine manifestations (e.g. Cushing's disease, carcinoid syndrome) are exceptional in MEN1 [8, 10]. Lymph node metastasis may occur but distant metastases are rare, small cell lung cancer is exceptional and L-NETs are not a major determinant of survival in MEN1 [8, 10, 36, 37]. Th-NETs are usually diagnosed in middle-aged adults with a strong male predominance (>90%) [8, 10, 11, 44], though the youngest reported case was 16 years old [45], and female patients accounted for 36% of the Japanese survey [46]. Familial clustering may occur [9, 44]. The importance of smoking as a risk factor [8, 44] has been recently mitigated [11, 46]. Prophylactic transcervical thymectomy during parathyroidectomy may be a protective tool [5, 10], especially in males or in the presence of familial clustering [11, 44], but should be performed in specialized centres to ensure complete removal of thymic remnants [5, 11]. MEN1 Th-NETs are aggressive and most affected patients die from their tumour, the median survival is 25–36% at 10 years [10, 11, 46].

3. Prognostic Factors in MEN1-NETs

The different systems of NET grading and staging defined in unselected NETs may not be fully applicable to MEN1-NETs due to potential tumour multifocality and MEN1 comorbidities, and the prognostic impact of a MEN1 setting may differ according to tumour phenotype. Yet, the most adverse prognostic factor in MEN1 GEP-NETs is the presence of liver and other distant metastasis [8].

MEN1 mutations: Menin is involved in a complex network of nuclear protein-protein interactions implicated in gene transcription, cell division and genomic stability, and several molecular partners have been identified along with their domains of interaction [8, 47]. Mutations affecting Jun-D and CHES-1 interaction domains have been associated with a higher risk of malignant NETs, respectively, Th-NETs [48] and P-NETs [49]. The *CDKN1B* V109G polymorphism has also been associated with more aggressive MEN1 neoplasia [50].

Immunohistochemical markers: Loss of the ATRX and/or DAXX expression was first reported in large MEN1-P-NETs (>3 cm) and associated with an altered lengthening telomere (ALT) phenotype [51], whereas the prognostic significance of other markers identified in sporadic NETs (e.g. Ki67 or the c-Kit/cytokeratin 19 expression phenotype [38]) has not been specifically addressed. Multicentre sample collection of MEN1-NETS would help clarifying this point and identifying additional prognostic factors.

4. Implications for the Clinical Management of MEN1 and/or NET Patients

Screening for NETs in MEN1 Patients

Screening recommendations are based on the penetrance of MEN1 neoplasia in mutation carriers, which already exceeds 50% by the age of 20 years and is close to 100% by the age of 50 years [5, 52]. If clinical evaluation may suggest hypoglycemia or peptic ulcer disease, annual assessment of basal fasting glucose, insulin, gastrin, glucagon, vasointestinal polypeptide (VIP), PP and chromogranin A is recommended, with abdominal CT or MRI every 1–2 years for the detection of NF-P-NETs and gastroscopy every 3 years for asymptomatic hypergastrinemia [5]. However, the cost-to-benefit ratio of systematic plasma marker determination has not been evaluated [16, 17], and the need for glucagon or VIP measurement in asymptomatic cases is unclear. If EUS is the most sensitive procedure for the detection of small (≤10 mm) GEP-NETs, SSTR imaging may further enhance its diagnostic accuracy if needed in a preoperative setting [9]. Chest CT is also recommended every 1–2 years [5], though this is a matter of debate [53]. In order to reduce the diagnostic burden, a simplified follow-up has been proposed after an initial workup, reducing the number of hormone assays and extending the interval between screenings to 3 years [53, 54]. Yet, if the early diagnosis of potentially aggressive NETs remains an essential piece of MEN1 follow-up, the choice of imaging modalities and timing may depend on available techniques as well as on patient's conditions and preferences [5].

Surgical Management and Outcome in MEN1-NETs

Surgery is essential in NETs and consensus guidelines have been established for sporadic cases based on proper staging, classification and grading [9, 25, 55]. The peculiarities of MEN1-NETs require further evaluation by a dedicated multidisciplinary team [5], though some controversies remain due to the lack of evidence-based recommendations [38]. As a general rule, the goal is to achieve the best results in terms of disease control and survival while preserving physiological functions and quality of life, keeping in mind the natural history of MEN1-NETs. Because the largest the extent of pancreatic surgery, the highest the risk of post-operative complications and long-term sequelae (diabetes mellitus, malabsorption and weight loss), the risk-to-benefit ratio is evaluated individually according to patient's age, conditions, tumour phenotype and extension and surgical expertise. If surgical removal of non-metastatic pancreatic gastrinomas >2 cm is commonly accepted, controversies remain for duodenal localizations because long-term post-operative control of ZES may be significantly worse in MEN1 than in sporadic cases [5, 38]. Post-operative remission and disease-free survival as low as 16 and 6% were observed at 5 years [56], though recent experience reported 30–70% short-term remissions depending on the surgical option [57]. Yet, non-surgical management of ZES is generally preferred unless medical treatment of hyperacidity is poorly effective or accepted by the patient [5, 38]. In contrast, surgical resection remains the first-line approach for non-metastatic MEN1 insulinomas [5, 38] with some technical controversies. Supporting previous experience, long-term post-operative remission was reported in >80% of a large series, with distal pancreatectomy giving the best results, though long-term complications occurred in 43.5% [40]. On the other hand, remission was also reported after tumour enucleation(s) or limited pancreatic resection, though late reoperations might be more frequent [58]. Thus, the benefits of extended pancreatic surgery should be balanced with post-operative risks, especially in young patients. In NF-P-NETs, surgery is advocated by MEN1 experts for tumours exceeding 1 cm [5] instead of 2 cm in sporadic cases [9]. Surgical resection of L-NETs is generally proposed if the tumour is resectable [5] with the aim of being curative while preserving as much lung tissue as possible [53]. The extent of surgery depends on tumour localisation and extension, with appropriate lymph node resection to detect metastasis [55], with no defined cut-off in tumour size for small asymptomatic L-NETs [5].

Pharmacological Management in MEN1-NETs

8

The aims of medical treatment are the control of hormone hypersecretion and tumour progression. Whereas SSA have long been used for the control of endocrine symptoms, their potential efficacy as antineoplastic drugs and the development of targeted therapies based on improved knowledge of tumorigenesis have modified the pharmacological approach of NETs [19, 20, 59]. First-generation SSA, sunitinib and mTor inhibitors have been approved in unselected NETs on the basis of controlled trials for advanced loco-regional and metastatic NETs [25]. There is experimental evidence in mice that pasireotide, a second-generation SSA, may reduce pituitary and NET growth while increasing survival [60]. Additional tools include systemic cytotoxic chemotherapy, loco-regional ablative therapies, debulking surgery [22] and PPRT with radiolabelled SSA [21]. However, no specific guidelines are available in MEN1 patients and specific reports are limited. New options may arise from experimental models, including gene therapy [61].

8.2 Conclusion

NETs are the most frequent tumours in MEN1 after primary HPT and malignant NETs are the main cause of mortality. While the early detection of potentially aggressive NETs is essential to improve life expectancy, the compromise between an acceptable and sustainable diagnostic schedule and screening efficacy remains an important issue in clinical practice. Consensus guidelines for NET management should be adapted to the MEN1 setting by expert multidisciplinary teams. Further research in MEN1 tumorigenesis, classification and identification of prognostic factors, as well as multicentre trials, may help improving life quality and expectancy in MEN1 patients.

Acknowledgements The authors thank Dr. Pasqualina Sannino, Neuromed, Pozzilli (IS) for PET nuclear imaging.

Bibliography

1. Cordella D, De Marco A, Eller-Vainicher C et al (2008) Screening of MEN1 gene in patients with either classic or variant MEN1 presentation. Paper presented at the 10th European Congress of Endocrinology, Berlin, Germany, 03–07 May 2008. In: Endocrine Abstracts 16: P282
2. Mayr B, Apenberg S, Rothämel T et al (1997) Menin mutations in patients with multiple endocrine neoplasia type 1. Eur J Endocrinol 137:684–687
3. Morelli A, Falchetti A, Martineti V et al (2000) MEN1 gene mutation analysis in Italian patients with multiple endocrine neoplasia type 1. Eur J Endocrinol 142:131–137
4. Vroonen L, Jaffrain-Rea ML, Petrossians P et al (2012) Prolactinomas resistant to standard doses of cabergoline: a multicenter study of 92 patients. Eur J Endocrinol 167:651–662. doi:10.1530/EJE-12-0236
5. Thakker RV, Newey PJ, Walls GV et al (2012) Clinical practice guidelines for multiple endocrine neoplasia type 1 (MEN1). J Clin Endocrinol Metab 97:2990–3011. doi:10.1210/jc.2012-1230
6. Vergès B, Boureille F, Goudet P et al (2002) Pituitary disease in MEN type 1 (MEN1): data from the France-Belgium MEN1 multicenter study. J Clin Endocrinol Metab 87:457–465. doi:10.1210/jcem.87.2.8145
7. Norton JA, Venzon DJ, Berna MJ et al (2008) Prospective study of surgery for primary hyperparathyroidism (HPT) in multiple endocrine neoplasia-type 1 and Zollinger-Ellison syndrome: long-term outcome of a more virulent form of HPT. Ann Surg 247:501–510. doi:10.1097/SLA.0b013e31815efda5
8. Pieterman CRC, Conemans EB, Dreijerink KMA et al (2014) Thoracic and duodenopancreatic neuroendocrine tumors in multiple endocrine neoplasia type 1: natural history and function of menin in tumorigenesis. Endocr Relat Cancer 21:121–142. doi:10.1530/ERC-13-0482
9. Falconi M, Eriksson B, Kaltsas G et al (2016) ENETS consensus guidelines update for the management of patients with functional pancreatic neuroendocrine tumors and non-functional pancreatic neuroendocrine tumors. Neuroendocrinology 103:153–171. doi:10.1159/000443171
10. De Laat JM, Pieterman CR, Van Den Broek MF et al (2014) Natural course and survival of neuroendocrine tumors of thymus and lung in MEN1 patients. J Clin Endocrinol Metab 99:3325–3333. doi:10.1210/jc.2014-1560
11. Singh Ospina N, Thompson GB, Nichols FC et al (2015) Thymic and bronchial carcinoid tumors in multiple endocrine neoplasia type 1: the Mayo Clinic experience from 1977 to 2013. Horm Cancer 6:247–253. doi:10.1007/s12672-015-0228-z
12. Brandi ML (2001) CONSENSUS: guidelines for diagnosis and therapy of MEN type 1 and type 2. J Clin Endocrinol Metab 86:5658–5671. doi:10.1210/jc.86.12.5658
13. Newey PJ, Jeyabalan J, Walls GV et al (2009) Asymptomatic children with multiple endocrine neoplasia type 1 mutations may harbor nonfunctioning pancreatic neuroendocrine tumors. J Clin Endocrinol Metab 94:3640–3646. doi:10.1210/jc.2009-0564
14. Gonçalves TD, Toledo RA, Sekiya T et al (2014) Penetrance of functioning and nonfunctioning pancreatic neuroendocrine tumors in multiple endocrine neoplasia type 1 in the second decade of life. J Clin Endocrinol Metab 99:E89–E96. doi:10.1210/jc.2013-1768
15. Goudet P, Dalac A, Le Bras M et al (2015) MEN1 disease occurring before 21 years old: a 160-patient cohort study from the Groupe d'Etude des Tumeurs endocrines. J Clin Endocrinol Metab 100:1568–1577. doi:10.1210/jc.2014-3659
16. De Laat JM, Pieterman CRC, Weijmans M et al (2013) Low accuracy of tumor markers for diagnosing pancreatic neuroendocrine tumors in multiple endocrine neoplasia type 1 patients. J Clin Endocrinol Metab 98:4143–4151. doi:10.1210/jc.2013-1800
17. Qiu W, Christakis I, Silva A et al (2016) Utility of chromogranin a, pancreatic polypeptide, glucagon and gastrin in the diagnosis and follow-up of pancreatic neuroendocrine tumours in multiple endocrine neoplasia type 1 patients. Clin Endocrinol 85:400–407. doi:10.1111/cen.13119
18. Ito T, Jensen RT (2016) Imaging in multiple endocrine neoplasia type 1: recent studies show enhanced sensitivities but increased controversies. Int J Endocr Oncol 3:53–66. doi:10.2217/ije.15.29
19. Baldelli R, Barnabei A, Rizza L et al (2014) Somatostatin analogs therapy in gastroenteropancreatic neuroendocrine tumors: current aspects and new perspectives. Front Endocrinol (Lausanne) 5:7. doi:10.3389/fendo.2014.00007

20. Kanakis G, Grimelius L, Spathis A et al (2015) Expression of somatostatin receptors 1-5 and dopamine receptor 2 in lung carcinoids: implications for a therapeutic role. Neuroendocrinology 101:211–222. doi:10.1159/000381061
21. Bison SM, Konijnenberg MW, Melis M et al (2014) Peptide receptor radionuclide therapy using radiolabeled somatostatin analogs: focus on future developments. Clin Transl Imaging 2:55–66. doi:10.1007/s40336-014-0054-2
22. Ramundo V, Del Prete M, Marotta V, Multidisciplinary Group for Neuroendocrine Tumors of Naples et al (2014) Impact of long-acting octreotide in patients with early-stage MEN1-related duodeno-pancreatic neuroendocrine tumours. Clin Endocrinol 80:850–855. doi:10.1111/cen.12411
23. Faggiano A, Tavares LB, Tauchmanova L et al (2008) Effect of treatment with depot somatostatin analogue octreotide on primary hyperparathyroidism (PHP) in multiple endocrine neoplasia type 1 (MEN1) patients. Clin Endocrinol 69:756–762. doi:10.1111/j.1365-2265.2008.03301.x
24. Marciello F, Di Somma C, Del Prete M et al (2014) Combined biological therapy with lanreotide autogel and cabergoline in the treatment of MEN-1-related insulinomas. Endocrine 46:678–681. doi:10.1007/s12020-013-0145-2
25. Pavel M, O'Toole D, Costa F et al (2016) ENETS consensus guidelines update for the management of distant metastatic disease of intestinal, pancreatic, bronchial neuroendocrine neoplasms (NEN) and NEN of unknown primary site. Neuroendocrinology 103:172–185. doi:10.1159/000443167
26. Maia MC, Muniz Lourenço D, Riechelmann R (2016) Efficacy and long-term safety of everolimus in pancreatic neuroendocrine tumor associated with multiple endocrine neoplasia type I: case report. Oncol Res Treat 39:643–645. doi:10.1159/000448699
27. Leotlela PD, Jauch A, Holtgreve-Grez H, Thakker RV (2003) Genetics of neuroendocrine and carcinoid tumours. Endocr Relat Cancer 10:437–450. doi:10.1677/erc.0.0100437
28. Zhang J, Francois R, Iyer R et al (2013) Current understanding of the molecular biology of pancreatic neuroendocrine tumors. J Natl Cancer Inst 105:1005–1017. doi:10.1093/jnci/djt135
29. de Laat JM, Tham E, Pieterman CR et al (2012) Predicting the risk of multiple endocrine neoplasia type 1 for patients with commonly occurring endocrine tumors. Eur J Endocrinol 167:181–187. doi:10.1530/EJE-12-0210
30. Anlauf M, Garbrecht N, Henopp T et al (2006) Sporadic versus hereditary gastrinomas of the duodenum and pancreas: distinct clinico-pathological and epidemiological features. World J Gastroenterol 12:5440–5446
31. Agarwal SK, Mateo CM, Marx SJ (2009) Rare germline mutations in cyclin-dependent kinase inhibitor genes in multiple endocrine neoplasia type 1 and related states. J Clin Endocrinol Metab 94:1826–1834. doi:10.1210/jc.2008-2083
32. Lee M, Pellegata NS (2013) Multiple endocrine neoplasia type 4. Front Horm Res 41:63–78. doi:10.1159/000345670
33. van Leeuwaarde RS, van Nesselrooij BP, Hermus AR et al (2016) Impact of delay in diagnosis in outcomes in MEN1: results from the Dutch MEN1 study group. J Clin Endocrinol Metab 101:1159–1165. doi:10.1210/jc.2015-3766
34. Lemos MC, Thakker RV (2008) Multiple endocrine neoplasia type 1 (MEN1): analysis of 1336 mutations reported in the first decade following identification of the gene. Hum Mutat 29:22–32. doi:10.1002/humu.20605
35. Concolino P, Costella A, Capoluongo E (2016) Multiple endocrine neoplasia type 1(MEN1): an update of 208 new germline variants reported in the last nine years. Cancer Genet 209:36–41. doi:10.1016/j.cancergen.2015.12.002
36. Goudet P, Murat A, Binquet C et al (2010) Risk factors and causes of death in men1 disease. A GTE (groupe d'etude des tumeurs endocrines) cohort study among 758 patients. World J Surg 34:249–255. doi:10.1007/s00268-009-0290-1
37. Ito T, Igarashi H, Uehara H et al (2013) Causes of death and prognostic factors in multiple endocrine neoplasia type 1: a prospective study: comparison of 106 MEN1/Zollinger-Ellison syndrome patients with 1613 literature MEN1 patients with or without pancreatic endocrine tumors. Medicine (Baltimore) 92:135–181. doi:10.1097/MD.0b013e3182954af1
38. Yates CJ, Newey PJ, Thakker RV (2015) Challenges and controversies in management of pancreatic neuroendocrine tumours in patients with MEN1. Lancet Diabetes Endocrinol 3:895–905. doi:10.1016/S2213-8587(15)00043-1

39. Sakurai A, Suzuki S, Kosugi S et al (2012) Multiple endocrine neoplasia type 1 in Japan: establishment and analysis of a multicentre database. Clin Endocrinol 76:533–539. doi:10.1111/j.1365-2265.2011.04227.x
40. Vezzosi D, Cardot-Bauters C, Bouscaren N et al (2015) Long-term results of the surgical management of insulinoma patients with MEN1: a Groupe d'étude des Tumeurs endocrines (GTE) retrospective study. Eur J Endocrinol 172(3):309–319. doi:10.1530/EJE-14-0878
41. Kann PH, Balakina E, Ivan D et al (2006) Natural course of small, asymptomatic neuroendocrine pancreatic tumours in multiple endocrine neoplasia type 1: an endoscopic ultrasound imaging study. Endocr Relat Cancer 13:1195–1202. doi:10.1530/EJE-07-0635
42. D'souza SL, Elmunzer BJ, Scheiman JM (2014) Long-term follow-up of asymptomatic pancreatic neuroendocrine tumors in multiple endocrine neoplasia type I syndrome. J Clin Gastroenterol 48:458–461. doi:10.1097/MCG.0000000000000062
43. Triponez F, Dosseh D, Goudet P et al (2006) Epidemiology data on 108 MEN1 patients from the GTE with isolated nonfunctioning tumors of the pancreas. Ann Surg 243:265–272. doi:10.1097/01.sla.0000197715.96762.68
44. Ferolla P, Falchetti A, Filosso P et al (2005) Thymic neuroendocrine carcinoma (carcinoid) in multiple endocrine neoplasia type 1 syndrome: the Italian series. J Clin Endocrinol Metab 90:2603–2609. doi:10.1210/jc.2004-1155
45. Goudet P, Murat A, Cardot-Bauters C et al (2009) Thymic neuroendocrine tumors in multiple endocrine neoplasia type 1: a comparative study on 21 cases among a series of 761 MEN1 from the GTE (Groupe des Tumeurs endocrines). World J Surg 33:1197–1207. doi:10.1007/s00268-009-9980-y
46. Sakurai A, Imai T, Kikumori T et al (2013) Thymic neuroendocrine tumour in multiple endocrine neoplasia type 1: female patients are not rare exceptions. Clin Endocrinol 78:248–254. doi:10.1111/j.1365-2265.2012.04467.x
47. Thakker RV (2014) Multiple endocrine neoplasia type 1 (MEN1) and type 4 (MEN4). Mol Cell Endocrinol 386:2–15. doi:10.1016/j.mce.2013.08.002
48. Thevenon J, Bourredjem A, Faivre L et al (2013) Higher risk of death among MEN1 patients with mutations in the JunD interacting domain: a Groupe d'etude des Tumeurs Endocrines (GTE) cohort study. Hum Mol Genet 22:1940–1948. doi:10.1093/hmg/ddt039
49. Bartsch DK, Slater EP, Albers M et al (2014) Higher risk of aggressive pancreatic neuroendocrine tumors in MEN1 patients with MEN1 mutations affecting the CHES1 interacting MENIN domain. J Clin Endocrinol Metab 99:E2387–E2391. doi:10.1210/jc.2013-4432
50. Circelli L, Ramundo V, Marotta V et al (2015) Multidisciplinary Group for NeuroEndocrine Tumours of Naples. Prognostic role of the CDNK1B V109G polymorphism in multiple endocrine neoplasia type 1. J Cell Mol Med 19:1735–1741. doi:10.1111/jcmm.12552
51. de Wilde RF, Heaphy CM, Maitra A et al (2012) Loss of ATRX or DAXX expression and concomitant acquisition of the alternative lengthening of telomeres phenotype are late eventsin a small subset of MEN-1 syndrome pancreatic neuroendocrine tumors. Mod Pathol 25:1033–1039. doi:10.1038/modpathol.2012.53
52. Machens A, Schaaf L, Karges W et al (2007) Age-related penetrance of endocrine tumours in multiple endocrine neoplasia type 1 (MEN1): a multicentre study of 258 gene carriers. Clin Endocrinol 67:613–622. doi:10.1111/j.1365-2265.2007.02934.x
53. Singh Ospina N, Maraka S, Montori V et al (2016) When and how should patients with multiple endocrine neoplasia type 1 be screened for thymic and bronchial carcinoid tumours? Clin Endocrinol 84:13–16. doi:10.1111/cen.12972
54. Waldmann J, Fendrich V, Habbe N et al (2009) Screening of patients with multiple endocrine neoplasia type 1 (MEN-1): a critical analysis of its value. World J Surg 33:1208–1218. doi:10.1007/s00268-009-9983-8
55. Caplin ME, Baudin E, Ferolla P et al (2015) Pulmonary neuroendocrine (carcinoid) tumors: European neuroendocrine tumor society expert consensus and recommendations for best practice for typical and atypical pulmonary carcinoids. Ann Oncol 26:1604–1620. doi:10.1093/annonc/mdv041
56. Norton JA, Fraker DL, Alexander HR et al (1999) Surgery to cure the Zollinger-Ellison syndrome. N Engl J Med 341:635–644. doi:10.1056/NEJM199908263410902
57. Imamura M, Komoto I, Ota S et al (2011) Biochemically curative surgery for gastrinoma in multiple endocrine neoplasia type 1 patients. World J Gastroenterol 17:1343–1353. doi:10.3748/wjg.v17.i10.1343

58. Bartsch DK, Albers M, Knoop R et al (2013) Enucleation and limited pancreatic resection provide long-term cure for insulinoma in multiple endocrine neoplasia type 1. Neuroendocrinology 98:290–298. doi:10.1159/000357779
59. Capurso G, Archibugi L, Delle Fave G (2015) Molecular pathogenesis and targeted therapy of sporadic pancreatic neuroendocrine tumors. J Hepatobiliary Pancreat Sci 22:594–601. doi:10.1002/jhbp.210
60. Walls GV, Stevenson M, Soukup BS et al (2016) Pasireotide therapy of multiple endocrine neoplasia type 1-associated neuroendocrine tumors in female mice deleted for an Men1 allele improves survival and reduces tumor progression. Endocrinology 157:1789–1798. doi:10.1210/en.2015-1965
61. Walls GV, Lemos MC, Javid M et al (2012) MEN1 gene replacement therapy reduces proliferation rates in a mouse model of pituitary adenomas. Cancer Res 72:5060–5068. doi:10.1158/0008-5472.CAN-12-1821

Prognostic Factors: Nuclear Medicine Imaging (FDG PET–Octreoscan/Gallium PET)

Maria Luisa De Rimini, Nicolina De Rosa, Anna Settembre, Gennaro Mazzarella, and Pietro Muto

On behalf of the ENETS Center of Excellence Multidisciplinary Group for Neuroendocrine Tumors in Naples, Italy

A. Colao et al. (eds.), *Neuroendocrine Tumors in Real Life*,
https://doi.org/10.1007/978-3-319-59024-0_9

Overview

Knowledge of receptor expression in neuroendocrine tumors (NET) is the key for therapy directed at tumor receptors. Receptor imaging (RI) for somatostatin receptor subtypes (SSTRs) expressing tumors offers complementary informations that enable the evaluation of the entire tumor burden and characterization of the heterogeneity of tumor receptor expression. RI allows to stratify patients responders and nonresponders to targeted treatment with somatostatin analogs.

^{18}F-FDG PET/CT has no primary indication in the study of NET until they are well differentiated and maintain slow growth and low metabolic activity. A positive metabolic scan correlates with a high Ki-67 and with poorly differentiated NET. It may indicate the disappearance of SSTRs on tumor cells, decreeing a worse outcome.

We report a case of a male affected with node metastasis from poorly differentiated high-grade neuroendocrine carcinoma of unknown primary site. Patient underwent SSTR ^{111}In-DTPA-pentetreotide (octreoscan) whole-body and SPECT/CT scan and metabolic ^{18}F-FDG PET scan. Octreoscan documented the loss of SSTR expression, while increased glucose metabolism at ^{18}F-FDG PET correlated with high Ki-67 expression and disease progression, suggesting the utility of chemotherapy.

Tumor RI has a strong impact in the patient workup, but, similarly, a positive metabolic ^{18}F-FDG PET can play a key role in NET management for its prognostic contribution, due to the variability in behavior of disease progression.

Clinical Case

This is the case of an old male, P.R. 80 years. Patient clinical history:

- Liver cirrhosis HCV correlated: CHILD–PUGH Class B8/AFP 5 ng/ml (normal range 0–8);
    - Cardiovascular hypertension.
    - Mild/moderate renal failure (creatinine 1.8 mg/dl).

Patient underwent clinical control because of the onset of fever associated with abdominal pain.

At hospital admission, an abdominal ultrasonography study showed multiple lymphadenopathy (max diameter, 40 mm).

These results suggested the need for further diagnostic investigations with CT and contrast enhancement CT (ce-CT).

A whole-body (WB) ^{18}F-FDG PET/CT scan was also associated for the evaluation of the metabolic burden of the lesions and looking for the primary lesion.

^{18}F-FDG PET/CT acquisition data and protocol are reported in ◘ Table 9.1, and ^{18}F-FDG PET/CT image *processing* is reported in ◘ Table 9.2.

PET/CT – *Semiquantitative Analysis*: Standard uptake value (SUV) has been calculated as the ratio of the uptake of ^{18}F-FDG (MBq/ml) in an area of interest, drawn on the AC images, and the administered activity normalized to the patient weight. The maximum SUV was obtained as standard reference of the ^{18}F-FDG PET study.

^{18}F-FDG PET/CT confirmed the diffuse, extensive, pathological metabolic involvement of abdominal, pelvic, and inguinal nodes, corresponding to CT morphological data, shown in ◘ Figs. 9.1, 9.2, and 9.3, by the correspondence of ^{18}F-FDG PET with the co-registered low-dose CT at fusion imaging and at comparison with the contrast enhancement CT (ce-CT).

High levels of chromogranin A (CgA) concentration were subsequently obtained: 340 U/L. As well known, CgA is a good general neuroendocrine serum marker with

Table 9.1 ^{18}F-FDG PET/CT acquisition protocol

Blood glucose before *injection*	90 mg/dl
^{18}F–FDG administered dose i.v.	2,5–4 MBq/kg
Scanner	*Siemens* PET/CT system – Biograph 16–3D
Co-registered low-dose CT for attenuation correction (AC) cross-sectional anatomy and fusion imaging analysis	100 mA sec
WB PET	From the top of the head to the middle third of the thigh
	Scan direction: cranio-caudal
	FOV 70 cm. 360°, 60 frames, time/projections, 45 s, 64 × 64 matrix
	Time duration/bed, 3 min

Table 9.2 ^{18}F-FDG PET/CT image *processing*

Reconstruction method	Truex Siemens HD PET
Iterative image reconstruction	Ordered-subset expectation maximization, 3 iterations, 21 subsets
	Image size 168; zoom 1
	Filter Gaussian; FWHM, 4.0
Reconstructed image reorientation	Three standard projection plans: transaxial, coronal, sagittal both for uncorrected and AC images

useful clinical applications in subjects with NET. High levels of CgA are strongly correlated with tumor volume and with the staging of the disease. Higher CgA is observed for metastatic disease compared to localized disease, and a correlation between CgA and survival in neuroendocrine tumors has been reported [1].

The evidence of increase of CgA levels suggested the utility of SSTR imaging, looking for neuroendocrine tumor. Patient underwent RI with ^{111}In-Octreoscan (OCT) whole-body and SPECT/CT scan.

^{111}In-OCT whole-body (WB) and SPET/CT acquisition data and protocol are reported in Table 9.3.

At ^{111}In-OCT scan results:

No evidence of pathological uptake related to SSTRs pathological expression of disease, as shown in the Figs. 9.4 and 9.5.

Patient underwent a left inguinal lymph node excision for pathology assessment of disease, showing the evidence of node metastasis from poorly differentiated high-grade neuroendocrine carcinoma. The tumor showed diffuse positivity for CD56 and for synaptophysin and Ki-67 = 90%. Pathology report is detailed in Fig. 9.6.

Patient PR was scheduled for chemotherapy, which was discontinued 4 months later, due to the severe worsening of the disease and the clinical status of the patient.

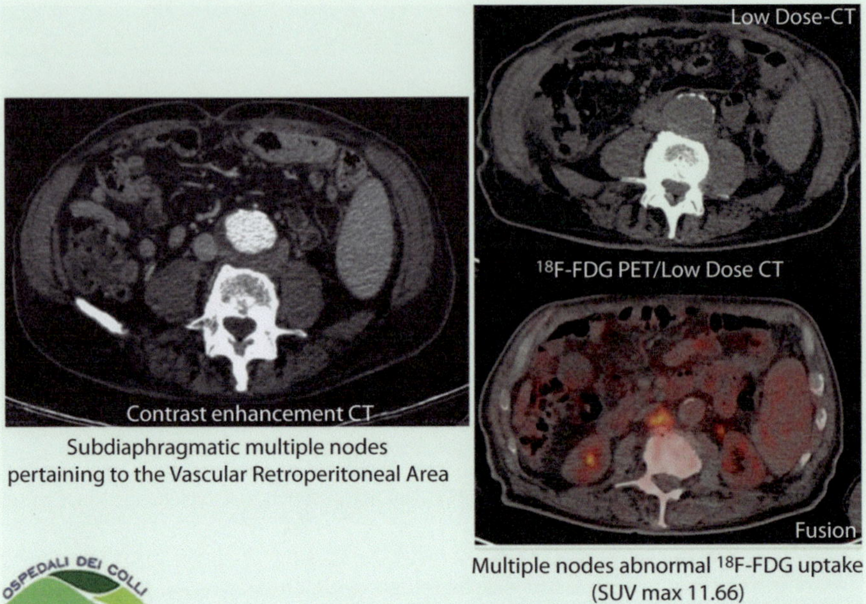

9

Fig. 9.1 Subdiaphragmatic multiple nodal lesions pertaining to the vascular retroperitoneal area are shown in transverse views, respectively at: diagnostic ce-CT (*left*), at co-registered low-dose nondiagnostic CT, and at 18F-FDG PET/CT fusion imaging (*right*)

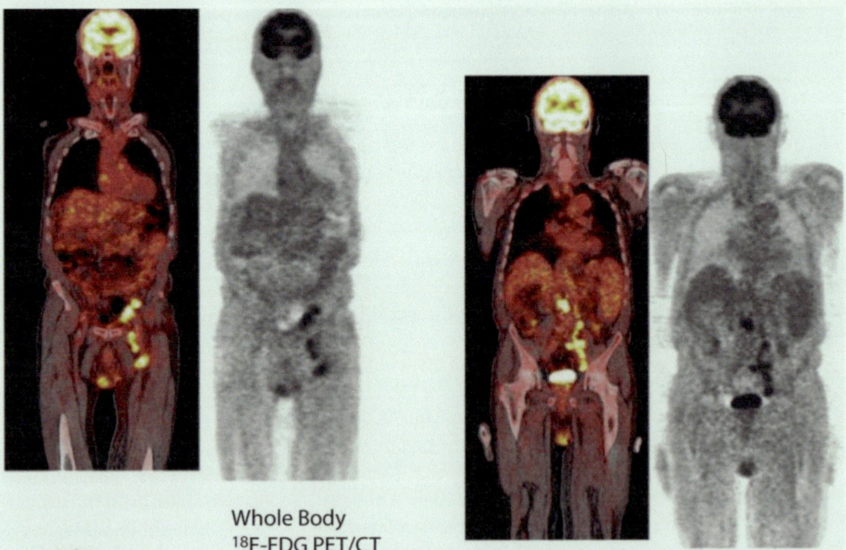

Fig. 9.2 Whole-body ^{18}F-FDG PET scan

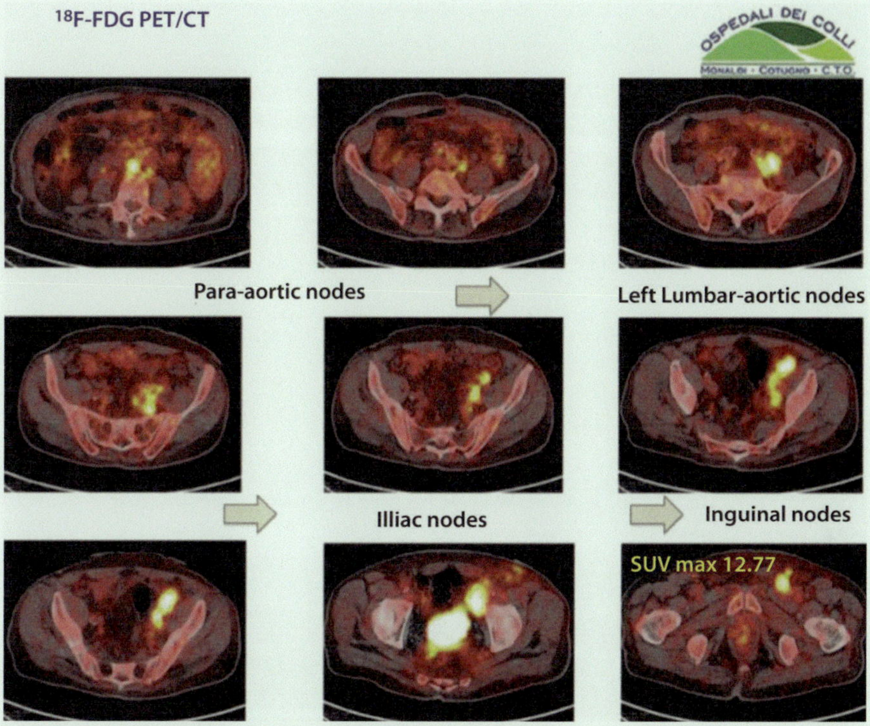

Fig. 9.3 Sequence of transverse reconstruction views at ^{18}F-FDG PET/CT fusion imaging show severe increase of radio tracer uptake, due to multiple node involvement

Table 9.3 ^{111}In-pentetreotide WB and SPECT/CT

^{111}In-OCT administered dose i.v.	200 MBq
Energy window	At 20% of ^{111}In photopeak (172 e 245 KeV)
Scanner	*GE gamma camera dual-head SPECT/CT system equipped with a medium-energy, high-resolution collimator (Discovery -NM/CT 670 Pro) 16 MSCT*
Planar images	Spots AP (plus LL and/or oblique): head, thorax, abdomen, pelvis up to 3/4 of the thigh
	500.000 cps/view or 10′/view
SPECT/CT	Patient position: supine, feet first
	FOV selected on the basis of clinical or planar diagnostic image indications
	360°, 60 frames, time/projections, 45 s, 64 × 64 matrix

Table 9.3 (continued)

Co-registered low-dose CT for attenuation correction (AC) and anatomical cross	10 mA sec 120 kV 3.75-mm slice thickness
Scan timing after radiotracer injection	Early (at 4 h) /delayed (at 24 h /optional 48–72 h), for planar and SPECT/CT scan
Reconstructed image reorientation	Three standard projection plans: transaxial, coronal, sagittal both for uncorrected and AC images

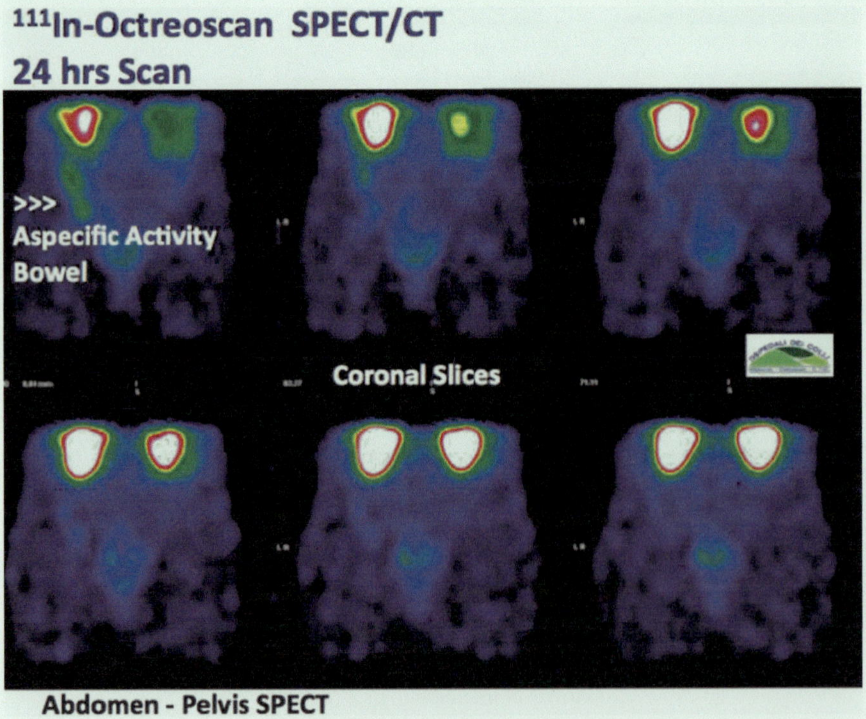

Fig. 9.4 24-h ^{111}In-OCT AC SPECT, abdominal coronal slices

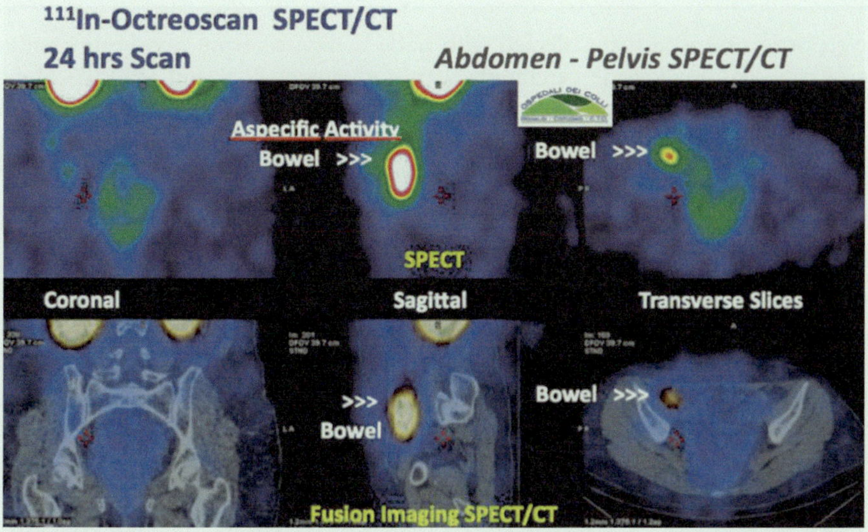

Fig. 9.5 24-h ^{111}In-OCT coronal and transaxial details of AC SPECT and SPECT/CT fusion images

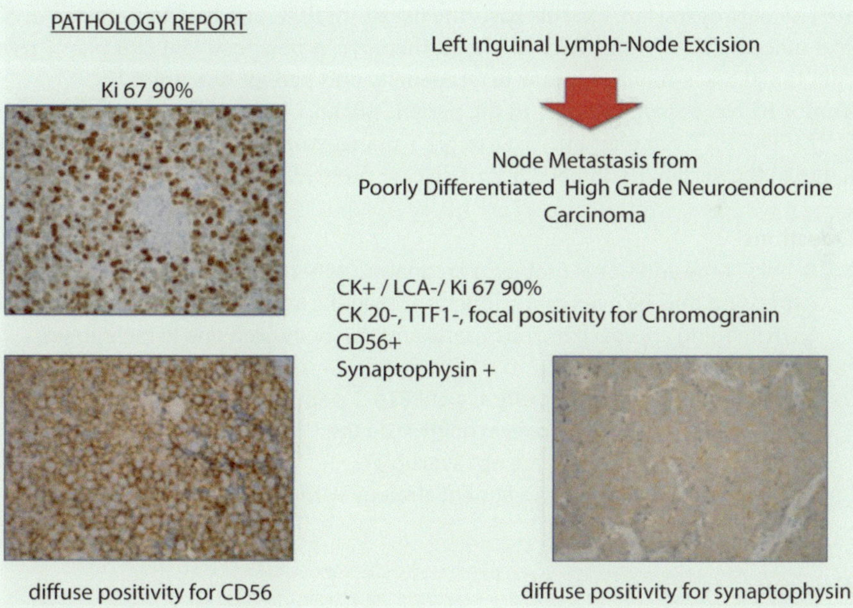

Fig. 9.6 Pathology report

9.1 Comments to the Case

We report a case of a male affected with node metastasis from poorly differentiated high-grade neuroendocrine carcinoma. ^{111}In-Octreoscan WB and SPECT/CT documented the loss of SSTR expression, while increased glucose metabolism at ^{18}F-FDG PET/CT correlated with high Ki-67 expression and disease progression, as confirmed in the pathology report.

Imaging results suggested the utility of chemotherapy according to the literature evidence of different patterns of NET at RI–SSTR and metabolic PET/CT.

The loss of SSTR expression has been found to coincide with a gain in glucose utilization in NET. ^{18}F FDG PET uptake reveals increased glucose metabolism only in less differentiated NET, with a direct proportionality to high Ki-67 expression in disease progression [5]. It has been shown a significantly higher median of ^{18}F FDG SUV max in patients with high-grade tumors, whereas patients with well-differentiated tumors demonstrate a higher uptake for ^{68}Ga-DOTA-TATE. ^{18}F-FDG PET/CT had no clinical impact on G1 NETs and a moderate impact on G2 NETs. However, in poorly differentiated NETs, ^{18}F-FDG PET/CT plays a significant clinical role in combination with (68) Gallium labeled somatostatin analogues (^{68}Ga peptides: DOTA-TOC, DOTA-NOC and DOTA-TATE). It has been demonstrated that ^{68}Ga-DOTA-TATE SUV max relates to grade and Ki-67 and can be used prognostically [6].

9

In NET patients, the presence of ^{18}F-FDG-positive tumors correlates strongly with a higher risk of progression. On this basis the use of ^{18}F FDG can lead to a change in NET clinical management from PRRT to chemotherapy; in perspective it can play a role in the functional assessment of tumor heterogeneity and patient outcomes [7].

Tumor RI has a strong impact in the patient workup, but, similarly, a positive metabolic ^{18}F-FDG PET can play a key role in NET management for its prognostic contribution, due to the variability in behavior of disease progression.

Questions

1. RI links some additional problems for analysis, where the evidence of SSTR expression may be even more important than the same presence of a receptor. SSTR imaging approach may be useful anyway, but which one RI techniques should we choose today?
2. Due to the most diagnostic efficacy of PET/CT peptides in the setting of patients and conditions defined above, in point 1, do the ^{111}In-OCT indication and utility still remain if PET peptides are not available?
3. Can imaging influence the treatment strategy with clinical impact?

Answers

1. Looking at tumor biology, ^{68}Ga-DOTA-octapeptide PET/CT actually takes the prominent role in the NET imaging, due to the high affinity to receptor binding, particularly effective in well-differentiated NET with high receptorial expression [5].

   Considering the SSTR expression variability, the diagnostic capability of PET/DOTA, even on low-density lesion SSTRs, is greater than the ^{111}In-OCT one, with increase in sensitivity (91–95%) and in specificity (82–97%) [6].

So, in the RI choice, we must take into account that the advantages compared to OCT scan are due to the best intrinsic spatial resolution of the PET scanner; the pharmacokinetic properties of the PET peptides affinity for receptor subtypes, considering that SSTRs are membrane receptors for which six subtypes have been identified by molecular analysis; and the best affinity to the peptide used in PRRT.

On this basis, the IR PET/CT is the technique with more specific competence in stratifying NET patients to predict and monitor response to targeted therapy.

2. Looking at a technological point of view, today we can overcome some limitations of ^{111}In-OCT. One of the main problems of SSTR imaging, for example, is the need to overcome the limit of spatial resolution that may invest the diagnosis of NET that generally appears as small lesions, with special reference to ^{111}In-OCT. The problem of size for the millimetric lesions is definitely improved by the use of tomographic scan (SPECT) and even more of multimodal systems. It has been demonstrated that combined modality imaging (both for SPECT/CT and PET/CT) increases the clinical impact of SSTR imaging and can be very effective in targeting NET. In a study that investigates liver metastases in 149 patients with GEP, the comparison between imaging procedures – SSTR SPECT/planar SSTR/conventional imaging procedure (CIP) – shows that combined SPECT technique to SSTR improves, respectively, sensitivity (SPECT, 92.3%; planar, 58.5%; CIP, 80%), VPN (SPECT, 94.4%; planar, 75.7%; CIP, 84.7%), and accuracy (SPECT, 96.6%; planar, 81.9%; CIP, 83.2%) [7].

   Moreover studies comparing SSTR-SPECT and SSTR-SPECT/CT techniques showed that, while the sensitivity remains substantially unchanged, the anatomical cross significantly improves the specificity (SSTR SPECT, 71%; SSTR SPECT/CT, 92.1% [8]).

   The main focus of SSTR imaging is NET, but it is well known that in addition to NET, they are expressed in a variety normal tissues. Multimodality also improves the ability to overcome the limit of the technique due to uptake of the radiocompound for receptor expression that is not connected to malignancy, as in the case of accessory spleen, or benign diseases, mainly in extra-abdominal seat.

   In summary, net of any consideration, the strong meaning to which we can refer and that makes the difference, when ^{111}In-OCT SSTR, whole-body, and SPECT/CT scans are compared to other techniques, is that adding the RI in the workup of patients with NET, it impacts in up to 30% of cases, conditioning correctly clinical and therapeutic management in one patient out of three [9].

3. ^{68}Ga-DOTA-peptide imaging has been shown to influence the management of patients, with a particular impact on initiation or continuation of PRRT or somatostatin analog medical therapy, based on the demonstration of somatostatin receptor expression. ^{68}Ga-DOTA-TATE has been shown to affect the management plan in 48% of NET patients [10].

   ^{18}F-FDG led to a change from PRRT to chemotherapy in 25% of patients with intermediate- or high-grade NETs [11], and, similarly, a recent study showed that ^{18}F-FDG findings affect 21% of patients, half of whom had G3 tumors. Moreover, the same study demonstrated that metastases observed by either tracer correlated with a shorter survival, and bone metastases correlate with the worst prognosis [6].

   At state, the availability of new treatment regimens needs for new prognostic and predictive biomarkers that can lead to better assessment of therapeutic response for individual patients [12].

Up to Date of the Topic

In the recent years, it has increased the need to deepen and spread in a multidisciplinary model the knowledge on neuroendocrine tumors and have standard references not only for classifying but also for sharing approaches to diagnosis and therapy. The understanding of great biological diversity and clinical complexity of NET makes necessary to detect markers and prognostic factors reproducible for new therapeutic pathways [13].

On this basis it takes place on a continuous thread between molecular imaging and molecular biology model of the tumor, so that the evidence of the target can spontaneously correlate with the molecular properties of it. In accordance with these expectations, molecular imaging correlates the kinetics of radiopharmaceuticals to specific metabolic and receptor targets, for diagnostic and therapeutic purposes, thus providing an ideal condition for approach to the disease as well as an effective example of theranostics.

Considering, once again, that the validity of a technique can be estimated looking at the capability that it manages itself in changing clinical and therapeutic management of a patient, the Nuclear Medicine of University College London Hospitals (UCLH), the national reference center of the United Kingdom for imaging of NET patients within the national health service, launched a transversal study by analyzing a database of patients undergoing ^{68}Ga-DOTA-TATE PET/CT (May 2005–August 2013). Histology, indications, and influence over management decisions were evaluated. The survival data were analyzed and correlated with the PET/CT results in a total of 1258 patients with known or suspected NET. The tumor grading was defined according to WHO classification and ENETS.

The results of the study documented high PPV of PET (99–100% for entero-pancreatic NET). The survival curves confirmed a better survival in patients showing negative PET scan, compared with the positive ones. In these last groups of patients, the survival curves showed direct correlation with the tumor grading. Moreover at PET scan, the evidence of bone metastases showed a significantly adverse prognostic weight, associated with significant reduction in survival when compared with the evidence of lymph node extension and liver metastases. In this study the AA report that the ^{68}Ga-DOTA-TATE PET/CT influences clinical management in a large percentage of NET patients, clearly directing the patient to address surgical therapy, chemotherapy, or PRRT [14]. Imaging plays a crucial role in the diagnosis and management of NETs, because the initial diagnostic workup and staging after histologic confirmation form the basis for the decision on whether to perform surgical resection or to initiate medical therapy. The small size of NETs makes it difficult for conventional anatomic imaging to visualize the primary tumor or its metastases, given that these modalities are unable to depict specific endocrine features; consequently, the diagnostic accuracy of functional imaging is significantly higher than that of conventional imaging. Finally, tumor heterogeneity cannot be fully assessed by tumor biopsy, and this is an area in which combined dual-tracer PET/CT, 68Ga-DOTA, and ^{18}F-FDG PET/CT offers distinct advantages even though referring clinicians rely mainly on the histologic grading [6].

Bibliography

1. Gut P et al (2016) Chromogranin A – unspecific neuroendocrine marker. Clinical utility and potential diagnostic pitfalls. Arch Med Sci 12(1):1–9
2. Adams S et al (1998) Limited value of fluorine-18 fluorodeoxyglucose positron emission tomography for the imaging of neuroendocrine tumours. Eur J Nucl Med 25:79–83
3. Panagiotidis E et al (2017) Comparison of the impact of ^{68}Ga-DOTATATE and ^{18}F-FDG PET/CT on clinical management in patients with neuroendocrine tumors. J Nucl Med 58:91–96
4. Nilica B et al (2016) Direct comparison of ^{68}Ga-DOTA-TOC and ^{18}F-FDG PET/CT in the follow-up of patients with neuroendocrine tumour treated with the first full peptide receptor radionuclide therapy cycle. Eur J Nucl Med Mol Imaging 43:1585–1592
5. Wild D et al (2003) DOTA-NOC, a high-affinity ligand of somatostatin receptor subtypes 2, 3 and 5 for labelling with various radiometals. Eur J Nucl Med Mol Imaging 30:1338–1347
6. Buchmann I el al (2007) Comparison of ^{68}Ga-DOTATOC PET and ^{111}In-DTPA-OCT (Octreoscan) SPECT in patients with neuroendocrine tumours. Eur J Nucl Med Mol Imaging 34(10):1617–1626
7. Gibril F et al (2004) Diagnostic uses of radiolabelled somatostatin receptor analogues in gastroenteropancreatic endocrine tumours. Digest Liver Dis 36(Suppl 1):S106–S120
8. Perri M et al (2008) Octreo-SPECT/CT imaging for accurate detection and localization of suspected neuroendocrine tumors. Q J Nucl Med Mol Imaging 52(4):323–333
9. Schillaci O et al (2014) SPECT/CT in neuroendocrine tumours. Clin Transl Imaging 2:477–489
10. Deppen SA, Blume J, Bobbey AJ et al (2016) ^{68}Ga-DOTATATE compared with ^{111}In- DTPA-octreotide and conventional imaging for pulmonary and gastroentero- pancreatic neuroendocrine tumors: a systematic review and meta-analysis. J Nucl Med 57:872–878
11. Kayani I et al (2008) Functional imaging of neuroendocrine tumors with combined PET/CT using ^{68}Ga-DOTATATE (DOTA-DPhe1,Tyr3- octreotate) and ^{18}F-FDG. Cancer 112:2447–2455
12. Hofman MS et al (2012) Changing paradigms with molecular imaging of neuro-endocrine tumors. Discov Med 14:71–81
13. Virgolini I (2015) Peptide receptor radionuclide therapy (PRRT): clinical significance of re-treatment? Eur J Nucl Med Mol Imaging 42:1949–1954
14. Skoura E et al (2016) The Impact of ^{68}Ga-DOTATATE PET/CT Imaging on Management of Patients with Neuroendocrine Tumors: Experience from a National Referral Center in the United Kingdom. J Nucl Med 57:34–40

Tumour Detection in Syndromic NET: Carcinoid Syndrome

Georgios K. Dimitriadis and Gregory Kaltsas

A. Colao et al. (eds.), *Neuroendocrine Tumors in Real Life*,
https://doi.org/10.1007/978-3-319-59024-0_10

Overview

Many gastro-enteropancreatic neuroendocrine tumours (GEP-NETs) secrete biologically active substances and can present with distinct clinical syndromes related to their oversecretion. In particular, carcinoid syndrome (CS) is a compendium of clinical manifestations including secretory diarrhoea, flushing and less commonly wheezing and dyspnoea secondary to overproduction of such compounds, mainly serotonin. Carcinoid syndrome is almost exclusively derived from small intestinal NETs that have metastasized to the liver and may also be associated with extensive fibrosis of heart valves and the mesenterium. Although the diagnosis is usually delayed due to the lack of tumour-specific symptoms, measurement of specific tumour metabolites such as 5-hydroxyindoloacetic acid facilitates the diagnosis. Conventional radiology and functioning imaging modalities using specific and occasionally non-specific tracers are used to identify the extent of disease and also provide information regarding prognosis and the application of specific treatment. The development though of diagnostic and predictive biomarkers that would allow for individualized workup and selection of specific treatments remains a priority in the field.

Clinical Case

A 56-year-old woman presented with a 6-year history of diarrhoea and flushing and recently developed shortness of breath. Initially flushing episodes lasted for a few minutes involving the upper part of her body and resolving spontaneously and were attributed to her menopause that happened at the same time until she developed episodes of diarrhoeas. These initially occurred a few times each day but gradually increased in frequency and volume. The patient underwent a series of investigations including full blood count, conventional biochemistry, thyroid function tests, microscopy and culture of the stool and a colonoscopy that revealed no pathology. Since she was also complaining of vague abdominal discomfort that was relieved with defecation without any associated weight loss, her symptoms were attributed to irritable bowel syndrome.

At presentation she was found dehydrated and had a postural drop of 20 mmHg in her blood pressure. On examination she was tachypnoeic and tachycardic, and her jugular venous pressure was elevated exhibiting prominent V waves. She had a pansystolic murmur that was more prominent on inspiration and bilateral ankle oedema. Her chest was clear, but her abdomen was distended, and on examination she was found to have an enlarged knobbly liver and ascites.

Initial management involved the use of diuretics, whereas an echogram of her heart revealed an enlarged right ventricle and severe tricuspid valve regurgitation. Following resuscitation and treatment of her heart failure, the patient underwent computerized tomography (CT) imaging of her chest, abdomen and pelvis. Several irregular hepatic arterial enhancing lesions involving both hepatic lobes with areas of calcification and necrosis were found, and there was also an area of mesenteric desmoplastic reaction. There were a number of enlarged lymph nodes in the ileocaecal junction, but no distinct lesion was seen in the ileum. There were no lesions in the chest or other obvious bony lesions.

Subsequent investigations revealed that her proBNP level at presentation was grossly elevated. As the provisional diagnosis of a neuroendocrine tumour probably originating from the ileum metastatic to the liver causing carcinoid syndrome and carcinoid heart disease was suspected, appropriate confirmatory biochemical and radiological investigations were undertaken. In an attempt to specifically identify the primary lesion, a CT enterography was performed that failed to identify a specific abnormality in the ileum.

10.1 Comments to the Case

This case is representative of the natural history of an undiagnosed small intestinal NET from symptom onset to the time of diagnosis. The delay in diagnosis is attributed to the lack of tumour-specific symptoms, the absence of highly sensitive and specific biomarkers that could be used to identify early-stage disease and the good performance status of the patients even in the presence of extensive disease [28]. CS is mostly encountered in small intestinal NETs metastasized to the liver although occasionally it can be found in patients with lung and ovarian NETs and in the presence of mesenteric metastases. The development of carcinoid heart disease (CHD), although recently less common than previously encountered, is the effect of non-metabolized secretory substances, mainly 5-hydroxytryptamine (5-HT or serotonin), causing fibrosis particularly of right-sided cardiac valves. The present case pinpoints the diagnostic pitfalls occurring from overlapping clinical manifestations seen in other gastrointestinal pathologies and some functioning NETs. It also highlights the importance of increased awareness from managing physicians due to the increased morbidity and mortality that can arise from delayed diagnosis or even misdiagnosis. It also reveals the need for developing sensitive and specific biomarkers that could facilitate early diagnosis and distinguish these tumours from other pathologies that could have an initial similar mode of presentation (◘ Fig. 10.1).

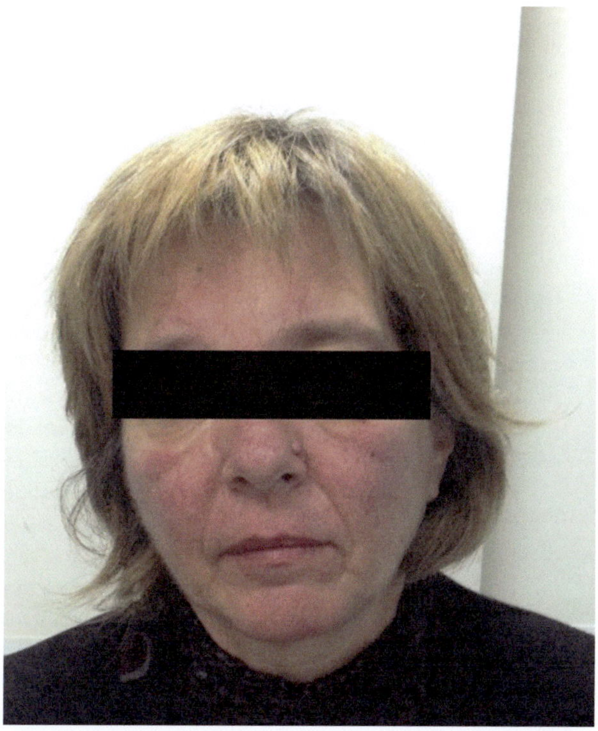

◘ **Fig. 10.1** Facial flushing from typical CS secondary to a small intestine NET

Questions

1. Are there any distinctive clinical features that could be used to distinguish the presence of carcinoid syndrome from pathologies presenting in a similar manner?
2. Which are the most common primary sites of origin?

Answers

1. Diagnosing CS in its early stages can be quite challenging due to the absence of specific symptoms. Most of CS symptoms are fairly common and can be similar to symptoms from conditions with overlapping characteristics. What might raise suspicion towards the presence of CS is usually the combination of flushing episodes and secretory diarrhoea.
2. CS is in most cases the result of hormonal oversecretion from a neuroendocrine tumour of the small intestine that has metastasized in the liver. Alternative primary sites that present with CS are bronchial and ovarian neuroendocrine tumours.

Up to Date of the Topic

Syndromic NET: *Carcinoid Syndrome*

The classical (typical) CS is encountered in 95% of cases and is characterized by cutaneous flushing (90%), gut hypermobility with diarrhoea (80%) and bronchospasm (15%) [13, 14, 27]. Additional manifestations include abdominal pain (40%), telangiectasia (25%), valvular heart disease (20–25%), wheezing (15%) and pellagra (5%) [19]. Serotonin is one of the major mediators of the symptoms of CS and is excreted in the urine metabolized to 5-HIAA. The diagnosis is usually suspected in the presence of synchronous diarrhoea and flushing episodes, which constitute the principal features of CS. In the early phases of the disease, the major mechanisms of diarrhoea are secretory along with gastrointestinal dysmotility; however, in later phases gut lymphangiectasia and bacterial overgrowth are also involved [19]. Diarrhoea is usually watery and can be of high volume, up to 6–8 L daily, can occur many times a day, is not related to foods and as it is secretory in nature tends to persist during the night. The flush consists of a pink to red colour and involves the face and upper trunk; it can last for a few minutes and occur many times per day without leaving a permanent discoloration and can be triggered following the consumption of alcohol or tyramine-containing foods [19]. Pellagra can rarely develop in CS as a result of a deficiency in niacin (also known as nicotinic acid or vitamin B3). In the case of CS, the development of pellagra is not secondary to inadequate intake of tryptophan, niacin or B vitamin cofactors, but rather due to an altered protein metabolism.

Atypical carcinoid syndrome (5%) is usually thought to be mediated by 5-hydroxytryptophan (5-HTP), histamine and other biogenic amines and consists of a flush that tends to be of protracted duration lasting for hours and of a purplish rather than the usual pink-red colour and occurs in the absence of triggering foods [22]. When the flush subsides, it may leave telangiectasia and hypertrophy of the skin, face and upper neck but can also involve the limbs, which may become acrocyanotic [19]. Occasionally, headache, lacrimation, hypotension, cutaneous oedema and bronchoconstriction may also occur.

Carcinoid crisis is the most immediate life-threatening complication and is characteristic of the excessive secretory component of the CS. It presents with hypotension, rarely hypertension and tachycardia predisposing to arrhythmias, bronchial wheezing, flushing and central nervous system dysfunction [19]. It can occur spontaneously or, more commonly, can be precipitated after anaesthesia, interventional procedures or medication (chemotherapy or radiopharmaceuticals causing tumour lysis and releasing large amounts of amines into the systemic circulation). The symptoms of CS may overlap with that of other gastrointestinal (GI) disorders including irritable bowel syndrome (IBS) (often presents with intermittent and chronic history of diarrhoea) or Crohn's disease (right quadrant abdominal pain, may present with perianal lesions), while flushing is a very common sign of menopause and, if wheezing is the only symptom, may be mistaken for asthma. However, the secretory nature of diarrhoea (not strictly related to food and nocturnal occurrence) should alarm caring physicians for the underlying diagnosis of CS.

Neuroendocrine tumours of the small intestine are the most common causes of CS that occurs in 20–30% of patients with liver metastases. The syndrome may also be encountered in patients with primary bronchial carcinoids or ovarian tumours or in the presence of extensive peritoneal metastases, when the secretory products exceed the capacity of inactivation by the liver or bypass the liver being released directly into the systemic circulation [13, 14, 27]. The less common atypical CS may be found with tumours originating from the former foregut mainly lung carcinoids [22, 27]. In up to 20% of cases, the primary tumour may not be identified (unknown primary) although in the majority of such cases unidentified ileal carcinoids are usually the cause.

Chromogranin A (CgA) is a 439 amino acid glycoprotein that is present in the secretory dense core granules of most neuroendocrine cells and still presents the biomarker of choice for the detection of most NETs including functioning gastrointestinal NETs [4]. The specificity of CgA in the diagnosis of NETs depends on the tumour type and burden as 100% specificities have been reported in patients with metastatic disease [29]. Elevated CgA was found to be more sensitive than high urinary 5-HIAA levels in patients with metastatic midgut lesions (87% vs 76%, respectively) [12]. In a study looking at a mixed series of 128 patients with NETs, increased levels were found in 29% and 67% of patients with locoregional metastatic disease, respectively [6]. The pragmatic prognostic value of CgA in making the diagnosis in patients with NETs has not been fully confirmed to date. However, false-positive elevation of CgA may commonly be encountered, and the European Neuroendocrine Tumor Society has reached a consensus regarding standard of care (SOC) regarding available CgA assays and interpretation of the results. CgA levels should be interpreted with caution in cases of impaired renal function, cardiac failure, Parkinson's disease, untreated hypertension, pregnancy and the use of certain medication [20]. Furthermore, steroid treatment or glucocorticoid excess can also up-regulate CgA mRNA expression. In cases of proton pump inhibitor use, these should be discontinued at least for 2 weeks before CgA is sampled. It is accepted that a recognized international standard for CgA assay is not currently available and variations in assay types may influence results. Therefore, reference laboratories should be preferred for CgA testing [20].

Small intestinal NETs produce serotonin and exhibit elevated 5-HIAA mostly measured as 24-h urinary levels [15, 20]. Urinary 5-HIAA has a 100% sensitivity and a 90% specificity for detecting CS and a 75% sensitivity and an almost 100% specificity for predicting a primary tumour in the jejuno-ileum, respectively [4, 20]. Some foods contain high levels of serotonin which may increase the levels of urinary 5-HIAA, and consumption should be avoided 3 days prior to urine collection: plums, pineapples, bananas, eggplants, tomatoes, avocados and walnuts [20]. ENETS standards of care divide them into two categories:

- Increasing 5-HIAA: acetanilide, phenacetin, glyceryl guaiacolate (found in many cough syrups), methocarbamol, reserpine, cisplatin, fluorouracil, melphalan, rauwolfia
- Decreasing 5-HIAA: chlorpromazine, heparin, imipramine, isoniazid, levodopa, monoamine oxidase inhibitors, methenamine, methyldopa, phenothiazines, promethazine, tricyclic antidepressants, chlorophenylalanine, corticotrophin, guanfacine, imipramine, isocarboxazid, isoniazid, levodopa, MAO inhibitors, moclobemide, octreotide

Most recently overnight serum and urinary 5-HIAA measurements have been shown to be equally sensitive and specific to 24-h urinary collections in substantiating the diagnosis and as are more easily performed are expected to represent the investigation of choice [1, 11]. Histamine metabolites are used for the diagnosis of the rare causes of atypical carcinoid syndrome.

The vast majority of NETs producing CS is derived from the small intestine. However, even small-sized tumours (<1 cm) may be associated with metastatic disease to the regional lymph nodes and the liver.

The use of cross-sectional conventional imaging by either triple-phase contrast-enhanced multi-slice CT or contrast-enhanced magnetic resonance imaging (MRI) represents the cornerstone of indirect abdominal initial staging as well as preoperative diagnosis [19]. Three reports on imaging of various NET metastases in the abdomen have revealed a mean sensitivity of 83% (range 61–100%) and specificity of 76% (range 71–80%) for CT scan, while a mean 93% (85–100%) sensitivity and an 88% (75–100%) specificity were obtained for MRI [20]. MRI scanning is currently considered the best modality in detecting hepatic infiltration regardless of contrast enhancement, but when CT is employed, examination in the portal-venous inflow phase is mandatory given the chance of not detecting some lesions [26]. These modalities are also used to evaluate the anatomy of the arteries and their relation to the tumours in CT/MRI angiography of the liver. Hepatic metastatic disease can be visualized with good results when utilizing contrast-enhanced ultrasound scanning [10]. The drawback of this method is that it is user dependent.

Colonoscopy can be used to identify tumours beyond the ileocaecal valve and into the colon. Assessment of lesions located at more proximal parts of the ileum or of the jejunum can be performed using advanced methods like enteroscopy including video capsule endoscopy (VCE) [5] or double-balloon enteroscopy [7] with good results. It would be fair to say though that their role in routine diagnostic assessment of gastrointestinal NETs has not yet been proven. Small bowel obstruction is an absolute contraindication for the use of VCE. CT or MR enterography is more effective in the case of small intestinal tumours and should be utilized where available. CT enterography has been reported to exert a mean sensitivity of 85% and a mean specificity of 97%, while for MR enterography, the same percentages are 87% and 100%, respectively [17, 26].

Somatostatin receptor imaging (111 Indium SRS) has approximately 90% sensitivity for primary/nodal G1-G2, small intestinal NETs and greater than 95% for liver metastases and remains a useful and widely available tool for initial staging as well as for follow-up. 68 Gallium-labelled positron emission tomography (PET) fused with contrast-enhanced CT (functional imaging) is more sensitive, particularly for the detection of small jejuno-ileal tumours or for distant metastases not detected by other direct or indirect imaging modalities. 68 Ga-DOTATOC PET/CT was found to be superior to ^{111}In SRS when searching for a primary NET in patients with unknown or suspected disease [25]. Radionuclide imaging can also be utilized for the detection of clinically suspicious metastatic bone disease, although conventional 99m-technetium whole-body bone scintigraphy still remains the modality of choice in detecting bone lesions [18]. In another study, whole-body MRI was found to be superior to 68 Ga-DOTATOC PET/CT in detecting bone metastases in patients with well-differentiated NETs [24]. The use of 68 Ga-DOTATATE PET/contrast-enhanced CT is associated with an increased diagnostic accuracy in the detection of extrahepatic particularly bone NET metastases compared to stand-alone contrast-enhanced CT [2]. The use of 18 fluorodeoxyglucose (FDG) PET is recommended in G3 NETs independent of the location of the tumour [3]. In a study of 104 patients with histopathologically proven NETs who underwent both ^{68}Ga-DOTATATE and ^{18}F-FDG PET/CT, no statistically significant differences in ^{18}F-FDG-derived SUVs were observed between different tumour grades although overall survival was found to decline rapidly with increasing histological grading [21]. Radionuclide imaging using newer traces, such as 11 carbon-5-hydroxytryptophan (5HTP) or 18 fluorodihydroxyphenylalanine (DOPA), has shown promising results but is not widely available to most healthcare professionals [16].

Often, an intestinal primary is difficult to detect by conventional imaging. Mesenteric lymph node metastases with accentuated desmoplastic reaction remain the most common imaging finding in patients with intestinal NETs. In this case, somatostatin receptor PET/CT is the most efficient imaging modality in the detection of an unknown primary [23]. Recent advances in tumour spatial and functional imaging along with circulating transcripts (mRNA) may represent the future strategy for real-time monitoring of disease progress and therapeutic efficacy. Surgery represents the best option for treating patients with GI NETs but cannot be widely applied in those with extensive disease.

Timely diagnosis is essential as when CHD becomes established is associated with increased morbidity and mortality. However, a significant number of patients with moderate to severe tricuspid regurgitation are either asymptomatic or have only mild symptoms [8]. NT-proBNP is currently considered to represent the best biomarker that exerts both diagnostic and prognostic significance for cardiac involvement. NT-proBNP, at the cut-off level of 260 pg/ml (31 pmol/l), appears to be the best biomarker to date for screening patients with CS in order to diagnose those with CHD [8]. Other biomarkers that have been used in the assessment of the disease include CgA and urinary 5-HIAA. Measurement of 24-hour urinary 5-HIAA excretion is a useful marker for determining those at risk of CHD when levels are

>300 µmol/24 h. Conventional cardiac echogram, transthoracic echogram and MRI cardiac imaging are used to delineate valvular lesions and extend cardiac decompensation. Several echographic grading systems have been developed; the most optimal for screening was the Westberg score, whereas other more complex systems were more suited to patients with established disease [9].

10.2 Conclusion

Carcinoid syndrome heralds the presence of widespread disease in patients with mostly small intestinal NETs. Although related symptoms can be non-specific, the combination of secretory diarrhoea and flushing exerts the highest diagnostic accuracy in making the diagnosis. When suspected 5-HIAA measurement in either the urine or plasma is currently the most sensitive and specific marker in establishing the diagnosis and can also be of prognostic significance. Identification of the primary and estimation of the extent of the disease and potential comorbidities such as carcinoid heart disease are of utmost primary importance in order to plan treatment and avoid local complications. Currently, gallium-labelled SRS is the best modality for staging the disease and may help identify the primary, whereas MRI is the method of choice for establishing the presence and extent of hepatic involvement and delineating abdominal pathology. Besides the application of many imaging modalities, small ileal NETs may still elude localization.

Bibliography

1. Adaway JE, Dobson R, Walsh J, Cuthbertson DJ, Monaghan PJ, Trainer PJ, Valle JW, Keevil BG (2015) Serum and plasma 5-hydroxyindoleacetic acid as an alternative to 24-h urine 5-hydroxyindoleacetic acid measurement. Ann Clin Biochem 53(Pt 5):554–560. doi:10.1177/0004563215613109
2. Albanus DR, Apitzsch J, Erdem Z, Erdem O, Verbung FA, Behrendt FF, Mottaghy FM, Heinzel A (2015) Clinical value of 68 DOTATATE -PET/CT compared to standard alone contrast enhanced CT for the detection of extra-hepatic metastases in patients with neuroendocrine tumors (NET). Eur J Radiol 84:1866–1872
3. Ambrosini V, Tomassetti P, Castellucci P, Campana D, Montini G, Rubello D, Nanni C, Rizzello A, Franchi R, Fanti S (2008) Comparison between 68Ga-DOTA-NOC and 18F-DOPA PET for the detection of gastro-entero-pancreatic and lung neuro-endocrine tumours. Eur J Nucl Med Mol Imaging 35:1431–1438
4. Ardill JE, Erikkson B (2003) The importance of the measurement of circulating markers in patients with neuroendocrine tumors of the pancreas and gut. Endocr Relat Cancer 10:459–462
5. Bailey AA, Debinski HS, Appleyard MN, Remedios ML, Hooper JE, Walsh AJ, Selby WS (2006) Diagnosis and outcome of small bowel tumors found by capsule endoscopy: a three center Australian experience. Am J Gastroenterol 101:2237–2243
6. Baudin E, Gigliotti A, Ducreux M et al (1998) Neuron-specific enolase and chromogranin A as markers of neuroendocrine tumors. Br J Cancer 78:1102–1107
7. Bellutti M, Fry LC, Schmitt J, Seemann M, Klose S, Malfertheiner P, Monkemuller K (2009) Detection of neuroendocrine tumors of the small bowel by double balloon enteroscopy. Dig Dis Sci 54:1050–1058
8. Bhattacharyya S, Davar J, Dreyfus G, Caplin ME (2007) Carcinoid heart disease. Circulation 116:2860–2865
9. Dobson R, Cuthbertson DJ, Jones J, Valle JW, Keevil B, Chadwick C, Poston GP, Burgess MI (2014) Determination of the optimal echocardiographic scoring system to quantify carcinoid heart disease. Neuroendocrinology 99(2):85–93

10. Dorffel Y, Wermke W (2008) Neuroendocrine tumors: characterization with contrast-enhanced ultrasonography. Ultraschall Med 29:506–514
11. Gedde-Dahl M, Thiis-Evensen E, Myklebust Tjølsen A, Skrede Mordal K, Vatn M, Bergestuen DS (2013) Comparison of 24-h and overnight samples of urinary 5-hydroxyindoleacetic acid in patients with intestinal neuroendocrine tumors. Endocr Connect 2:50–54. doi:10.1530/EC-12-0077
12. Janson ET, Holmberg L, Stridsberg M et al (1997) Carcinoid tumors: analysis of prognostic factors and survival in 301 patients from a referral center. Ann Oncol 8:685–690
13. Kaltsas GA, Besser GM, Grossman AB (2004) The diagnosis and medical management of advanced neuroendocrine tumors. Endocr Rev 25:458–511. doi:10.1210/er.2003-0014
14. Kaltsas G, Rockall A, Papadogias D, Reznek R, Grossman AB (2004) Recent advances in radiological and radionuclide imaging and therapy of neuroendocrine tumours. Eur J Endocrinol 151:15–27
15. Kema IP, Meijer WG, Meiborg G, Ooms B, Willemse PH, de Vries EG (2001) Profiling of tryptophan-related plasma indoles in patients with carcinoid tumors by automated, on-line, solid-phase extraction and HPLC with fluorescence detection. Clin Chem 47:1811–1820
16. Koopmans KP, de Vries EG, Kema IP, Elsinga PH, Neels OC, Sluiter WJ, van der Horst-Schrivers AN, Jager PL (2006) Staging of carcinoid tumors with 18F-DOPA PET: a prospective, diagnostic accuracy study. Lancet Oncol 7:728–734
17. Masselli G, Polettini E, Casciani E, Bertini L, Vecchioli A, Gualdi G (2009) Small-bowel neoplasms: prospective evaluation of MR enteroclysis. Radiology 251:743–750
18. Meijer WG, van der Veer E, Jager PL, van der Jagt EJ, Piers BA, Kema IP, de Vries EG, Willemse PH (2003) Bone metastases in carcinoid tumors: clinical features, imaging characteristics, and markers of bone metabolism. J Nucl Med 44:184–191
19. Niederle B, Pape UF, Costa F, Gross D, Kelestimur F, Knigge U, Öberg K, Pavel M, Perren A, Toumpanakis C, O'Connor J, O'Toole D, Krenning E, Reed N, Kianmanesh R, Vienna Consensus Conference participants (2016) ENETS consensus guidelines update for neuroendocrine neoplasms of the jejunum and ileum. Neuroendocrinology 103(2):125–138. doi:10.1159/000443170. Epub 2016 Jan 12
20. O'Toole D, Grossman A, Gross D, Delle Fave G, Barkmanova J, O'Connor J, Pape UF, Plockinger U (2009) ENETS consensus guidelines for the standards of care in neuroendocrine tumors: biochemical markers. Neuroendocrinology 90:194–202
21. Panagiotidis E, Alshammari A, Michopoulou S, Skoura E, Naik K, Maragkoudakis E, Mohmaduvesh M, Al-Harbi M, Belda M, Caplin ME, Toumpanakis C, Bomanji J (2017) Comparison of the Impact of 68Ga-DOTATATE and 18F-FDG PET/CT on Clinical Management in Patients with Neuroendocrine Tumors. J Nucl Med 58(1):91–96
22. Papadogias D, Makras P, Kossivakis K, Kontogeorgos G, Piaditis G, Kaltsas G (2007) Carcinoid syndrome and carcinoid crisis secondary to a metastatic carcinoid tumor of the lung: a therapeutic challenge. Eur J Gastroenterol Hepatol 19(12):1154–1159
23. Prasad V, Ambrosini V, Hommann M et al (2010) Detection of unknown primary neuroendocrine tumors (CUP-NET) using (68) Ga-DOTA-NOC receptor PET/CT. Eur J Nucl Med Mol Imaging 37:67e77
24. Schraml C, Schwenzer NF, Sperling O, Aschoff P, Lichy MP, Müller M, Brendle C, Werner MK, Claussen CD, Pfannenberg C (2013) Staging of neuroendocrine tumours: comparison of [^{68}Ga]DOTATOC multiphase PET/CT and whole-body MRI. Cancer Imaging 5;13:63–72
25. Schreiter NF, Bartels AM, Froeling V, Steffen I, Pape UF, Beck A, Hamm B, Brenner W, Rottgen R (2014) Searching for primaries in patients with neuroendocrine tumors (NET) of unknown primary and clinically suspected NET: evaluation of Ga-68 DOTATOC PET/CT and in-111 DTPA octreotide SPECT/CT. Radiol Oncol 48(4):339–347
26. Sundin A, Vullierme MP, Kaltsas G, Plöckinger U, all other Mallorca Consensus Conference participants (2009) ENETS consensus guidelines for the standards of care in neuroendocrine tumors: radiological examinations. Neuroendocrinology 90:167–183. doi:10.1159/000184855
27. Tomassetti P, Migliori M, Lalli S, Campana D, Tomassetti V, Corinaldesi R (2001) Epidemiology, clinical features and diagnosis of gastroenteropancreatic endocrine tumors. Ann Oncol 12(Suppl 2):S95–S99
28. Vinik A, Silva MP, Woltering EA, Go VL, Warner R, Caplin M (2009) Biochemical testing for neuroendocrine tumors. Pancreas 38(8):876–889
29. Zatelli MC, Torta M, Leon A et al (2007) Chromogranin A as a marker of neuroendocrine neoplasia: an Italian multicenter study. Endocr Relat Cancer 14:473–482

Tumor Detection in Syndromic NET: Zollinger-Ellison Syndrome

Roberta Modica, Luigi Camera, Vincenzo Napolitano, Manuela Avellino, Rosa Fonti, Silvana Del Vecchio, Leonardo De Luca, Annamaria Colao, and Antongiulio Faggiano

On behalf of the ENETS Center of Excellence Multidisciplinary Group for Neuroendocrine Tumors in Naples, Italy

A. Colao et al. (eds.), *Neuroendocrine Tumors in Real Life*,
https://doi.org/10.1007/978-3-319-59024-0_11

Overview

The Zollinger-Ellison syndrome (ZES) is a clinical disorder characterized by recurrent peptic ulcers due to hypergastrinemia induced by a gastrinoma, a gastrin-secreting neuroendocrine tumor. ZES is sporadic in 60–75% of cases, whereas in the remaining patients, it is associated with multiple endocrine neoplasia type 1 (MEN1), an autosomal dominant disorder resulting in hyperplasia and/or tumors of endocrine and non-endocrine organs. Here we present a case of a 40-year-old female, presented with recurrent epigastric pain and acid reflux, uncontrolled with proton pump inhibitors. A MEN1-related ZES was hypothesized on the basis of early age of onset and the evidence of multifocal tumors within the pancreas and duodenum, despite the absence of primary hyperparathyroidism. The diagnostic workup included endoscopic ultrasound, contrast-enhanced multi-detector computed tomography, and somatostatin-receptor scintigraphy.

Clinical Case

11

A 40-year-old female presented to our institution in January 2005 complaining of recurrent epigastric pain. The patient had suffered from upper abdominal pain, acid reflux, heartburn, and nausea since 2000. In 2002, gastroscopy had revealed hiatal hernia and erosive gastritis, with multiple ulcers, which was only partially improved with proton pump inhibitor (PPI) therapy. The patient's medical and family histories were unremarkable. On physical examination, she had mild direct tenderness in the epigastric region and left upper quadrant of the abdomen, with normal bowel sounds. Routine biochemical testing was normal except mild anemia. Due to these findings, Zollinger-Ellison syndrome (ZES) was suspected, and hormonal testing was carried out. Serum gastrin levels were above the normal limit 1215 pg/mL (normal range 30–100 pg/mL), although PPI withdrawal was not initially performed due to the high risk of gastric bleeding. Subsequently, during hospitalization, PPI were stopped, and symptoms were carefully monitored, thus allowing measurement of gastrin levels after 7 and 10 days of withdrawal, which did not vary significantly (1080 and 990 pg/mL, respectively). Multiple imaging studies were then performed. Endoscopic ultrasound (EUS) revealed multiple small (<1 cm) hypoechoic lesions within the pancreatic head and body and other smaller lesions, with the same characteristics, within the duodenal wall (◘ Fig. 11.1a). Both the pancreatic and the duodenal lesions were confirmed at the contrast-enhanced multidetector computed tomography (CT) (◘ Fig. 11.1b). The 111In-DTPA-octreotide (octreoscan) showed one focal epigastric uptake of the tracer (◘ Fig. 11.2). Possible MEN1-associated diseases were evaluated revealing normal calcium and parathyroid hormone levels, as well as pituitary hormones. Nevertheless, based on the early age of tumor development and multifocality, a genetic test for MEN1 was performed. Detection of a germline MEN1 mutation confirmed the genetic syndrome. The patient underwent surgery in 2006, since clinical symptoms were not fully controlled with PPI. No evidence of metastatic disease had been found on preoperative studies. Laparotomic pylorus-preserving Whipple pancreaticoduodenectomy was performed to remove the gastrinomas. Pathologic examination revealed a diagnosis of well-differentiated neuroendocrine tumor (NET) both in the pancreatic and duodenal lesions. Tumor cells had acidophilic cytoplasm and round nucleoli, arranged in tubular and organoid patterns. The largest duodenal lesion was 5.2 mm in size

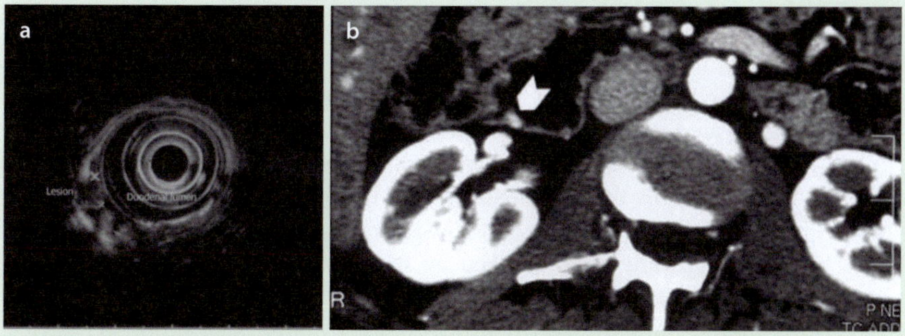

Fig.11.1 **a** Endoscopic ultrasound showing a 5.2 mm hypo-echoic intra-mural nodule within the duodenal wall. **b** Contrast-enhanced multi-detector computed tomography shows a hyper-vascular nodule within the duodenal wall (*arrow head*). The duodenal lumen is distended by water

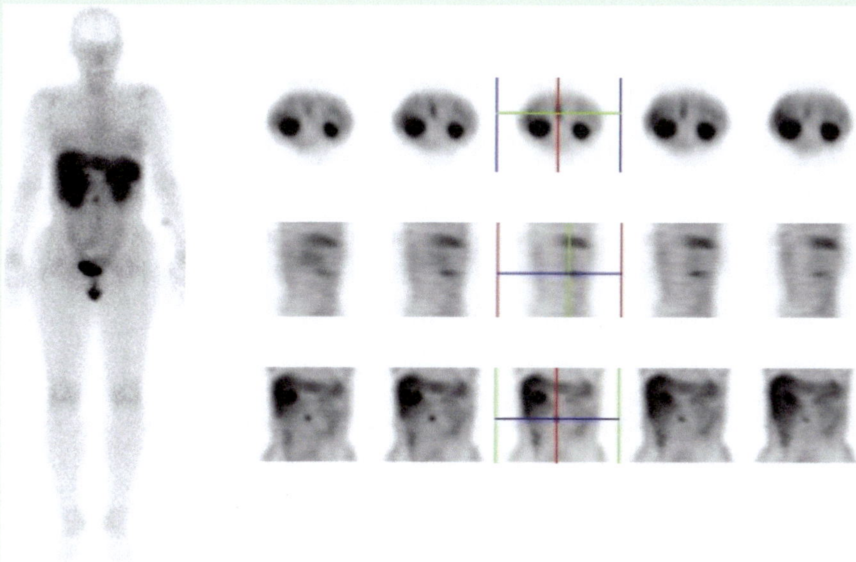

Fig. 11.2 Octreoscan showing focal tracer uptake in the epigastric region

and was positive for gastrin immunostaining. The postoperative level of serum gastrin was within the normal range. One year later hypercalcemia associated to low serum levels of phosphates and high parathyroid hormone levels occurred, leading to a diagnosis of primary hyperparathyroidism (PHPT). The patient was regularly followed up for MEN1 manifestations. Due to occurrence of renal and bone damage, she underwent total parathyroidectomy and subsequently required replacement therapy with calcium and calcitriol for development of hypoparathyroidism. During the follow-up, serum gastrin levels resulted within the normal range, while a new pancreatic NET was detected at the imaging evaluation. This nonfunctioning tumor was stable under therapy with somatostatin analogues (SSA).

11.1 Comments to the Case

ZES is a clinical syndrome characterized by hypergastrinemia derived from gastrinoma, a gastrin-secreting NET, most often located within the duodenal wall or the pancreatic head. Chronic elevated gastrin levels stimulate gastric acid hypersecretion resulting in chronic or recurrent or refractory peptic ulcer disease and/or chronic diarrhea. Diagnosis of ZES requires the demonstration of hormonal hypersecretion with inappropriate fasting hypergastrinemia with acid gastric fluid. As in the case reported, the patient's history is typically characterized by recurrent abdominal pain, peptic ulcer disease, or severe reflux esophagitis and/or diarrhea or by acid-related symptoms which may fail to respond to standard treatment regimens [1, 2]. PPI can suppress gastric acid hypersecretion and control related symptoms; conversely, their widespread use can hide symptoms of ZES. Thus diagnosis of ZES is frequently delayed a mean of 5 years, just what happened to our patient, whose symptoms had begun 5 years before diagnosis. ZES is common in MEN1, as gastrinoma is the most frequent functional NET in this subset of patients [3, 4]. In our patient ZES diagnosis was supported by the tenfold increase of serum gastrin levels, persisting elevated after PPI withdrawal, together with the demonstration of duodenal tumor on imaging. Furthermore, in this case the presence of multiple lesions, located in the pancreas and duodenum, arose the suspicion of MEN1, though in the absence of any other pathological findings.

Questions

1. Which biochemical test allows the diagnosis of gastrinoma?
2. What is the most effective imaging modality to identify gastrinomas?
3. Can the ZES precede primary hyperparathyroidism as the first manifestation of MEN1?

Answers

1. ZES diagnosis requires the combination of fasting hypergastrinemia and elevated gastric acid secretion [5]. Fasting serum gastrin is usually the first biochemical test to be performed, but there is no absolute level of elevated gastrin, which undoubtedly allows the diagnosis of ZES. In a small percentage of patients, gastrin levels can even be normal, and there is a high variability among different assays. Furthermore, a number of other clinical conditions, as chronic atrophic gastritis, *Helicobacter pylori* infection, and chronic renal failure, may alter gastrin levels. The widespread use of PPI makes diagnosis more difficult, as it increases fasting gastrin levels and alters the assessment of gastric acid secretion. In most patients with suspected ZES, the gastric pH is abnormally elevated under PPI. Conversely, PPI withdrawal can be harmful [6]. Evaluation of gastric acid secretion is rarely performed; thus gastrin provocative tests, with secretin or glucagon, can be used although with limited availability and reliability [2].
2. The localization of gastrinoma can be extremely difficult, as they can be very small, though different imaging modalities are currently available. Contrast-enhanced multi-detector CT scan and magnetic resonance imaging (MRI) represent the standard of choice for tumor localization and staging, since gastrinomas are highly vascular tumors [7]. EUS can guide fine needle aspiration and allows

precise assessment of the tumor growth; thus it is especially useful in MEN1 patients with multiple, small NET. Noteworthy contrast-enhanced multi-detector CT has been shown to be complementary to EUS in the identification of pancreatic-duodenal NET in MEN1 [8, 9]. With regard to functional imaging, recent data show higher sensitivity of 68Gallium PET in MEN1, compared with octreoscan, and 68Gallium-DOTATOC-PET/CT is being increasingly used [10–12].

3. Parathyroid tumors, pathologically identified as hyperplasia or adenoma, and related PHPT represent the most common and frequent features of MEN1, occurring in about 95% of patients, usually occurring as the first manifestation, while gastroenteropancreatic (GEP)-NET occurs in approximately 40–70% of patients [13]. Data from the German MEN1 database show that PHPT was the most frequent presentation (41%), but also GEP-NET and pituitary adenomas presented as the first presentation of MEN1 in 22% and 21% of patients, respectively [14]. In a cohort of 160 young MEN1 patients, PHPT was the most frequent disease, but interestingly it occurred as the first symptom in only 56% of them [15]. In a recent Italian study, which included 475 MEN1 patients, PHPT was the first MEN1 manifestation in 291 cases (67% of all patients with overt MEN1 and 71.85% of patients with MEN1-related PHPT), while GEP-NETs were the first MEN1 manifestation in 81 cases (18.6% of all patients with overt MEN1 and 35.2% of patients with MEN1-related GEP-NET). In 16 cases GEP-NETs were the only manifestation of MEN1, while they were associated with other lesions in 214 cases. Among functioning tumors, gastrinoma was the most common with 61 (26.6% of total GEP-NETs) cases [16]. These data highlight PHPT is not always the initial biological or clinical abnormality to appear in MEN1; thus ZES should be suspected as the first manifestation of the genetic syndrome.

Up to Date of the Topic

ZES and gastrinoma can still represent a clinical challenge both for diagnosis and treatment. The incidence of gastrinoma is approximately 0.1–3 persons per million each year in most geographical areas, with a slight female preponderance. To date the real incidence is difficult to identify as there can be an overlap with peptic ulcer disease, and the correct diagnosis may be delayed by the widespread use of PPI that can elevate serum gastrin levels, the cornerstone of biochemical diagnosis. Gastrinoma is most commonly diagnosed in patients aged between 20 and 50 years, although it can arise at any age and commonly arise in the "gastrinoma triangle," comprising the head of the pancreas and the first and second parts of the duodenum [1]. ZES is sporadic in 60–75% of cases, and in the remaining patients, it is associated with MEN1. Both sporadic and MEN1-related gastrinomas may have an aggressive biologic behavior and develop distant metastasis, mainly to the liver. Sporadic ZES is usually due to isolated duodenal or pancreatic gastrinoma, while MEN1 patients commonly have multiple, small (<1.5 cm) gastrinomas arising in the duodenum [4, 17]. Clinical symptoms of ZES overlap with idiopathic peptic ulcer or gastroesophageal reflux, and there are not any unique features which characterize patients with ZES. Fasting serum gastrin is typically elevated, but in a small percentage of patients, gastrin levels can even be normal, and there is a high variability among different assays. The combination of fasting hypergastrinemia and elevated gastric acid secretion allows the diagnosis of ZES. Fasting elevated gastrin levels can be detected in various clinical conditions, as chronic renal failure and chronic atrophic gastritis, but the most common cause is the widespread use of PPI [7]. Thus, it is recommended to stop PPI before establishing the diagnosis of ZES, but their withdrawal can be harmful. If gastrin is >10 times increased with a gastric pH <2.1, ZES is confirmed. If gastrin is <10 times increased with a gastric pH >2.1, which occurs in 66% of ZES patients, a secretin test and measurement of basal acid output should be performed to exclude other diseases. Endoscopic measurement of gastric acid output can be performed using either pH paper or a pH meter. Gastrin provocative tests commonly imply secretin or seldom glucagon, but they are not widely available and require PPI withdrawal too. Secretin test requires intravenous administration of 2 μg/kg bodyweight secretin; an increase in gastrin levels of more than 100 pg/ml is considered positive, whereas a rise of 200 pmg/mL is virtually diagnostic [1, 2, 5, 6]. A number of imaging modalities are currently available to identify gastrinomas, but tumor detection often remains difficult. The early detection of lesions is important to establish diagnosis, to plan surgery, when feasible, and even to monitor the tumor growth. Noteworthy MEN1 patient requires lifelong imaging monitoring with variable intervals; thus concerns arise about the radiation risk, especially in younger patients. Current guidelines indicate either contrast-enhanced multi-detector CT or magnetic resonance imaging (MR) as the standard of choice for tumor localization and staging [7]. However, MR is size dependent, and it can represent a major concern in gastrinomas that are frequently small and multiple in MEN1. EUS can guide fine needle aspiration and allows precise assessment of the tumor growth; thus it is especially useful in MEN1 patients with multiple, small NET. EUS has high sensitivity even for lesions <5 mm, but it is operator dependent and invasive. Furthermore nodular lesions in the pancreatic tail can be missed. Thus contrast-enhanced multi-detector CT and EUS are complementary in identifying pancreatic and duodenal NET [8, 9]. With regard to functional imaging, recent data show that 68Gallium PET in MEN1 is more sensitive than octreoscan, which has been the most widely used and standardized technique [10]. 68Gallium-DOTATOC-PET/CT is being increasingly used, due to its high sensitivity and specificity, the advantage in terms of radiation dose to the patient, and the reduction of the length of the exam, compared with octreoscan [11]. Nevertheless its routine use in screening of MEN1 patients has been questioned, but it allows to obtain significant information in patients with suspected or known metastatic disease [18]. Currently the availability of imaging modality often influences the choice of the clinician. Prospective comparative studies should better define sensitivity and specificity of the different imaging modalities, as well as their possible long-term risk and reliability, together with their optimal sequencing use in specific subset of patients. Noteworthy the prompt and correct identification of ZES can influence treatment, although the optimal management is still debated. Usually medical therapy with PPI to reduce gastric acid secretion represents the first-line therapy, due to their efficacy and cost-effectiveness. Often high PPI doses may be required, although some concerns about their long-term use, as the rebound of acid hypersecretion if stopped, a possible increased risk of gastric cancer, malabsorption of nutrients, fractures, and small intestinal bacterial overgrowth [6, 19, 20]. In sporadic ZES, 40–70% of patients already have lymph node metastases at surgery, and even in patients with MEN-1, gastrinomas have a very high risk to develop metastasis. Thus surgical cure requires an aggressive resection such as a pancreaticoduodenectomy. Surgery in sporadic gastrinomas is curative in about 60% of patients, but all ZES patients without MEN1 who do not have a medical contraindication should undergo surgical exploration. The role of surgical resection is more controversial in MEN1, due to the complex risk/benefit assessment. Extensive surgery may be curative, though it is not routinely recommended [1, 5, 7]. SSA (octreotide and lanreotide) appear an interesting option particularly in MEN1 since the management of gastrinoma should address both the control of symptoms due to the hormone hypersecretion and the gastrinoma itself. However to date there is no indication in routine use of SSA in ZES [21, 22].

In conclusion, ZES is a clinical syndrome determined by gastrinomas mainly located in the duodenum and pancreas, whose symptoms may be closely similar to idiopathic peptic disease. Biochemical diagnosis and tumor detection can be challenging, but it is crucial to achieve an early identification, in order to plan the best management strategy and avoid metastatic progression.

Bibliography

1. Epelboym I, Mazeh H (2014) Zollinger-Ellison syndrome: classical considerations and current controversies. Oncologist 19(1):44–50
2. Ito T, Cadiot G, Jensen RT (2012) Diagnosis of Zollinger-Ellison syndrome: increasingly difficult. World J Gastroenterol 18(39):5495–5503
3. Gibril F, Schumann M, Pace A, Jensen RT (2004) Multiple endocrine neoplasia type 1 and Zollinger-Ellison syndrome: a prospective study of 107 cases and comparison with 1009 cases from the literature. Medicine (Baltimore) 83(1):43–83
4. Ito T, Igarashi H, Uehara H, Jensen RT (2013) Pharmacotherapy of Zollinger-Ellison syndrome. Expert Opin Pharmacother 14(3):307–321
5. Jensen RT (2004) Gastrinomas: advances in diagnosis and management. Neuroendocrinology 80(Suppl 1):23–27
6. Singh Ospina N, Donegan D, Rodriguez-Gutierrez R, Al-Hilli Z, Young WF Jr. (2016) Assessing for multiple endocrine neoplasia type 1 in patients evaluated for Zollinger-Ellison Syndrome-Clues to a safer diagnostic process. Am J Med.. pii: S0002-9343(16)31249-9. doi:10.1016/j.amjmed.2016.11.035. [Epub ahead of print]
7. Falconi M, Eriksson B, Kaltsas G, Bartsch DK, Capdevila J, Caplin M, Kos-Kudla B, Kwekkeboom D, Rindi G, Klöppel G, Reed N, Kianmanesh R, Jensen RT (2016) Vienna consensus conference participants. ENETS consensus guidelines update for the Management of Patients with functional pancreatic neuroendocrine tumors and non-functional pancreatic neuroendocrine tumors. Neuroendocrinology 103(2):153–171
8. Norton JA, Jensen RT (2004) Resolved and unresolved controversies in the surgical management of patients with Zollinger-Ellison syndrome. Ann Surg 240(5):757–773
9. Camera L, Paoletta S, Mollica C, Milone F, Napolitano V, De Luca L, Faggiano A, Colao A, Salvatore M (2011 Jun) Screening of pancreaticoduodenal endocrine tumours in patients with MEN 1: multidetector-row computed tomography vs. endoscopic ultrasound. Radiol Med 116(4):595–606
10. Froeling V, Elgeti F, Maurer MH, Scheurig-Muenkler C, Beck A, Kroencke TJ, Pape UF, Hamm B, Brenner W, Schreiter NF (2012) Impact of Ga-68 DOTATOC PET/CT on the diagnosis and treatment of patients with multiple endocrine neoplasia. Ann Nucl Med 26(9):738–743
11. Lastoria S, Marciello F, Faggiano A, Aloj L, Caracò C, Aurilio M, D'Ambrosio L, Di Gennaro F, Ramundo V, Camera L, De Luca L, Fonti R, Napolitano V, Colao A (2016) Role of (68)Ga-DOTATATE PET/CT in patients with multiple endocrine neoplasia type 1 (MEN1). Endocrine 52(3):488–494

12. Ito T, Jensen RT (2016) Imaging in multiple endocrine neoplasia type 1: recent studies show enhanced sensitivities but increased controversies. Int J Endocr Oncol 3(1):53–66
13. Thakker RV, Newey PJ, Walls GV, Bilezikian J, Dralle H, Ebeling PR, Melmed S, Sakurai A, Tonelli F, Brandi ML (2012) Endocrine Society. Clinical practice guidelines for multiple endocrine neoplasia type 1 (MEN1). J Clin Endocrinol Metab 97(9):2990–3011
14. Schaaf L, Pickel J, Zinner K, Hering U, Höfler M, Goretzki PE, Spelsberg F, Raue F, von zur Mühlen A, Gerl H, Hensen J, Bartsch DK, Rothmund M, Schneyer U, Dralle H, Engelbach M, Karges W, Stalla GK, Höppner W (2007) Developing effective screening strategies in multiple endocrine neoplasia type 1 (MEN 1) on the basis of clinical and sequencing data of German patients with MEN 1. Exp Clin Endocrinol Diabetes 115(8):509–517
15. Goudet P, Dalac A, Le Bras M, Cardot-Bauters C, Niccoli P, Lévy-Bohbot N, du Boullay H, Bertagna X, Ruszniewski P, Borson-Chazot F, Vergès B, Sadoul JL, Ménégaux F, Tabarin A, Kühn JM, d'Anella P, Chabre O, Christin-Maitre S, Cadiot G, Binquet C, Delemer B (2015) MEN1 disease occurring before 21 years old: a 160-patient cohort study from the Groupe d'étude des Tumeurs endocrines. J Clin Endocrinol Metab 100(4):1568–1577
16. Giusti F, Cianferotti L, Boaretto F, Cetani F, Cioppi F, Colao A, Davì MV, Faggiano A, Fanciulli G, Ferolla P, Ferone D, Fossi C, Giudici F, Gronchi G, Loli P, Mantero F, Marcocci C, Marini F, Masi L, Opocher G, Beck-Peccoz P, Persani L, Scillitani A, Sciortino G, Spada A, Tomassetti P, Tonelli F, Brandi ML (2017) Multiple endocrine neoplasia syndrome type 1: institution, management, and data analysis of a nationwide multicenter patient database. Endocrine. doi: 10.1007/s12020-017-1234-4 [Epub ahead of print]
17. Anlauf M, Garbrecht N, Henopp T, Schmitt A, Schlenger R, Raffel A, Krausch M, Gimm O, Eisenberger CF, Knoefel WT, Dralle H, Komminoth P, Heitz PU, Perren A, Klöppel G (2006) Sporadic versus hereditary gastrinomas of the duodenum and pancreas: distinct clinico-pathological and epidemiological features. World J Gastroenterol 12(34):5440–5446
18. Albers MB, Librizzi D, Lopez CL, Manoharan J, Apitzsch JC, Slater EP, Bollmann C, Kann PH, Bartsch DK (2017) Limited value of Ga-68-DOTATOC-PET-CT in routine screening of patients with multiple endocrine neoplasia type 1. World J Surg 41(6):1521–1527. doi:10.1007/s00268-017-3907-9. [Epub ahead of print]

19. Jensen RT (2006) Consequences of long-term proton pump blockade: insights from studies of patients with gastrinomas. Basic Clin Pharmacol Toxicol 98(1):4–19
20. Corleto VD, Festa S, Di Giulio E, Annibale B (2014) Proton pump inhibitor therapy and potential long-term harm. Curr Opin Endocrinol Diabetes Obes 21(1):3–8
21. Auernhammer CJ, Göke B (2007) Medical treatment of gastrinomas. Wien Klin Wochenschr 119(19–20):609–615
22. Massironi S, Zilli A, Conte D (2015) Somatostatin analogs for gastric carcinoids: for many, but not all. World J Gastroenterol 21(22):6785–6793

Tumor Detection in Syndromic NET: Hypoglycemic Hyperinsulinemic Syndrome

Elisa Cosaro and Maria Vittoria Davi

A. Colao et al. (eds.), *Neuroendocrine Tumors in Real Life*,
https://doi.org/10.1007/978-3-319-59024-0_12

Overview

Hypoglycemic hyperinsulinemic syndrome is characterized by inappropriate increased levels of insulin in the presence of low plasma glucose concentrations. In adults, it is caused in most cases by an insulinoma and less frequently by nesidioblastosis or autoimmune hypoglycemia. After biochemical diagnosis, imaging techniques are performed to localize the insulinoma and plan the best surgical approach. The most used noninvasive radiological techniques are abdomen ultrasonography (US), computed tomography scan, or magnetic resonance imaging, the choice depending on their availability and on the local radiologist's expertise. In case of negative or discordant results, endoscopic US and/or selective arterial calcium stimulation test with hepatic venous sampling can be performed to localize the tumor or to diagnose nesidioblastosis. Nowadays, nearly 98% of insulinomas are detected with the preoperative tests plus intraoperative US.

Clinical Case

12

In 2014, a 40-year-old obese man was referred for evaluation of hypoglycemic episodes associated with tachycardia, sweating, and tremor that occurred during fast and resolved after eating. The patient was admitted for a 72-h supervised fast that was stopped after 8 h when he developed symptoms of hypoglycemia. At the time glucose was 46 mg/dl, insulin 11.3 mcU/mL, and C-peptide 2.63 ng/ml. Administration of IV dextrose resulted in prompt resolution of his symptoms with normalization of glucose level. The insulin antibodies were negative. The patient subsequently underwent conventional radiological diagnostic procedures, such as abdomen computed tomography (CT) and magnetic resonance imaging (MRI), which failed to detect the insulinoma (◘ Fig. 12.1). Consequently, he underwent endoscopic ultrasound (EUS) which showed an uncertain 5-mm nodule in the tail of the pancreas. Given the inconclusive results of the imaging tests, the patient was submitted to a selective arterial calcium stimulation test (SACST), which showed a twofold hepatic vein insulin increase after injection of calcium at the splenic artery, 1.6-fold increase at gastroduodenal artery, and no increase at superior mesenteric artery. MEN1 diagnosis was excluded by genetic testing. The patient underwent a laparoscopic left splenopancreatectomy after doing an intraoperative US that revealed a 1.5 cm nodule at the body-tail of the pancreas (◘ Fig. 12.2). The pathological report was consistent with the diagnosis of a G2-NET, with Ki67 of 3% and insulin positivity at immunochemistry. The long-term follow-up showed normal glucose levels proving that surgery had been successful.

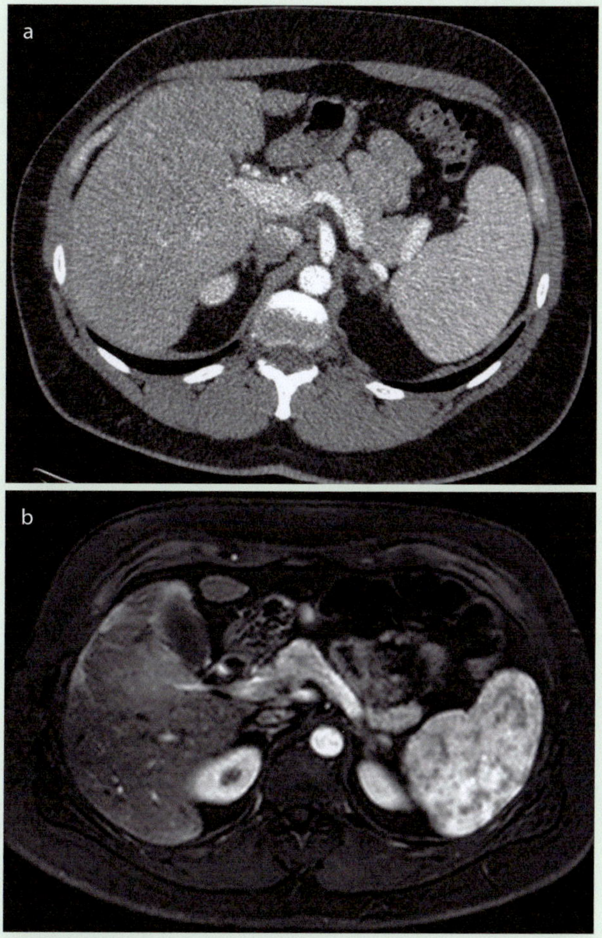

Fig. 12.1 **a** CT and **b** MR: on pancreatic phase the pancreatic lesion is not visible and was missed preoperatively

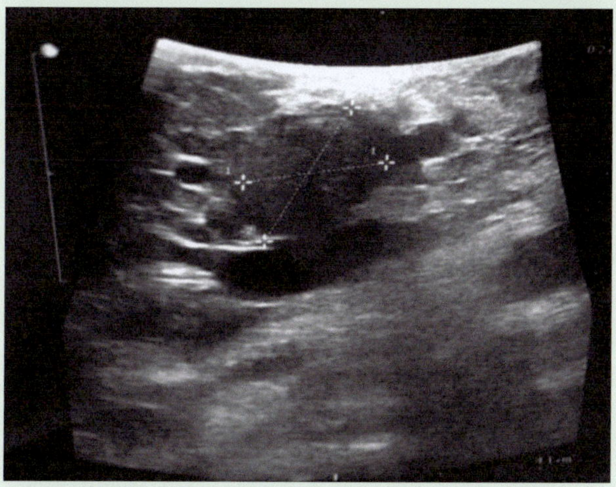

Fig. 12.2 Intraoperative US: small hypoechoic nodule with well-defined margins is visible at the pancreatic body near to the pancreatic isthmus

12.1 Comments to the Case

The Whipple triad, which includes symptoms consistent with hypoglycemia, a low plasma glucose concentration, and resolution of symptoms after the plasma glucose concentration is raised, was established. As a consequence, a fasting test was performed to differentiate between insulin-mediated or non-insulin-mediated hypoglycemia. The laboratory data were compatible with insulinoma, according to the following cutoff established by the Endocrine Society guidelines: insulin of ≥ 3 μU/ml ($\geq$ 18 pmol/l), C-peptide ≥ 0.6 ng/ml ($\geq$ 0.2 nmol/l) in the presence of glycemia <55 mg/dl [1]. The negative insulin antibodies excluded the diagnosis of autoimmune hypoglycemia, a disease that rarely occurs in the Caucasian population and that generally presents a high level of insulin, usually greater than 100 mcU/mL. The localization of the tumor meant that the best surgical approach, i.e., enucleation vs pancreatic resection in open or laparoscopic surgery, can be planned. The conventional radiological imaging failed to detect the tumor, as in about 30% of insulinomas that show an «atypical» vascular pattern resulting in iso- or even hypoattenuating lesions with respect to adjacent pancreatic parenchyma. In the present case in which the EUS also gave an uncertain result, SACTS played an important role in regionalizing the source of insulin hypersecretion at the body-tail of the pancreas. Furthermore, the intraoperative (I)US was useful in defining the exact site of the tumor, which appeared as a hypoechoic lesion, and its relationship with adjacent vascular structures and with the pancreatic duct for choice of the appropriate surgical approach. Laparoscopic distal splenopancreatectomy instead of enucleation was carried out because of the tumor proximity to the pancreatic duct.

Questions

12

1. What is the best localization procedure to start the diagnostic workup of a suspected insulinoma?
2. In the case of MEN1 patients, what is the best diagnostic procedure?

Answers

1. There is not one best localization procedure. The choice of imaging procedures depends on the expertise of the radiologist and the availability of equipment.
2. According to recent literature, given the multiplicity of insulinomas in MEN1 patients, EUS is the best procedure due to its high sensitivity in detecting small lesions of the pancreas. It is also useful because it allows a biopsy to be performed to confirm the diagnosis.

Up to Date of the Topic

Hypoglycemic hyperinsulinemic syndrome (HHS) is characterized by inappropriate increased levels of insulin in the presence of low plasma glucose concentrations. In adults, it is caused in most cases by an insulinoma and less frequently by nesidioblastosis that can occur as a feature of the noninsulinoma pancreatogenous hypoglycemia syndrome (NIPHS) or of post-gastric bypass hypoglycemia. Furthermore, in the differential diagnosis, we must consider the possibility of the insulin autoimmune hypoglycemia that occurs in patients who have antibodies directed to endogenous insulin (Hirata's syndrome) and also the self-administration of a beta cell secretagogue, such as a sulfonylurea or repaglinide [1–3].

HHS should be suspected in patients in whom Whipple's triad is documented. Once Whipple's triad has been confirmed, diagnostic evaluation is usually recommended in a healthy-appearing patient, whereas it is not required in an ill or medicated patient in whom hypoglycemia may be easily recognized as part of the underlying illness or its treatment [1]. Measurement of insulin and C-peptide is mandatory during a spontaneous episode of hypoglycemia or a provoked one by tests such as supervised fast or mixed meal test to differentiate between insulin-mediated or non-insulin-mediated hypoglycemia. In a series of 170 patients, 99% had a positive fast test within 72 h [4]. Insulin antibodies should also be measured in all cases of HHS. Autoimmune hypoglycemia is a rare disorder in Caucasian race, whereas it is more common in East Asian populations. It results from the unregulated release of insulin bound to the antibodies independent of the prevailing serum glucose [5]. A correct diagnosis is important to avoid unnecessary invasive diagnostic procedures or surgical intervention of pancreatic resection. Only when the biochemical diagnosis of HHS is confirmed and the presence of insulin antibodies is excluded, should imaging diagnostic tests be performed in order to detect the insulinoma [6]. Localization tests include noninvasive procedures, such as abdominal US, CT, and MRI and invasive procedures such as endoscopic US (EUS) and SACST. The mean sensitivity of abdomen US is less than 70% and depends on several factors, such as operator's expertise, tumor diameter, and patient's habitus [7]. Given that the majority of insulinomas are smaller than 2 cm, they can easily be missed by US. A significant improvement in the diagnosis and localization of insulinoma has been obtained by contrast-enhanced US (CEUS) with a sensitivity of up to 89.2% [8]. The intravenous administration of sonographic contrast may help in the identification of the lesion as it typically appears at CEUS as a hypervascular lesion [9]. The multidetector CT (MDCT) scan is generally considered the first imaging technique to localize the insulinoma due to its high detection rate, wide availability, and short examination time. Its sensitivity ranges between 83 and 95.3% [10–12]. On CT, insulinomas are usually isodense to normal parenchyma on baseline scan and appear as brightly enhancing lesions that demonstrate rapid washout in the portal and late venous phases [13]. Less than 20% of insulinomas show an «atypical» appearance, as result of arterial hypovascularity due to the presence of abundant fibrous stroma. The information obtained with MRI is similar to that obtained by CT with the advantage that the patient is spared radiation exposure. However, the examination time is longer compared to CT, and it is less available among the centers. On MRI, the majority of insulinomas displays low signal intensity on T1-weighted fat-suppressed images and high signal intensity on T2-weighted images. During the contrast-enhanced study, the lesion typically shows hypervascularity during the arterial phase and subsequent washout during late venous phase [13, 14]. Its sensitivity is variable reaching 95–100% in some studies [15, 16]. Diffusion-weighted sequences may help in the identification of these tumors based on its sensitivity and contrast resolution [17].

EUS is an effective tool for detecting insulinomas with higher sensitivity at the head and body of the pancreas (92.6% and 78.9%, respectively) compared to the tail (40%) [18, 19]. EUS can be superior to CT/MRI to detect small pancreatic NETs in patients with MEN1 in whom the possibility of multiple lesions is high. Thus, some authors recommend EUS as the first-choice pancreas imaging technique in patients with MEN1 [20]. The drawbacks of this procedure are the limited availability, invasiveness, and requirement of skill endoscopist.

SACTS is indicated in the case of negative or inconclusive results of conventional imaging procedures to localize or regionalize occult insulinomas with a sensitivity of up to 92.8% [21–23]. It may also be useful in differentiating an insulinoma from nesidioblastosis with high specificity in patients with HHS [23]. The procedure consists of catheterization of the right hepatic vein via the inferior vena cava after puncture of the femoral vein and catheterization with selected injection of calcium into the GDA, SMA, and SA. An increase in hepatic vein insulin of at least two- to three-fold at 20, 40, and 60 seconds after injection of calcium will regionalize the source of excess insulin secretion to the head of the pancreas (GDA), the uncinate (SMA), and head-body (SA). In about 25% of surgically confirmed insulinomas, biochemical results were positive in more than one arterial distribution as a result of aberrant arterial anatomy [24].

As regards nuclear medicine imaging, due to the low expression of somatostatin receptor (SSTR) type 2 in benign insulinomas, SSTR scintigraphy (Octreoscan) detection rate has been reported relatively low, of up to 47% [26]. 68Ga-DOTANOC PET/CT has also limited utility for localizing the insulinoma in patients with clinical and biochemical suspicion of HHS [27].

Recently, ^{111}In-DOTA-exendin-4 SPECT-CT has been shown to be highly sensitive (≥ 95% sensitivity) in detecting insulinomas, targeting the glucagon-like peptide-1 receptors (GLP-1R) highly expressed in these tumors [27]. ^{68}Ga-DOTA-exendine-4 PET-CT has been reported as having a higher spatial resolution and lower radiation burden compared with ^{111}In-DOTA-exendin-4 SPECT-CT [28]. Thus, this technique could become a promising tool in detecting insulinomas if its high sensitivity is confirmed in larger series.

12

Finally, IUS plays an important role in identifying the insulinoma, its relationship with the pancreatic duct and blood vessels for a correct surgical approach (enucleation or resection) [29].

12.2 Conclusions

Only after the biochemical diagnosis of insulinoma has been confirmed, should the imaging techniques be performed to localize the tumor and plan the best surgical approach. The most frequently used noninvasive localization procedures are abdomen CT scan or MRI that detect the insulinoma in about 90% of cases. EUS can help to find small tumors mainly in the head and body of the pancreas and confirm the diagnosis with fine needle biopsy. In the case of negative or inconclusive results of these imaging techniques, SACS test with hepatic venous sampling can be considered in the diagnostic workup of HH to regionalize the insulin hypersecretion and/or to diagnose nesidioblastosis.

Bibliography

1. Cryer PE, Axelrod L, Grossman AB, Heller SR, Montori VM, Seaquist ER, Service FJ (2009) Endocrine Society SO evaluation and management of adult hypoglycemic disorders: an Endocrine Society clinical practice guideline. AU J Clin Endocrinol Metab 94(3):709
2. Service FJ (1999) Classification of hypoglycemic disorders. Endocrinol Metab Clin N Am 28(3):501
3. Davi MV, Pia A, Guarnotta V, Pizza G, Colao A, Faggiano A, NIKE Group (2017) The treatment of hyperinsulinemic hypoglycaemia in adults: an update. J Endocrinol Investig 40:9–20
4. Placzkowski KA, Vella A, Thompson GB et al (2009) Secular trends in the presentation and management of functioning insulinoma at the Mayo Clinic,1987–2007. J Clin Endocrinol Metab 94:1069–1073
5. Lupsa BC, Chong AY, Cochran EK, Soos MA, Semple RK, Gorden P (2009) Autoimmune forms of hypoglycemia. Medicine (Baltimore) 88(3):141–153
6. Davi' MV, Falconi M (2009) Pancreas: Insulinoma--new insights into an old disease. Nat Rev Endocrinol 5:300–302
7. Mehrabi A, Fischer L, Hafezi M, Dirlewanger A, Grenacher L, Diener MK, Fonouni H, Golriz M, Garoussi C, Fard N, Rahbari NN, Werner J, Büchler MW (2014) A systematic review of localization, surgical treatment options, and outcome of insulinoma. Pancreas 43(5):675–686
8. An L, Li W, Yao KC, Liu R, Lv F, Tang J, Zhang S (2011) Assessment of contrast-enhanced ultrasonography in diagnosis and preoperative localization of insulinoma. Eur J Radiol 80(3):675–680
9. D' Onofrio M, Mansueto G, Vasori S, Falconi M, Procacci C (2003) Contrast-enhanced ultrasonographic detection of small pancreatic insulinoma. J Ultrasound Med 22(4):413–417
10. Zhao YP, Zhan HX, Zhang TP et al (2011) Surgical management of patients with insulinomas: result of 292 cases in a single institution. J Surg Oncol 103:169–174
11. Jyotsna VP, Rangel N, Pal S et al (2006) Insulinoma: diagnosis and surgical treatment. Retrospective analysis of 31 cases. Indian J Gastroenterol 25:244–247
12. Gouya H, Vignaux O, Augui J et al (2003) CT, endoscopic sonography, and a combined protocol for preoperative evaluation of pancreatic insulinomas. AJR Am J Roentgenol 181:987–992
13. Graziani R, Brandalise A, Bellotti M, Manfredi R, Contro A, Falconi M, Boninsegna L, Pozzi MR (2010) Imaging of neuroendocrine gastroenteropancreatic tumours. Radiol Med 115(7):1047–1064
14. Thoeni RF, Mueller-Lisse UG, Chan R, Do NK, Shyn PB (2000) Detection of small, functional islet cell tumors in the pancreas: selection of MR imaging sequences for optimal sensitivity. Radiology 214(2):483–490
15. Ichikawa T, Peterson MS, Federle MP et al (2000) Islet cell tumor of the pancreas: biphasic CT versus MR imaging in tumor detection. Radiology 216:163–171
16. Menegaux F, Schmitt G, Mercadier M (1993) Pancreatic insulinomas. Am J Surg 165:243–248
17. Caramella C, Dromain C, De Baere T, Boulet B, Schlumberger M, Ducreux M, Baudin E (2010) Endocrine pancreatic tumours: which are the most useful MRI sequences? Eur Radiol 20(11):2618–2627
18. Sotoudehmanesh R, Hedayat A, Shirazian N et al (2007) Endoscopic ultrasonography (EUS) in the localization of insulinoma. Endocrine 31:238–241
19. Joseph AJ, Kapoor N, Simon EG, Chacko A, Thomas EM, Eapen A, Abraham DT, Jacob PM, Paul T, Rajaratnam S, Thomas N (2013) Endoscopic ultrasonography--a sensitive tool in the preoperative localization of insulinoma. Endocr Pract 19(4):602–608
20. van Asselt SJ, Brouwers AH, van Dullemen HM, van der Jagt EJ, Bongaerts AH, Kema IP, Koopmans KP, Valk GD, Timmers HJ, de Herder WW, Feelders RA, Fockens P, Sluiter WJ, de Vries EG, Links TP (2015) EUS is superior for detection of pancreatic lesions compared with standard imaging in patients with multiple endocrine neoplasia type 1. Gastrointest Endosc 81(1):159–167
21. Doppman JL, Miller DL, Chang R, Shawker TH, Gorden P, Norton JA (1991) Insulinomas: localization with selective intraarterial injection of calcium. Radiology 178(1):237–241
22. Guettier JM, Kam A, Chang R, Skarulis MC, Cochran C, Alexander HR, Libutti SK, Pingpank JF, Gorden P (2009) Localization of insulinomas to regions of the pancreas by intraarterial calcium stimulation: the NIH experience. J Clin Endocrinol Metab 94(4):1074–1080

23. Thompson SM, Vella A, Thompson GB, Rumilla KM, Service FJ, Grant CS, Andrews JC (2015) Selective arterial calcium stimulation with hepatic venous sampling differentiates Insulinoma from nesidioblastosis. J Clin Endocrinol Metab 100(11):4189–4197
24. Thompson SM, Vella A, Service FJ, Grant CS, Thompson GB, Andrews JC (2015) Impact of variant pancreatic arterial anatomy and overlap in regional perfusion on the interpretation of selective arterial calcium stimulation with hepatic venous sampling for preoperative localization of occult insulinoma. Surgery 158(1):162–172
26. Mirallie E, Pattou F, Malvaux P et al (2002) Value of endoscopic ultrasonography and somatostatin receptor scintigraphy in the preoperative localization of insulinomas and gastrinomas. Experience of 54 cases. Gastroenterol Clin Biol 26:360–366
27. Sharma P, Arora S, Karunanithi S, Khadgawat R, Durgapal P, Sharma R, Kandasamy D, Bal C, Kumar R (2016) Somatostatin receptor based PET/CT imaging with 68Ga-DOTA-Nal3-octreotide for localization of clinically and biochemically suspected insulinoma. Q J Nucl Med Mol Imaging 60(1):69–76
27. Christ E, Wild D, Ederer S, Béhé M, Nicolas G, Caplin ME, Brändle M, Clerici T, Fischli S, Stettler C, Ell PJ, Seufert J, Gloor B, Perren A, Reubi JC, Forrer F (2013) Glucagon-like peptide-1 receptor imaging for the localisation of insulinomas: a prospective multicentre imaging study. Lancet Diabetes Endocrinol 1:115–122
28. Antwi K, Fani M, Nicolas G, Rottenburger C, Heye T, Reubi JC, Gloor B, Christ E, Wild D (2015) Localization of hidden Insulinomas with 68Ga-DOTA-Exendin-4 PET/CT: a pilot study. J Nucl Med 56:1075–1078
29. Grover AC, Skarulis M, Alexander HR, Pingpank JF, Javor ED, Chang R, Shawker T, Gorden P, Cochran C, Libutti SK (2005) A prospective evaluation of laparoscopic exploration with intraoperative ultrasound as a technique for localizing sporadic insulinomas. Surgery 138:1003–1008

Tumor Staging: Bronchi

Pier Luigi Filosso, Francesco Guerrera, Matteo Roffinella, Paolo Solidoro, and Alberto Sandri

A. Colao et al. (eds.), *Neuroendocrine Tumors in Real Life*,
https://doi.org/10.1007/978-3-319-59024-0_13

Overview

Peripheral bronchopulmonary carcinoids (BCs) are oftentimes totally asymptomatic and incidentally diagnosed, while centrally located ones are usually discovered through the symptoms caused by the obstruction of the central airway. Contrast CT scan represents the gold standard radiological imaging for the preoperative workup, while FDG-PET scan is still controversial. Bronchoscopy, generally negative in the peripheral forms, makes possible to detect the lesion and to biopsy the tumor, in case of central BCs. Surgery represents the mainstay of treatment, and anatomical resections associated with systemic lymphadenectomy should be performed. Postoperative long-term clinical and radiological follow-up is mandatory, especially in case of biologically aggressive tumoral forms: local relapses or distant metastases are, in fact, reported even many years after the first operation.

Clinical Case

A 42-year-old totally asymptomatic woman was admitted in our hospital after the incidental diagnosis of two bilateral pulmonary nodules through a chest X-ray occasionally performed. She was not an active smoker, and she worked as an administrative employee in an International Company. Bronchoscopy was negative; a generic «carcinoma not otherwise specified» diagnosis was achieved through a transthoracic fine-needle aspiration biopsy in the right-sided nodule. FDG-PET scan revealed a 4.8 SUV uptake in the right node (▣ Fig. 13.1) and a 2.3 SUV in the left one.

13

The patient underwent an anterolateral right thoracotomy; through a small wedge resection, the nodule was resected and a frozen section revealed a *neuroendocrine neoplasia* (the pathologists were unable to differentiate between an atypical or a typical carcinoid). Therefore, the patient received a right lower lobectomy. Through an accurate residual lung palpation, other three nodules were also found in the upper lobe, and all were resected with two limited wedge resections. Definitive histological diagnosis revealed multifocal pT4N0 atypical carcinoid. Postoperative octreoscan was performed, revealing an elective uptake at the left-sided nodule. Twenty days after the first intervention, the patient underwent to a small left anterolateral thoracotomy, through which a left lower lobe segmental resection with systematic lymphadenectomy was performed. Definitive histology revealed another multifocal (three nodules in the same segment, pT3N0) atypical carcinoid. A strict clinical/radiological follow-up was started, and the patient is alive and disease-free 6 years after the interventions.

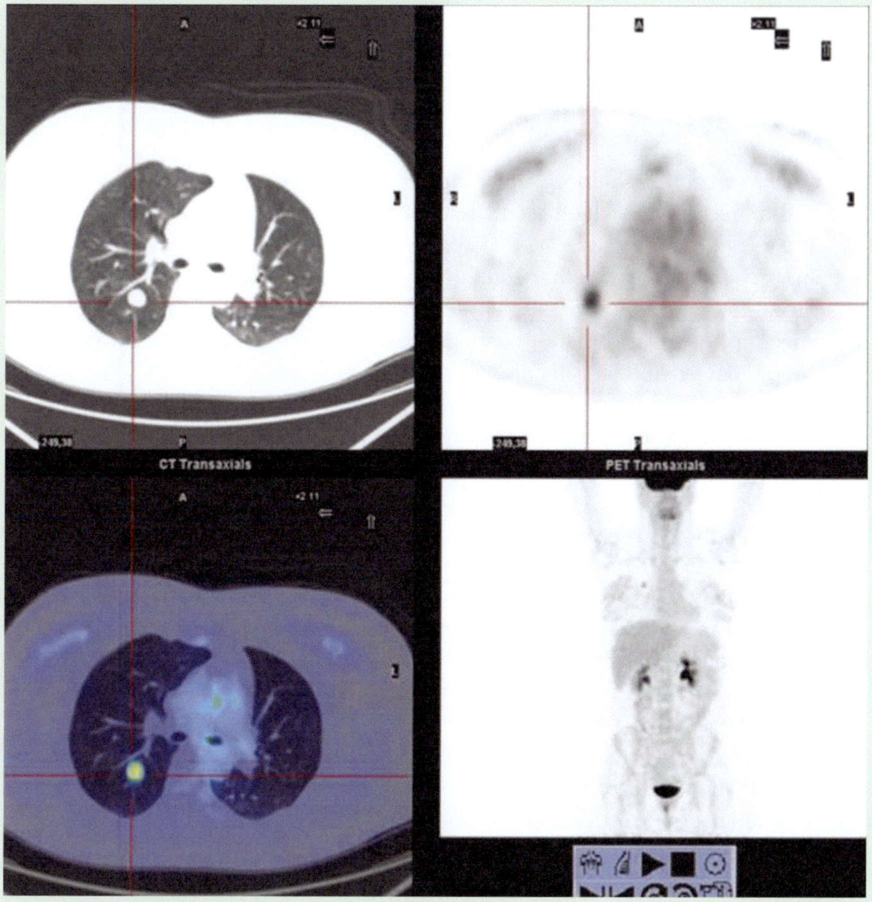

Fig. 13.1 Clinical case report: preoperative FDG-PET scan: SUV 4.8 elective uptake at the right- sided lung nodule

13.1 Comments to the Case

This is a real unusual clinical case of bronchopulmonary carcinoid, and it presents several matters of discussion.

Questions

1. How a lung neuroendocrine tumor may be diagnosed?
2. Is there a role for a preoperative PET scan?
3. Which lung resection should be performed?
4. Is clinical/radiological follow-up always recommended?

Answers

1. Especially in case of a peripheral lesion, a bronchopulmonary carcinoid may be totally asymptomatic, and incidentally discovered, generally through a chest X-ray performed for other reasons. Moreover, bronchoscopy may be negative, particularly when the lesion is small and peripheral. Very often, a preoperative correct cyto/histological tumor confirmation is quite impossible, due to the difficulty to recognize the peculiar features (e.g., the presence and number of mitosis and/or necrosis) which differentiate typical from atypical carcinoids.
2. The role of preoperative FDG-PET scan is still controversial: however, in case of a suspect undiagnosed solitary pulmonary nodule, it should be always performed.
3. An anatomical resection (segmentectomy/lobectomy) and systematic lymphadenectomy are usually recommended. An increased risk of tumor recurrence has been reported in case of incomplete resections.
4. A long-term clinical and radiological follow-up is mandatory, especially in case of biologically aggressive tumoral forms. Local relapses or distant metastases are, in fact, reported even many years after the first operation.

Up to Date of the Topic

Preoperative diagnostic workup. One-third of patients with bronchopulmonary carcinoids (BCs) are asymptomatic, and the neoplasm is incidentally discovered, while performing a radiological examination for other reasons. In case of centrally located lesions (■ Fig. 13.2), symptoms may include obstructive pneumonia, atelectasis, and wheezing, caused by the obstruction of the central airway. Prolonged treatments for pneumonia or asthma are occasionally observed in central forms and often precede the eventual tumor diagnosis [1, 2]. Functioning carcinoids are relatively infrequent (no more than 10–15% of cases); the most common associated hormonal syndrome is the ectopic adrenocorticotropic hormone (ACTH) secretion, the so-called Cushing's syndrome (CS). In approximately 1% of all CS patients, the ectopic ACTH secretion is caused by a bronchopulmonary carcinoid [3]. Other less frequent hormonal

13

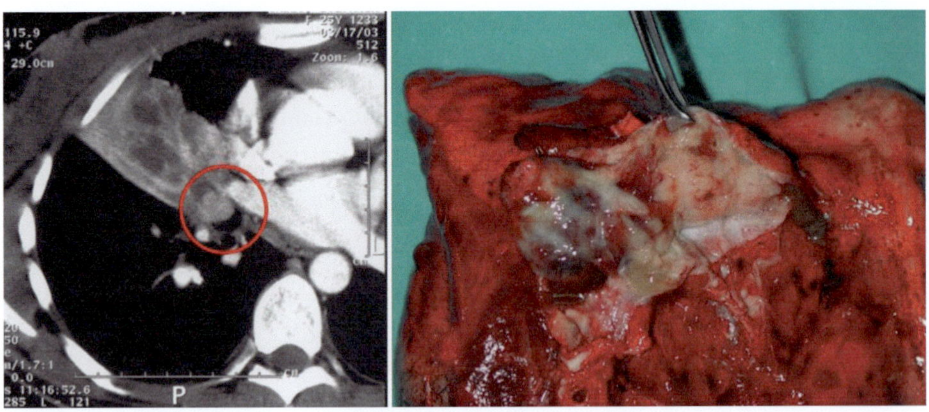

■ **Fig. 13.2** Centrally located right-sided typical carcinoid: CT scan and surgical specimen. The *red* circle shows the endobronchial tumor component which causes atelectasis

syndromes are due to ectopic secretion of growth hormone (GH), antidiuretic hormone (ADH), and parathyroid hormone (PTH) [3, 5]. The authors of this chapter have also recently observed a very rare clinical case of BC associated with myasthenia gravis. In less than 5% of the cases, BCs may be associated with multiple endocrine neoplasia type 1 (MEN 1) syndrome [6, 7].

From the epidemiological point of view, there is an equal distribution between male and female in BCs, and they may occur at any age, even if typical carcinoid is one of the most frequent tumors in childhood [8]. BCs' incidence has increased over the past 30 years, probably due to the large diffusion of lung cancer screening programs and the increased use of more sensitive and specific neuroendocrine tumor markers in routine histopathology; Hauso *and Coll* [8] recently reported that bronchopulmonary carcinoids were the most common neuroendocrine tumor in the USA.

The gold standard radiological imaging for the preoperative patient's evaluation is the contrast CT scan [9]. The typical appearance of a peripheral form is a round or ovoid lung nodule with smooth or lobular margins [10, 11] (◘ Fig. 13.3), which does not differ from other small peripheral primary lung cancers. Atelectasis, air trapping, and/or remarks of obstructive pneumonia, lung abscess/bronchiectasis are the most common signs of a tumor with a central location and an endobronchial growth (◘ Fig. 13.2). A correct mediastinal evaluation is also of paramount importance, since lymph nodal metastases (◘ Fig. 13.4) may be possible even at presentation [4].

Nuclear medicine plays an important role in the preoperative workup for patients with bronchopulmonary carcinoids. The role of FDG-PET scan is still debated and controversial, since it is reported to be negative in low proliferative tumors (generally typical carcinoid) (◘ Fig. 13.5) and often positive in case of more aggressive ones (atypical carcinoid). Therefore, it has been advocated that PET scan may be useful to determine BC's biological behavior [12, 13].

^{111}In-pentetreotide/octreotide scintigraphy (octreoscan) has been historically used to detect BCs and also to evaluate possible lymph nodal involvement, since more than 80% of them express somatostatin-type receptor-2 and receptor-5 ($SSTR_2$ and $SSTR_5$) [14]; this nuclear medicine examination has shown high specificity and

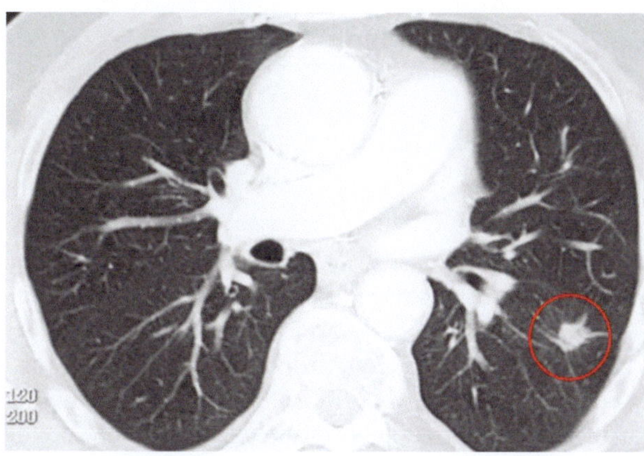

◘ **Fig. 13.3** Thoracic CT scan showing a left-sided typical carcinoid (*red circle*)

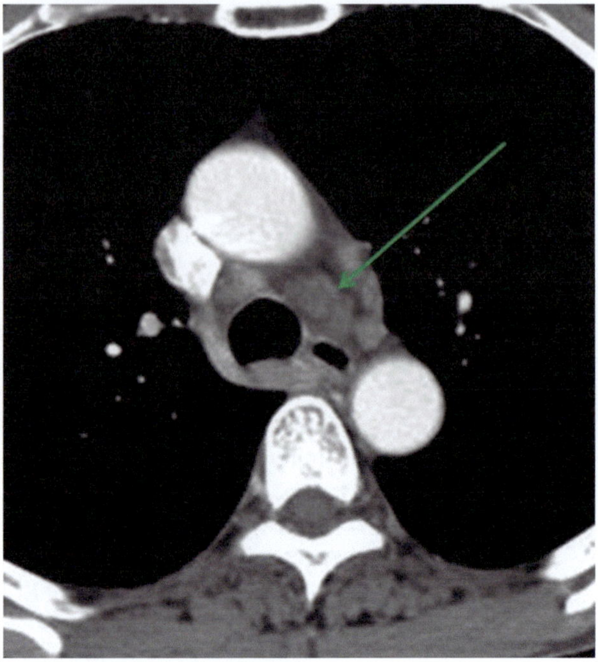

Fig. 13.4 Thoracic CT scan showing left mediastinal lymph nodal involvement (*green arrow*) in an atypical carcinoid

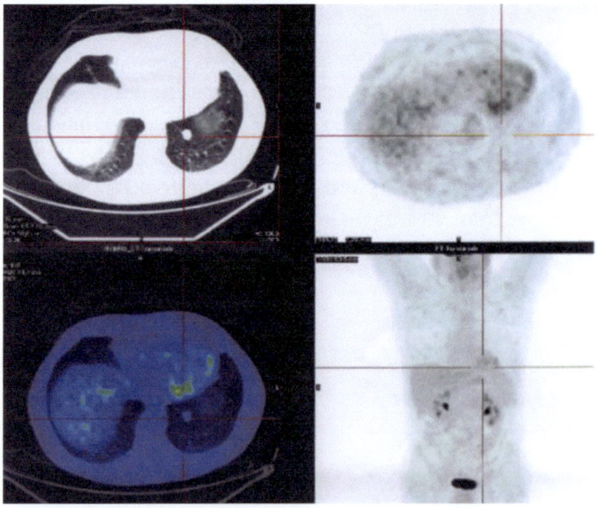

Fig. 13.5 FDG-PET scan is usually negative in low proliferating neoplasms (in this case, tumor definitive diagnosis revealed a typical carcinoid

13

sensitivity (87% and 9%, respectively). Moreover, an octreoscan positivity may also predict a positive response to peptide receptor radiotargeted therapy (PRRT) [15]. The development of new nuclear medicine tracers (e.g., ^{68}Gallium) has recently improved the diagnostic procedures dedicated to low-grade tumors detection. Their higher affinity for $SSTR_2$ receptors, an improved bio-distribution associated with an increased tumor uptake, resulted in a superior resolution of this tracer, compared to

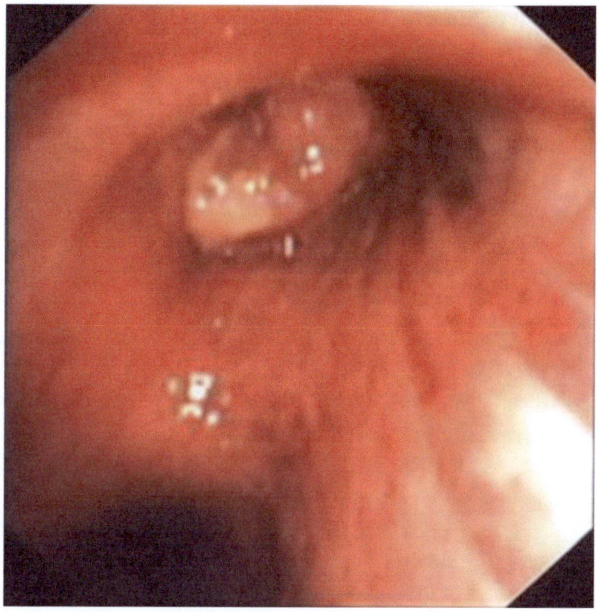

Fig. 13.6 Typical endobronchial BC endoscopic appearance

octreoscan [16, 17]. However, the availability of this tracer to more experienced institutions, only, may limit its diffusion into the routine clinical practice.

Other diagnostic techniques are requests to achieve BC definitive diagnosis, as well as to have a correct preoperative tumor staging.

Bronchoscopy is usually indicated in case of tumor with central location. A direct vision of the lesion is possible, and a smooth reddish-brown growth, sometimes covered by mucosa is the typical endoscopic tumor appearance (Fig. 13.6). In such patients, a correct diagnosis of carcinoid is achieved in about 70% of cases, when a proper bioptic specimen is obtained [18]. BC biopsy is generally safe, even if bleeding (usually self-limiting) has been seldom described, particularly in case of richly vascularized lesions. This complication rate is about 1.5%, while major bleeding rate, requiring a prompt surgical intervention, was reported in less than 0.5% of the cases. When the risk of bleeding is strongly suspected, a rigid bronchoscopy could be taken into account: through this procedure, a large tumor biopsy can be performed and the possible complication can be safely managed. Several studies have reported difficulty to obtain a correct differentiation between typical and atypical carcinoid, since for this a large specimen of well-preserved tumor is requested. Sometimes, a generic diagnosis of «carcinoma» or «squamous cell carcinoma,» or, more frequently, «small cell carcinoma» is found, depending on the difficulty to retrieve immunohistochemical analyses on small tumor's specimens. The ability to diagnose a peripheral BC through a transthoracic fine-needle aspiration biopsy is approximately 40% [19, 20]; the ability to differentiate the carcinoid subtype in this procedure is 10–20% lower [21, 22].

Full functional respiratory test should be carried out in all surgical cases, especially to determine the possible association of carcinoid with asthma or chronic obstructive pulmonary disease (COPD) [23–25]. In particular, cardiac stress tests and lung perfusion scanning are requested in case of suspected or planned pneumonectomy.

Brain CT scan or MRI are not routinely performed in BC's preoperative diagnostic workup, since brain metastases development is an uncommon event also in poorly differentiated neuroendocrine carcinomas. These diagnostic procedures are conversely requested in case of clinical symptoms or suspicion.

Postoperative Surveillance and Follow-Up. Since BCs are usually characterized by an indolent biological behavior, long-term postoperative surveillance is recommended. Post-resectional tumor relapses may occur approximately in 20% of ACs and in 5% TCs [2, 26]; the risk of recurrence is strictly dependent from the histologic tumor subtype, the presence of lymph nodal metastases, and the completeness of resection [5, 9, 26]. Recurrences mostly occur within 10 years in TCs [2, 27, 28] and within 5 years in ACs [2, 27, 29], even if very late relapses (also after 20 years) have been seldom reported [30, 31].

Most recurrences are distant (liver, adrenal gland, bone), and it is not clear how a specific follow-up schedule may alter the outcome. Therefore, a follow-up limited to the chest seems not to be effective to detect possible distant metastases development; the utility of other imaging techniques is still matter of debate [5, 9, 26].

According to the European Neuroendocrine Tumor Society (ENETS) expert consensus and practice guidelines [9], chest CT scan and chromogranin A (CgA) blood measurement should be performed at 3 and 6 months after surgery and then every 12 months for the first 3 years, in case of TCs. After this period, an annual CgA and CT scan are recommended every 3 years. In ACs, CT imaging, and CgA blood dosage should be performed 3 months after surgery and then every 6 months, for 5 years. Annual CT scan should be carried out, afterward.

13.2 Conclusions

In conclusion, BC's clinical presentation is strictly dependent from its location in the lung. It may be totally asymptomatic in case of peripheral form, while recurrent pneumonia, asthma, and hemoptysis are the most common symptoms when the lesion presents with an endobronchial growth.

Contrast thoracic CT scan is actually the gold standard radiological imaging in the preoperative patient's workup. Atelectasis, air trapping, and signs of obstructive pneumonia are commonly observed in case of central BCs; a round or ovoid lung nodule is the typical appearance of peripheral lesions.

Bronchoscopy is usually indicated in case of centrally-located tumor: in such patients, a correct diagnosis of carcinoid is achieved in about 70% of cases. The ability to obtain BC diagnosis in peripheral lesions, through a transthoracic biopsy, is approximately 40%.

Long-term clinical and radiological postoperative surveillance is recommended: post-resectional tumor recurrences may, in fact, occur in about 20% ACs and 5% TCs. The risk of recurrence is strictly dependent from the tumor histological subtype, the presence of lymph nodal metastases, and the completeness of resection.

Bibliography

1. Godwin JD 2nd (1975) Carcinoid tumors: an analysis of 2837 cases. Cancer 36:560–569
2. Detterbeck FC (2010) Management of Carcinoid Tumors. Ann Thorac Surg 89:998–1005
3. Isidori AM, Kaltsas GA, Grossman AB (2006) Ectopic ACTH syndrome. Front Horm Res 35:143–156
4. Filosso PL, European Society of Thoracic Surgeons (ESTS), Neuroendocrine Tumors of The Lung Working-Group, Steering Committee, Asamura H, Brunelli A, Filosso PL, Garcia-Yuste M, Lim E, Papagiannopoulos K, Sarkaria I, Thomas P (2014) Knowledge of pulmonary neuroendocrine tumors: where are we now? Thorac Surg Clin 24:ix–xii
5. Öberg K, Hellman P, Ferolla P, Papotti M, ESMO Guidelines Working Group (2012) Neuroendocrine bronchial and thymic tumors: ESMO clinical practice guidelines for diagnosis, treatment and follow-up. Ann Oncol 23(Suppl 7):vii120–vii123
6. Thakker RV, Newey PJ, Walls GV, Bilezikian J, Dralle H, Ebeling PR, Melmed S, Sakurai A, Tonelli F, Brandi ML (2012) Clinical practice guidelines for multiple endocrine neoplasia type 1 (MEN1). J Clin Endocrinol Metab 97:2990–3011
7. Brandi ML, Gagel RF, Angeli A, Bilezikian JP, Beck-Peccoz P, Bordi C, Conte-Devolx B, Falchetti A, Gheri RG, Libroia A, Lips CJ, Lombardi G, Mannelli M, Pacini F, Ponder BA, Raue F, Skogseid B, Tamburrano G, Thakker RV, Thompson NW, Tomassetti P, Tonelli F, Wells SA Jr, Marx SJ (2001) Guidelines for diagnosis and therapy of MEN type 1 and type 2. J Clin Endocrinol Metab 86:5658–5671
8. Hauso O, Gustafsson BI, Kidd M, Waldum HL, Drozdov I, Chan AK, Modlin IM (2008) Neuroendocrine tumor epidemiology: contrasting Norway and North America. Cancer 113:2655–2664
9. Caplin ME, Baudin E, Ferolla P, Filosso P, Garcia-Yuste M, Lim E, Oberg K, Pelosi G, Perren A, Rossi RE, Travis WD (2015) ENETS consensus conference participants: pulmonary neuroendocrine (carcinoid) tumors: European neuroendocrine tumor society expert consensus and recommendations for best practice for typical and atypical pulmonary carcinoids. Ann Oncol 26:1604–1620
10. Jeung MY, Gasser B, Gangi A, Charneau D, Ducroq X, Kessler R, Quoix E, Roy C (2002) Bronchial carcinoid tumors of the thorax: spectrum of radiologic findings. Radiographics 22:351–365
11. Meisinger QC, Klein JS, Butnor KJ, Gentchos G, Leavitt BJ (2011) CT features of peripheral pulmonary carcinoid tumors. AJR Am J Roentgenol 197:1073–1080
12. Abgral R, Leboulleux S, Déandreis D, Aupérin A, Lumbroso J, Dromain C, Duvillard P, Elias D, de Baere T, Guigay J, Ducreux M, Schlumberger M, Baudin E (2011) Performance of (18) fluorodeoxyglucose-positron emission tomography and somatostatin receptor scintigraphy for high Ki67 (≥10%) well-differentiated endocrine carcinoma staging. J Clin Endocrinol Metab 96:665–671
13. Kubota K, Okasaki M, Minamimoto R, Miyata Y, Morooka M, Nakajima K, Sato T (2014) Lesion-based analysis of (18)F-FDG uptake and (111)in-Pentetreotide uptake by neuroendocrine tumors. Ann Nucl Med 28:1004–1010
14. Righi L, Volante M, Tavaglione V, Billè A, Daniele L, Angusti T, Inzani F, Pelosi G, Rindi G, Papotti M (2010) Somatostatin receptor tissue distribution in lung neuroendocrine tumours: a clinicopathologic and immunohistochemical study of 218 'clinically aggressive' cases. Ann Oncol 21:548–555
15. Bodei L, Cremonesi M, Kidd M, Grana CM, Severi S, Modlin IM, Paganelli G (2014) Peptide receptor radionuclide therapy for advanced neuroendocrine tumors. Thorac Surg Clin 24:333–349
16. Haug AR, Cindea-Drimus R, Auernhammer CJ, Reincke M, Beuschlein F, Wängler B, Uebleis C, Schmidt GP, Spitzweg C, Bartenstein P, Hacker M (2014) Neuroendocrine tumor recurrence: diagnosis with 68Ga-DOTATATE PET/CT. Radiology 270:517–525
17. Ambrosini V, Morigi JJ, Nanni C, Castellucci P, Fanti S (2015) Current status of PET imaging of neuroendocrine tumours ([18F]FDOPA, [68Ga]tracers, [11C]/[18F]-HTP). Q J Nucl Med Mol Imaging 59:58–69
18. Escalon J, Detterbeck F (2009) Carcinoid tumors. In: Shields T, JI LC, Reed C, Feins R (eds) General thoracic surgery 7th edition. Lippincott Williams & Wilkins, Philadelphia, pp 1539–1554
19. Mezzetti M, Raveglia F, Panigalli T, Giuliani L, Lo Giudice F, Meda S, Conforti S (2003) Assessment of outcomes in typical and atypical carcinoids according to latest WHO classification. Ann Thorac Surg 76:1838–1842

20. Rea F, Rizzardi G, Zuin A, Marulli G, Nicotra S, Bulf R, Schiavon M, Sartori F (2007) Outcome and surgical strategy in bronchial carcinoid tumors: single institution experience with 252 patients. Eur J Cardiothorac Surg 31:186–191
21. Frierson HF Jr, Covell JL, Mills SE (1987) Fine needle aspiration cytology of atypical carcinoid of the lung. Acta Cytol 31:471–475
22. Nicholson SA, Ryan MR (2000) A review of cytologic findings in neuroendocrine carcinomas including carcinoid tumors with histologic correlation. Cancer 90(3):148–161
23. Banki F (2010) Pulmonary assessment for general thoracic surgery. Surg Clin North Am 90:969–984
24. Fibla JJ, Brunelli A, Cassivi SD, Deschamps C (2012) Aggregate risk score for predicting mortality after surgical biopsy for interstitial lung disease. Interact Cardiovasc Thorac Surg 15:276–279
25. Falcoz PE, Puyraveau M, Thomas PA, Decaluwe H, Hürtgen M, Petersen RH, Hansen H, Brunelli A (2016) ESTS database committee and ESTS minimally invasive interest group: video-assisted thoracoscopic surgery versus open lobectomy for primary non-small-cell lung cancer: a propensity-matched analysis of outcome from the European Society of Thoracic Surgeon database. Eur J Cardiothorac Surg 49:602–609
26. Filosso PL, Ferolla P, Guerrera F, Ruffini E, Travis WD, Rossi G, Lausi PO, Oliaro A (2015) European Society of Thoracic Surgeons lung neuroendocrine tumors working-group steering committee: multidisciplinary management of advanced lung neuroendocrine tumors. J Thorac Dis 7(Suppl 2):S163–S171
27. Filosso PL, Rena O, Donati G, Casadio C, Ruffini E, Papalia E, Oliaro A, Maggi G (2002 Feb) Bronchial carcinoid tumors: surgical management and long-term outcome. J Thorac Cardiovasc Surg 123:303–309
28. Thomas CF Jr, Tazelaar HD, Jett JR (2001) Typical and atypical pulmonary carcinoids : outcome in patients presenting with regional lymph node involvement. Chest 119:1143–1150
29. Filosso PL, Rena O, Guerrera F, Moreno Casado P, Sagan D, Raveglia F, Brunelli A, Welter S, Gust L, Pompili C, Casadio C, Bora G, Alvarez A, Zaluska W, Baisi A, Roesel C (2015) Thomas PA; ESTS NETs-WG steering committee: clinical management of atypical carcinoid and large-cell neuroendocrine carcinoma: a multicentre study on behalf of the European Association of Thoracic Surgeons (ESTS) neuroendocrine Tumours of the lung working group. Eur J Cardiothorac Surg 48:55–64
30. El Jamal M, Nicholson AG, Goldstraw P (2000) The feasibility of conservative resection for carcinoid tumours: is pneumonectomy ever necessary for uncomplicated cases? Eur J Cardiothorac Surg 18:301–306
31. García-Yuste M, Matilla JM, Cueto A, Paniagua JM, Ramos G, Cañizares MA, Muguruza I (2007) Spanish multi-centric study of neuroendocrine Tumours of the lung for the Spanish Society of Pneumonology and Thoracic Surgery (EMETNE-SEPAR): typical and atypical carcinoid tumours: analysis of the experience of the Spanish multi-centric study of neuroendocrine Tumours of the lung. Eur J Cardiothorac Surg 31:192–197

Tumour Staging: Ileum

Tahir Akbar, Rajaventhan Srirajaskanthan, and John K. Ramage

A. Colao et al. (eds.), *Neuroendocrine Tumors in Real Life*,
https://doi.org/10.1007/978-3-319-59024-0_14

Overview

Ileal neuroendocrine tumours are one of the most common gastro-enteropancreatic neuroendocrine tumours (GEP-NETs), making up to 28% of all GEP-NETs. Small bowel NETs are the most common type of small bowel tumour; 45% of these lesions occur in the distal ileum. Small bowel neuroendocrine tumours commonly present in the sixth to seventh decade [1]; however, they can occur at any time of life. In up to 30% of cases, these lesions are multiple [2], with some case series reporting this to be as high as 40% [3]. When diagnosed, ileal NETs are frequently larger than 2 cm and have spread to regional lymph nodes.

In this article, we will review the different staging methods of GEP-NETs and incorporate the tumour, node and metastases (TNM) staging systems developed by the European Neuroendocrine Tumour Society (ENETS) and American Joint committee on Cancer (AJCC). The importance of radiology in staging will be discussed extensively, including the difficulties with each resource and the challenges in accurately staging and locating the primary site of disease. We will look at the role of histology in the grading of tumours, with focus on the mitotic and proliferation indices.

Clinical Case

A 48-year-old female presented with symptoms of right upper quadrant abdominal pain for 4 months. There was no weight loss and anorexia, with no symptoms of flushing, diarrhoea or palpitations. Clinical examination was normal.

Investigations

A liver ultrasound revealed five hyperechoic lesions, the largest of these measuring 2.6 cm. A computed tomography (CT) scan of her chest, abdomen and pelvis diagnosed metastatic liver disease of unknown primary. In search of a primary malignancy, she had a normal oesophago-gastro-duodenoscopy and colonoscopy.

Magnetic resonance imaging (MRI) of the liver prior to biopsy revealed multiple lesions, with increased T2 signal and low T1 signal. With injection of contrast, the lesions appeared as hypervascular raising the possibility of an underlying neuroendocrine tumour.

Histology from the liver biopsy demonstrated a well-differentiated G1 NET with positive immunohistochemistry (IHC) stains for chromogranin A (CgA), synaptophysin and neuron-specific enolase (NSE). CK7, CK20, EMA, oestrogen and progesterone receptors and S100 were negative. There were no mitoses seen per 10 HPF and Ki67 index was <1%. The plasma CgA level was 94 ng/mL (normal range 39 ng/mL).

A fluorodeoxyglucose (FDG) positron emission tomography (PET)/CT showed no evidence of uptake above or below the diaphragm.

An octreoscan (◘ Fig. 14.1) revealed increased uptake in the superior aspect of the liver lesion, with no further uptake in the abdomen.

In search for a primary site of the GEP-NET, she went on to have a capsule endoscopy which revealed five small polyps within the distal terminal ileum (◘ Fig. 14.2).

Treatment

This lady proceeded to surgery and underwent a right hemicolectomy with extended ileal resection for removal of the primary tumours and wedge resection of the solitary liver metastases (◘ Fig. 14.3). 400 mm of distal ileum was removed and 14 disc-shaped tumours were found ranging from 5 to 10 mm. This was more than the five spotted on the capsule endoscopy. The small bowel carcinoid had a typical insular pattern with round cells. The tumour was infiltrating the submucosa, muscularis propria and subserosa. No definite vascular invasion was seen; however, two regional lymph

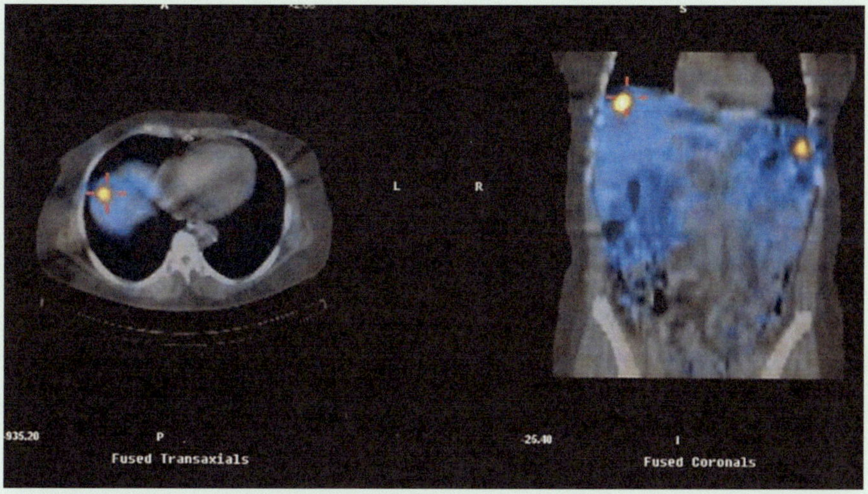

Fig. 14.1 NM octreotide scan with SPECT: this shows one of the areas of increased focal tracer concentration noted in the superior aspect of the liver. The area on the spleen is physiological with no tumour uptake

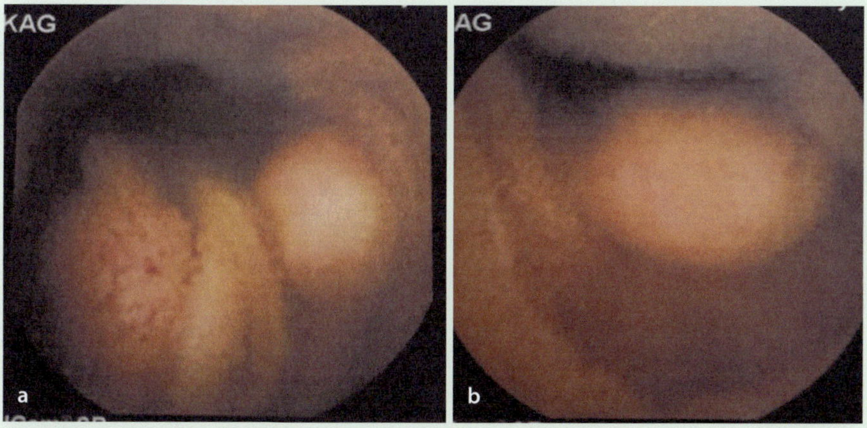

Fig. 14.2 Pictures from a wireless capsule study of the small bowel. Image at 2 h 52 min showed a nodule (*left*) and a second nodule at 3 h 18 min (*right*). Distance between the nodules is 1–2 cm

nodes showed metastatic neuroendocrine tumour. In the liver, there were multiple deposits in the right lobe and five deposits on the left lobe. Three deposits were found in segment 3 and further deposits were found in segment 4a and 4b. These were removed by wedge resection, and the patient returned at a later time for a right hepatectomy. The histology was consistent with metastatic neuroendocrine tumour. Staging by AJCC TNM and ENETS stage was stage 4, pT3(m), N1, M1. WHO and ENETS grade classification was Grade 1.

She continues to have normal CgA levels 5 years post resection, and CT of the chest/abdomen/pelvis shows no evidence of disease recurrence.

Final staging of this disease was T3(m)N1 M1.

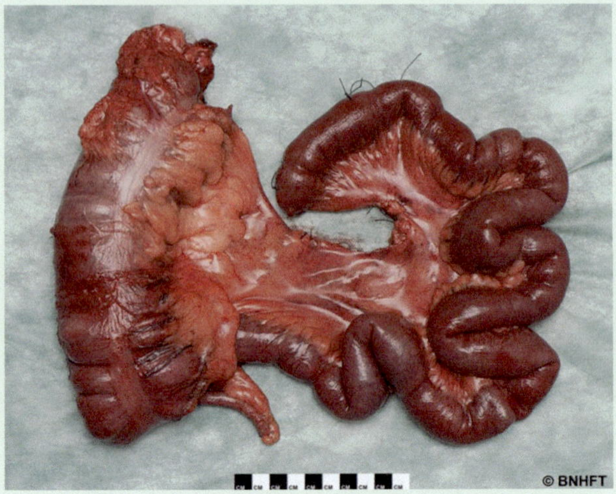

Fig. 14.3 Specimen sample of the surgical ileal resection

14.1 Comments to the Case

This case demonstrates the difficulty with staging in this condition and the challenges and approaches taken in finding ileal NET. In this case, a capsule endoscopy was needed. FDG PET/CT, octreoscan, CT and MRI imaging did not reveal the primary site. Therefore, it is important to have access to a wide range of imaging techniques to ensure the most accurate staging of the disease.

Questions

1. What is the most accurate way of staging small bowel neuroendocrine tumour (NET) metastases?
2. How should we make sure that there are no further NET primaries in the small bowel if one has been removed?

Answers

1. The most accurate way of staging well-differentiated small bowel NET metastases is ^{68}Ga-DOTATATE PET [4]. For poorly differentiated tumours, FDG PET is more likely to be positive [5]. Some patients may have a mixed population of tumour cells, where some tumours are more positive on each modality; hence, imaging the same patients with both types of PET tracer may be an advantage [6]. Many patients will be staged by CT and octreoscan which will be less accurate.
2. Most patients will have had axial imaging with CT or MRI prior to surgery, and this may show up more than one tumour. However, many will be missed unless enteroclysis is used [7], which is not a technique commonly employed since it can be challenging for patients. At surgery it is important that multiple primary

tumours are considered. If an open laparotomy is performed, then the small bowel should be palpated to look for further primaries [8]. However, if there is a laparoscopic resection (e.g. laparoscopic right hemicolectomy), then the patient should ideally have further imaging of the residual small bowel which may be by wireless capsule endoscopy to ensure that the rest of the bowel is normal.

Up to Date of the Topic

Imaging Techniques in Staging Ileal NETs

Staging would normally start with CT and MRI imaging. MRI may be more sensitive than CT for the detection of small liver metastases [9, 10]. However, CT may be better for the evaluation of peritoneal and mesenteric disease[8].

It should ideally involve the use of gallium-DOTA-TOC/-NOC/-TATE PET if available, having the highest sensitivity and specificity [11], but this technique is not widely used as yet. PET scanning with specific tracers such as 11C-5HTP, ^{18}F-DOPA or ^{18}F-DG may be used but is mainly experimental at present [12, 13, 14, 15]. As in the case described above, endoscopy or the use of capsule endoscopy can be of additional value in determining a primary site of the lesion. However, one of the common risks of this procedure is capsule retention. The incidence of capsule retention ranges from 0% to 13%, with the most common site of detainment in the ileum [16, 17]. A study of 937 patients reported an incidence of 0.75% of patients worldwide who required surgical intervention to remove a retained capsule [18]. Therefore, in high-risk groups a patency capsule should be used prior to the main test, as it is shown to be a safe and effective method of demonstrating whether a capsule will pass safely [19].

Biochemical analysis of relevant biomarkers such as plasma CgA and urine 5-hydroxyindoleacetic acid (5-HIAA) should complement imaging.

Imaging Challenges

Computed Tomography (CT)

The biggest challenge with CT staging in Ileal NETs is identifying the primary tumour site [20]. In one case series of 52 patients, it was only found once in a patient with an ileal tumour causing intussusception into the caecum [21]. The use of CT is recommended to identify metastatic disease, with an important role at staging, as it is normally good at identifying any mesenteric mass. However, neuroendocrine hepatic metastases may be difficult to identify and delineate on CT as they may be isointense to the liver on portal venous phase imaging (PVP), mimicking a haemangioma. A triple-phase CT of pre-contrast, hepatic arterial-dominant phase and PVP imaging is necessary as the lesion may only be seen on one of the three phases [22].

Magnetic Resonance Imaging (MRI)

Routine MRI may not identify the primary tumour site as standard MRI protocols used do not offer superiority over CT in assessing small bowel lesions. A dedicated small bowel MRI or MRI enteroclysis may be more accurate, but the latter are not widely available. On imaging, NETs manifest as asymmetric wall thickening with signal isointensity on T1-weighted images and iso-hypersensitivity on T2-weighted images [23]. The use of MR imaging like CT is important in staging for metastatic disease, with mesenteric involvement and liver metastasis identified accurately [24]. Whole-body MRI has been used and is under evaluation.

Somatostatin Receptor Scintigraphy (Octreoscan)
Octreoscan is recommended as a first-line staging for investigation for GEP-NETs. An ^{111}In-labelled somatostatin analogue, pentetreotide, concentrates in GEP-NETs containing somatostatin receptor subtypes 2 and 5, making it suitable for the imaging of tumours containing those somatostatin receptor subtypes. It is highly sensitive and specific for GEP-NETs and has similar specificity for both functioning and non-functioning tumours [25]. A limitation of SSRS is reduced sensitivity in smaller lesions, which is an issue for many ileal lesions, and reduced sensitivity in those exhibiting low receptor density [26]. In ileal lesions, 123I-mIBG scintigraphy is less sensitive than ^{111}In scintigraphy and therefore does not have a first-line role [27].
PET/CT
PET/CT alongside octreoscan and CT imaging forms the staging techniques used to diagnose ileal NETs. Several somatostatin analogues have been developed, including DOTA octreotide (DOTATOC) and DOTA octreotate (DOTATATE), which bind to SSTR (somatostatin receptor) 2 and SSTR5[18]. FDG PET will be more positive in poorly differentiated tumours and the DOTATATE/NOC more positive in well-differentiated cases. An ideal may be to have imaging using both, but costs and availability are a major concern.

In a study of 24 patients with ileal NETs, DOTATE PET-CT changed the surgical management in at least 20% of these cases, therefore showing its importance in preoperative staging [28]. In a study of 27 patients, ^{18}F–F DOPA had a sensitivity of 96% in detecting region-based disease, compared to 72% of CT and SSRS combined [29]. In a further review of 23 patients, 18F-DOPA-PET was superior to both SSRS and CT in sensitivity in detecting GEP-NETs [30]. These latter techniques are still in a research phase.

Tumour, Node and Distant Metastasis Staging
The first World Health Organization (WHO) classification for neuroendocrine tumours in 1980 used the term carcinoid for most of the tumours. Carcinoids were divided into enterochromaffin cell carcinoids, gastrin cell carcinoids and unspecified carcinoids. The 1980 classification did not take into account the heterogeneity of these tumours, not recognising, for example, the difference of carcinoid of the stomach and ileum [31]. In the 2000 classification, neuroendocrine tumours were divided into well-differentiated endocrine tumours, well-differentiated endocrine carcinomas and poorly differentiated endocrine carcinomas. This however did not differentiate based on proliferation markers and did not allow for prognostication in advanced disease [32].

In 2007, The European Neuroendocrine Tumour Society (ENETS) developed the TNM classification (▪ Table 14.1) for the first time in staging of NETS, bringing staging in NETs in line with other tumours. Staging in this new consensus differed for the primary site. The TNM method of staging was supported by the American Joint Committee on Cancer (AJCC). Although the AJCC developed a different TNM staging for some sites, they endorsed the ENETS TNM staging for ileal NETs.

The 2010 WHO classification acknowledged the ENETS grading system for neuroendocrine neoplasms of the gastrointestinal tract, separating well-differentiated

Table 14.1 ENETS/AJCC TNM staging of ileal NETs [37]

Stage	Tumour stage	Histology	Nodes	Metastasis
1	T1	Tumour invades lamina propria or submucosa, and size 1 cm or less	N0 (no regional lymph nodes metastasis)	M0 (no distant metastasis)
2a	T2	Tumour invades muscularis propria or size greater than 1 cm	N0	M0
2b	T3	Tumour invades muscularis propria into subserosal tissue without penetration of overlying serosa	N0	M0
3a	T4	Tumour invades serosa or other organs or adjacent structures	N0	M0
3b	Any T		N1 (regional lymph node metastasis)	
4	Any T		Any N	M1 (distant metastasis)

There is no definition for tumour in situ for the ileum as no precursor has been identified

tumours into low-grade (G1) and intermediate-grade (G2) categories. All poorly differentiated neuroendocrine tumours are high-grade (G3) neuroendocrine carcinomas according to this classification. The WHO, in this classification, also endorsed the staging of neuroendocrine neoplasms using the specified TNM staging, based on the AJCC modification of this system.

Survival in Relation to Stage of Disease

A study looking at 138 patients assessed survival in relation to stage of disease [33] (Fig. 14.4). They found no difference in survival between stage 2 and stage 3 but a difference between stage 2 and those with stage 4. There was a significant improvement in survival for patients with G1 compared to those with G2 NETs. In a further study of 115 cases, there was a lack of statistically significant differences between stages 1/2 and stage 3 for midgut NETs [34]. In a large series of 215 patients, TNM classification was able to differentiate significantly between different tumour stages (stages 1–3 vs. stage 4) [35]. In a review of 425 patients, the team was able to demonstrate a prognostic difference between each stage [36]. In a larger study of 1072, the ENETS staging system was superior to the WHO 2010 classification in predicting prognosis. The WHO classification was unable to differentiate between stages 2 and 3 and was not accurate in predicting survival [37].

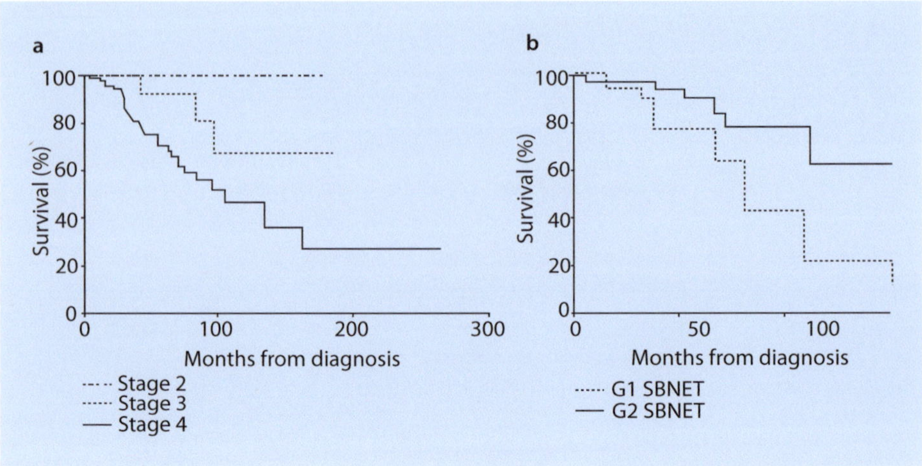

Fig. 14.4 **a** Cumulative small bowel NET survival according to TNM staging. **b** Cumulative small bowel NET survival curve assessing histological grade (Adapted from: Rajaventhan Srirajaskanthan et al. [33])

Table 14.2 The 2010 WHO classification of GEP-NETs [37]

Differentiation	Grade	Mitotic count *	Ki-67 index	WHO
Well differentiated	Low grade (G1)	<2 per 10 HPF	≤2%	Grade 1
	Intermediate grade (G2)	2–20 per 10 HPF	3–20%	Grade 2
Poorly differentiated	High grade (G3)	>20 per HPF	>20%	Grade 3

14.2 Conclusions

14

Many improvements have been made recently in the staging of ileal NET, and this has led to more logical surgical strategies. The inclusion of histological grading into the staging process has improved prognostic accuracy, and it is clear that «T» staging alone does not differentiate prognosis between all groups. Other factors such as multiple tumours, involvement of mesenteric vessels and hormone secretion also need to be considered in relation to prognosis and therapy (Table 14.2).

Bibliography

1. Pinchot SN, Holen K, Sippel RS et al (2008) Carcinoid tumors. Oncologist 13:1255–1269
2. Yamaguchi T, Manabe N, Tanaka S, Fukumoto A, Shimamoto M, Nakao M et al (2005) Multiple carcinoid tumours of the ileum preoperatively diagnosed by enteroscopy with the double-balloon technique. Gastrointest Endosc 62:315–318

3. Klöppel G (2007) Tumour biology and histopathology of neuroendocrine tumours. Best Pract Res Clin Endocrinol Metab 21(1):15–31
4. Geijer H, Breimer LH (2013) Somatostatin receptor PET/CT in neuroendocrine tumours: update on systematic review and meta-analysis. Eur J Nucl Med Mol Imaging 40(11):1770–1780
5. Kwee TC, Basu S, Saboury B, Ambrosini V, Torigian DA, Alavi A (2011) A new dimension of FDG-PET interpretation: assessment of tumor biology. Eur J Nucl Med Mol Imaging 38:1158–1170
6. Nilica B et al (2016) Direct comparison of 68Ga-DOTA-TOC and 18F-FDG PET/CT in the follow-up of patients with neuroendocrine tumour treated with the first full peptide receptor radionuclide therapy cycle. Eur J Nucl Med Mol Imaging 43:1585–1592
7. Kamaoui I, De-Luca V, Ficarelli S, Mennesson N, Lombard-Bohas C, Pilleul F (2010) Value of CT enteroclysis in suspected small-bowel carcinoid tumors. AJR Am J Roentgenol 194:629–633
8. Boudreaux JP, Klimstra DS, Hassan MM et al (2010) The NANETS consensus guideline for the diagnosis and management of neuroendocrine tumors: well-differentiated neuroendocrine tumors of the Jejunum, Ileum, Appendix, and Cecum. North American Neuroendocrine Tumor Society (NANETS). Pancreas 39:753–766
9. Dromain C, de Baere T, Baudin E et al (2003) MR imaging of hepatic metastases caused by neuroendocrine tumors: comparing four techniques. Am J Roentgenol 180(1):121–128
10. Debray MP, Geoffroy O, Laissy JP et al (2001) Imaging appearances of metastases from neuroendocrine tumours of the pancreas. Br J Radiol 74:1065–1070
11. Öberg K, Knigge U, Kwekkeboom D, Perren A (2012) Neuroendocrine Gastroenteropancreatic Tumours: ESMO clinical practice guidelines. Ann Oncol 23(Suppl 7):vii124–vii130
12. Rockall AG, Reznek RH (2007) Imaging of neuroendocrine tumours (CT/MR/US). Best Pract Res Clin Endocrinol Metab 21:43–68
13. Sundin A, Vullierme MP, Kaltsas G et al (2009) ENETS consensus guidelines for the standards of Care in Neuroendocrine Tumors: radiological examinations. Neuroendocrinol 90:167–183
14. Koopmans KP, Neels OC, Kema IP et al (2008) Improved staging of patients with carcinoid and islet cell tumors with 18F-dihydroxy-phenyl-alanine and 11C-5-hydroxy-tryptophan positron emission tomography. J Clin Oncol 26:1489–1495
15. Binderup T, Knigge U, Loft A et al (2010) 18F-fluorodeoxyglucose positron emission tomography predicts survival of patients with neuroendocrine tumors. Clin Cancer Res 16:978–985
16. Cave D, Legnani P, de Ranchis R et al (2005) ICCE consensus for capsule retention. Endoscopy 37:1065–1067
17. Cheon JH, Kim YS, Lee IS et al (2007) Can we predict spontaneous capsule passage after retention? A nationwide study to evaluate the incidence and clinical outcomes of capsule retention. Endoscopy 39:1046–1052
18. Barkin J, Friedman S (2002) Wireless capsule endoscopy requiring surgical intervention: the world's experience. Am J Gastroenterol 97:A907
19. Römmele C, Brueckner J, Messmann H, Gölder SK (2016) Clinical experience with the PillCam patency capsule prior to video capsule endoscopy: a real-world experience. Gastroenterol Res Pract 2016:9657053
20. Sugimoto E, Lorelius LE, Eriksson B, Oberg K (1995) Midgut carcinoid tumours. CT appearance Acta Radiol 36:367–371
21. Wiener-Carrillo I, González-Alvarado C, Cervantes-Valladolid M, Echaverry-Navarrete D, Zubieta-O'Farrill G, Gudiño-Chávez A (2014) Intussusception secondary to a carcinoid tumor in an adult patient. Int J Surg Case Rep 5(5):265–267
22. Paulson EK, McDermott VG, Keogan MT et al (1998) Carcinoid metastases to the liver: role of triple-phase helical CT. Radiol 206:143–150
23. GoreRM BJW, Mehta UK, Newmark GM, Yaghmai V (2005) GI carcinoid tumours: appearance of the primary and detecting metastases. Best Pract Res Clin Endocrinol Metab 19(2):245–263
24. Scarsbrook AF, Thakker RV, Wass JA, Gleeson FV, Phillips RR (2006) Multiple endocrine neoplasia: spectrum of radiologic appearances and discussion of a multitechnique imaging approach. Radiographics 26:433–451
25. Maroun J, Kocha W, Kvols L et al (2006) Guidelines for the diagnosis and management of carcinoid tumours. Part 1: the gastrointestinal tract. A statement from a Canadian National Carcinoid Expert Group. Curr Oncol 13(2):67–76

26. Ramage et al (2012) Guidelines for the management of gastroenteropancreatic neuroendocrine (including carcinoid) tumours (NETs). Gut 61:6e32. doi:10.1136/gutjnl-2011-300831
27. Kaltsas GA, Mukherjee JJ, Grossman AB (2001) The value of radiolabelled MIBG and octreotide in the diagnosis and management of neuroendocrine tumours. Ann Oncol 12(Suppl 2):S47e50
28. Ihan H, Fendler WP, Cyran CC et al (2015) Impact of Ga-DOTATATE PET/CT on the surgical management of primary neuroendocrine tumors of the pancreas or ileum. Ann Surg On- col 22:164–171
29. Yakemchuk VN, Jager PL, Chirakal R, Reid R, Major P, Gulenchyn KY (2012) PET/CT using 18F-FDOPA provides improved staging of carcinoid tumor patients in a Canadian setting. Nucl Med Commun 33(3):322–330
30. Koopmans KP J, Neels OC, Kema IP, Elsinga PH, Sluiter WJ, Vanghillewe K, Brouwers AH, Jager PL, de Vries EG (2008) Improved staging of patients with carcinoid and islet cell tumors with 18F-dihydroxy-phenyl-alanine and 11C-5-hy-droxy-tryptophan positron emission tomography. J Clin Oncol 26:1489–1495
31. KlöppelG PA, Heitz PU (2004) The gastroenteropancreatic neuroendocrine cell system and its tumors: the WHO classification. Ann N Y Acad Sci 1014:13–27
32. Ferrone CR, Tang LH, Tomlinson J et al (2007) Determining prognosis in patients with pancreatic endocrine neoplasms: can the WHO classification system be simplified? J Clin Oncol 25:5609–5615
33. R Srirajaskanthan, A Ahmed, A Prachialias et al (2013) ENETS TNM staging predicts prognosis in small bowel neuroendocrine tumours. ISRN Oncology 420795:7 pages. doi: 10.1155/2013/420795
34. Jann H, Roll S, Couvelard A et al (2011) Neuroendocrine tumors of midgut and hindgut origin: tumor-node-metastasis classification determines clinical outcome. Cancer 117(15):3332–3341
35. Pape UF et al (2008b) Prognostic relevance of a novel TNM classification system for upper gastroenteropancreatic neuroendocrine tumors. Cancer 113:256–265
36. Strosberg JR, Cheema A, Weber J et al (2011) Prognostic validity of a novel American Joint Committee on Cancer staging classification for pancreatic neuroendocrine tumors. J Clin Oncol 29:3044–3049
37. Rindi G, Falconi M, Klersy C et al (2012) TNM staging of neoplasms of the endocrine pancreas: results from a large international cohort study. J Natl Cancer Inst 104:764–777

Tumor Staging: Pancreas

Roberta Elisa Rossi and Sara Massironi

A. Colao et al. (eds.), *Neuroendocrine Tumors in Real Life*,
https://doi.org/10.1007/978-3-319-59024-0_15

Overview

In patients with pancreatic neuroendocrine tumor (pNET), the assessment of the tumor extent and location and the evaluation of any possible local and/or distant metastases are both required to decide on the proper treatment.

We have reviewed the current evidence on the staging techniques in pNET settings, and we have reported a pertinent case report.

A search was performed on PubMed for the terms: pancreatic neuroendocrine tumors, staging, imaging, endoscopic ultrasound, and nuclear imaging. We searched for all the relevant articles published in PubMed between 1990 and 2016.

Ultrasound endoscopy (EUS) is particularly advantageous in the detection of small, often multifocal pNETs. Of note, as in our case, EUS is extremely useful in the preoperative setting to establish whether a lesion is feasible for surgical resection as it can visualize adjacent vessels and lymphadenopathy. In fact, the invasion of close vessels (e.g., the superior mesenteric artery) represents a contraindication to surgery. Finally, a complete histological assessment of the tumor usually by EUS-guided fine needle aspiration, including the detection of the mitotic Ki-67 index, is needed to tailor the proper treatment to an individual patient. Conventional radiology [i.e., computed tomography (CT) scan and magnetic resonance imaging (MRI)] is used to assess the extent of the tumor and the possible location of the primary lesion. Nuclear imaging [somatostatin receptor scintigraphy (SRS) and, more recently, positron emission tomography (PET) scanning based on 68Ga-radiolabeled somatostatin analogs (Ga-68 PET)] aims at identifying distant metastases – particularly bone metastases which represent a poor prognostic factor and a contraindication to surgery – and somatostatin analog (SSA) receptors prior to medical therapy or peptide radioreceptor therapy (PRRT).

EUS, conventional radiology, and nuclear imaging are all key techniques in the staging of pNETs and should be considered complementary in order to tailor the therapeutic strategy according to a tumor's and patient's features.

Clinical Case

A 73-year-old man was referred to our unit in 2013 with a recent medical history of severe weight loss, episodes of hypoglycemia, and deep venous thrombosis. His past medical history included cholecystectomy for gallbladder empyema, right inguinal hernia repair, and benign hypertrophic prostate.

On suspicion of a glucagonoma, plasma glucagon levels were measured: they resulted to be increased at 3385 pg/mL (normal values <150). A computed tomography (CT) scan was performed, and a solid lesion, 60 x 43 mm, was found sited at the head of the pancreas and biopsied during an ultrasound endoscopy (EUS): it was confirmed to be a well-differentiated neuroendocrine tumor (NET), chromogranin A, and glucagon positive. The Ki-67 proliferative index was 18% (G2 NET, according to WHO 2010 [1]). The tumor was assessed as inoperable due to the invasion of both the superior mesenteric artery and vein. Nuclear imaging [(PET/CT with 68gallium-labeled somatostatin analogs (Ga-68 PET)] was positive on the pancreas, but did not show any neuroendocrine metastases. The patient was therefore treated with octreotide LAR 30 mg every 28 days and then started on peptide radioreceptor therapy (PRRT) with neo-adjuvant purposes (five cycles). EUS was repeated: it showed a dimensional reduction of the lesion (currently 43 x 32 mm) without any infiltration of the superior mesenteric artery or vein. The case was then discussed in a multidisciplinary team: the team agreed on the feasibility of a potentially curative surgical approach. The patient is currently alive and listed for surgery.

15.1 Comments to the Case

This case highlights the importance of a multidisciplinary approach to pancreatic NETs (pNETs) and the complementary role of imaging and endoscopic techniques in the management pathway.

Firstly, the primary pNET was detected by CT scan, which did not find distant metastases as confirmed by Ga-68 PET.

EUS played a pivotal role both in the final diagnosis of the primary tumor by biopsy and in its grading characterization. Furthermore, it was extremely useful in the preoperative setting as it allowed to establish the invasion of close vessels, which made the tumor inoperable.

Ga-68 PET also helped to identify SSA receptors in order to start the patient on SSA medical therapy and radiolabeled SSAs.

Finally, EUS was repeated to assess the tumor response to radio-targeted therapy and showed a dimensional reduction of the lesion without vessel infiltration, which made the tumor feasible for the curative surgical approach (◘ Figs. 15.1 and 15.2).

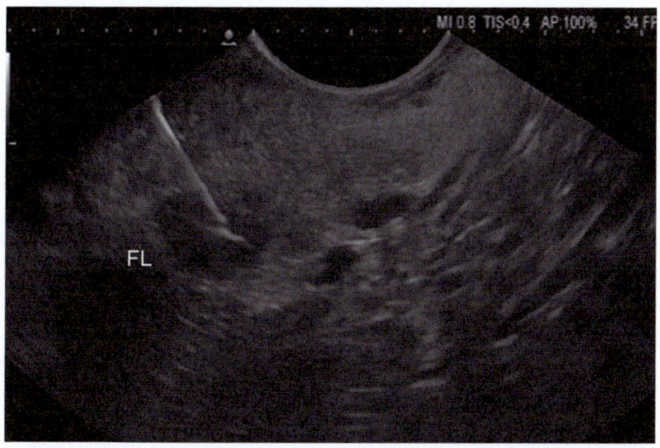

◘ **Fig. 15.1** Ultrasound endoscopy with fine needle aspiration of a solid lesion, sited at the head of the pancreas

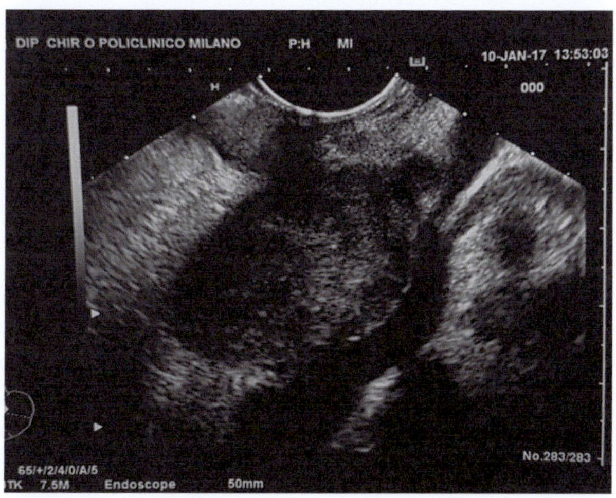

◘ **Fig. 15.2** Ultrasound endoscopy showing invasion of both the superior mesenteric vein and artery by a 60 × 43 mm solid lesion, sited at the head of the pancreas

Questions

1. Which is the role of EUS in the staging process of pNETs?
2. Is there any difference in the diagnostic accuracy between EUS, CT, and magnetic resonance imaging (MRI)?
3. Should nuclear imaging tests always be performed in the staging of pNETs?

Answers

1. EUS has a decisive role in the staging of pNETs, particularly in the local staging of pNETs. In particular, in the preoperative setting, EUS can provide additional useful information (e.g., the distance from the vessels and the pancreatic duct, the Ki-67 proliferation index) toward the best therapeutic management. Furthermore, the possibility of EUS-guided FNA tattooing of pancreatic lesions may be extremely helpful.
2. EUS appears to be more accurate than conventional radiological imaging as it can properly study the distance from the vessels and the pancreatic duct, which is a piece of necessary information to be provided in the preoperative setting. Moreover, any adjacent lymphadenopathy can be easily seen and evaluated through EUS. Of note, EUS is well suited to the identification of small pancreatic lesions, as small as 2–5 mm (e.g., insulinomas), which are not usually detected by conventional radiological or nuclear imaging. The presence and extent of liver metastases and lymph node metastases are among the most important prognostic factors for patients with pNETs. CT and MRI can be used as alternative modalities in the staging process for the detection of distant metastases. However, MRI may be superior, in direct comparison to CT, in the detection of liver metastases.
3. Nuclear imaging, particularly Ga-68 PET scan, should always be performed in the staging process as it is accurate in identifying distant metastases, particularly bone metastases. Furthermore, nuclear imaging allows the detection of SSA receptors in order to select those patients who may be suitable to medical therapy or radiolabeled SSAs.

Up to Date of the Topic

Pancreatic Neuroendocrine Tumor: Staging

Pancreatic neuroendocrine tumors (pNETs) are rare neoplasms, which constitute approximately 2% of all pancreatic tumors with a recently increasing incidence [2]. Their clinical incidence is reported to be of 1–5 new cases per year in a 100,000 population, with a prevalence of 10/100,000 population [3]. These heterogeneous neoplasms include functioning tumors, which secrete a variety of peptide hormones, and nonfunctioning tumors, which often show metastases, mainly liver metastases, at the time of diagnosis. The most common metastatic locations are the liver and peripancreatic lymph nodes followed by the lungs and bones; bone metastases are osteoplastic in most cases [4]. In patients with pNETs, the assessment of the tumor extent and location and the evaluation of prognostic factors and the individual patient's performance status and comorbidities are required to define the proper treatment [4–6].

The staging of pNETs is based on TNM evaluation. A TNM consensus has been proposed on NETs by the European Neuroendocrine Tumor Society (ENETs)

(▫ Table 15.1), and in one large comparative study of 1072 pNET patients, both the American Joint Committee on Cancer (AJCC) and ENETS TNM classifications were found to be independent predictors of survival at multivariate analysis. However, the ENETS TNM classification proved superior to and more accurate than the AJCC TNM classification [7].

In evaluating the local extent of the primary tumor, it is important to establish the tumor dimension, any invasion of close vessels, nerves, and lymph nodes. The

▫ **Table 15.1** A tumor-node-metastasis (TNM) staging system for pancreatic neuroendocrine tumors (pNETs) [7]

T primary tumor		
ENETs TNM		**AJCC/UICC TNM**
T1	Confined to pancreas, <2 cm	Confined to pancreas, <2 cm
T2	Confined to pancreas, 2–4 cm	Confined to pancreas, >2 cm
T3	Confined to pancreas, >4 cm, or invasion of the duodenum or bile duct	Peripancreatic spread, but without major vascular invasion (truncus coeliacus, A. Mesent. Sup.)
T4	Invasion of adjacent organs or major vessels	Major vascular invasion

N lymph nodes	
Nx	Lymph nodes cannot be evaluated
N0	Tumor cells are absent from regional lymph nodes
N1	The presence of lymph node metastases
M presence of distant metastasis	
M0	No distant metastasis
M1	Some metastasis to distant organs (beyond regional lymph nodes)

TNM staging			
I	T1	N0	M0
IIa	T2	N0	M0
IIb	T3	N0	M0
IIIa	T4	N0	M0
IIIb	Any T	N1	M0
IV	Any T	Any N	M1

AJCC American Joint Committee on Cancer, *ENETS* European Neuroendocrine Tumor Society, *UICC* Union for International Cancer Control dimension of the primary tumor is crucial to decide on how to manage it; in fact, for small pNETs noninvasive approaches (i.e., wait and watch or SSAs) have been accepted [8]. Moreover, the evaluation of the tumor extent and the identification of the exact site of the primary tumor and any metastatic lymph nodes are necessary to decide whether a curative surgical approach is possible. In the case of localized primary tumor, without vascular or neurologic invasion, a local curative treatment (i.e., surgical resection) is possible, whereas in those cases with invasion of vessels or where distant metastases are present at the initial diagnosis, other treatment options with palliative intent need to be taken into account.

In evaluating the local extent of a pNET, standard abdominal ultrasound, EUS, computed CT scan, and MRI study are frequently used [4, 5]. However, EUS is the most accurate technique for the local staging of pNETs as it can properly study any local vascular and node involvement and the distance of the lesion from the pancreatic duct.

For evaluating any distant spreading, besides CT scan and MRI, somatostatin receptor scintigraphy (SRS) or, even better, PET scanning based on 68Ga-radiolabeled SSAs should be routinely performed in order to evaluate the extent of metastatic disease [4, 5, 9–11]. The use of SRS or Ga68-PET aims both at identifying distant metastases – particularly bone metastases which represent a poor prognostic factor and a contraindication to surgery [12] – and detecting SSA receptors prior to medical therapy or radiolabeled SSAs.

Furthermore, a complete histological assessment of the tumor by biopsy, including the detection of the mitotic Ki-67 index, is needed prior to treatment as well-differentiated pNETs show a different behavior from poorly differentiated pNETs with a consequently different therapeutic approach [13, 14].

▪ Ultrasound Endoscopy

The close proximity of the pancreas to the gastric and duodenal walls particularly lends itself to detailed examination by EUS. The head of the pancreas and the uncinate process can be visualized transduodenally, whereas the neck, body, and tail are seen through the stomach wall. The pancreatic parenchyma, ducts, and vascular structures can be well visualized. Of note, any adjacent celiac, peripancreatic, para-aortic, and periportal lymphadenopathy can also be seen and evaluated. Unlike other imaging tools such as CT, MRI, and SRS, EUS is well suited to the identification of small pancreatic lesions as small as 2–5 mm [15, 16].

EUS is particularly advantageous in the detection of both small insulinomas, which are usually not seen by SRS, and multifocal pNETs [17]. Furthermore, EUS-guided fine needle aspiration (FNA) allows to collect a histologic sample for a final diagnosis. Sensitivities of 61%–84% and overall accuracy of up to 92.5% have been reported for EUS-FNA in diagnosing pNETs [18–20]. Such high sensitivity together with the low incidence of complications makes EUS-FNA the procedure of choice to achieve the final diagnosis [21]. Of note, EUS-FNA allows not only to establish the neuroendocrine nature of a pancreatic lesion but also to obtain relevant prognostic data (e.g., the Ki-67 proliferative index) to guide the therapeutic strategy [22–24].

Several studies on the accuracy of EUS, particularly in the detection of insulinomas, have been published with detection rates ranging from 79% to 94% [25–27]. In a recent meta-analysis, Puli et al. found that EUS has excellent sensitivity and specificity to localize pNETs approaching 100%. Of note, in a subgroup analysis, EUS showed high sensitivity and specificity to detect any insulinoma or gastrinoma in the pancreas [28]. A study on 52 patients reported a sensitivity of 89.5% and accuracy of 83.7% for EUS in the detection of insulinomas. The authors found that the accuracy depends on the location of the tumor and is greatest for tumors in the pancreatic head [29]. In addition, EUS-guided FNA may detect malignant lymph nodes or liver metastases. Finally, the determination of the Ki-67 proliferative index may give prognostic information that is useful to guide further therapeutic decisions.

Regarding small (i.e., ≤2 cm) nonfunctioning well-differentiated pNETs, a wait-and-watch approach has been recently suggested in selected cases [8, 30, 31]. EUS is extremely important in this specific setting to establish the Ki-67 index as this information is crucial to the management decision process [32]. Moreover, EUS can help in the serial follow-up of these patients to detect any growth or suspicious features necessitating surgical resection.

Furthermore, EUS is extremely useful in the preoperative setting for local staging, in particular to establish whether a lesion is feasible for surgical resection as it can visualize adjacent vessels and any lymphadenopathy. In fact, the invasion of close vessels (e.g., the superior mesenteric or splenic artery) represents a contraindication to surgery. Moreover, EUS can establish the distance between the tumor lesion and the main pancreatic duct in order to define the best surgical approach (enucleation vs. resection) [32].

Another emerging application of EUS to both functioning and nonfunctioning pNETs is the performance of EUS-guided fine needle tattooing (EUS-FNT) of the lesion in order to facilitate its precise localization during surgery, particularly in the case of a laparoscopic approach [33–36].

Conventional Imaging

Imaging plays a crucial role in the detection of clinically suspected pNETs as well as for staging in patients diagnosed with pNETs. Conventional imaging modalities include US, CT, and MRI.

The presence and extent of liver metastases are among the most important prognostic factors for patients with pNETs. Recently, the presence of lymph node metastases as well as the extent of the lymph node metastases or the number of positive lymph nodes have been suggested as important prognostic factors [37].

CT is considered to be a good diagnostic tool for the detection of a primary pNET with sensitivity and specificity at approximately 73% and 96%, respectively [4]. Of note, whole-body CT scanning is a well-established method for the staging of NETs [38] with reported sensitivity and specificity for the detection of liver metastases at approximately 82% and 92%, respectively [4]. CT imaging should be performed with multi-detector CT scanners and allowing for a slice thickness of less than 1.5 mm and multi-planar reconstructions [38].

A recent study on 109 patients with surgically proven pNETs (NET G1 = 66, NET G2 = 31, NEC = 12) who underwent multi-detector CT (MDCT) evaluated the staging accuracy of this technique for pNETs: it showed that MDCT accurately depicts the tumor stage with accuracy at 85%–88% for determining the T stage and at 83%–89% for node metastases. In addition, MDCT proved useful to the prediction of tumor grade as uncommon findings (i.e., ill-defined, heterogeneously enhanced and hypo-vascular appearance and duct dilation) were more common in higher-grade tumors [39].

MRI is considered to be an excellent imaging modality for the detection of pNETs thanks to its multi-parametric approach and good-contrast resolution [40]. MRI is also used for the staging of pNETs. It can be used alternatively or in addition to CT imaging when there is clinical suspicion of a pNET that cannot be detected with CT imaging alone or when results are unclear [38]. The MRI diagnostic performance in detecting primary tumors in the pancreas shows sensitivity and specificity at approximately 93% and 88%, respectively [4]. Of note, MRI has shown to be superior, in direct comparison with CT, in the detection of liver metastases with a detection rate of up to 95% [41].

Sequences should include in- and opposed-phase T1-weighted (T1 W) imaging, T2-weighted (T2 W) imaging with and without fat suppression in axial and coronal orientation, dynamic contrast-enhanced T1 W 3D sequences with fat suppression [unenhanced, arterial (delay, 20s), portal venous (55 s), venous (90s), and delayed phase (120 s)], as well as MRCP (best after contrast application) [38].

Diffusion-weighted imaging (DWI) is a functional MRI technique which provides qualitative and quantitative data, for instance, to identify any area of restricted water diffusion as in tumors. A recent retrospective study including 25 patients investigated the added value of DWI in pNET evaluation and compared MRI to 68Ga-DOTANOC positron emission tomography/computed tomography (PET/CT) results [40]. The authors found that conventional MRI, DW-MRI, and 68Ga-DOTANOC PET/CT can be alternative tools for pNET detection. Diffusion-weighted MRI should be considered for patients with clinical suspicion but negative conventional imaging findings or for those cases where other techniques are not feasible. However, the consensus on the three techniques seems the best approach. Furthermore, DWI and hepato-specific contrast material for liver MRI are useful as liver metastases from pNETs are usually very small [42–44]. Again, DWI or hepatobiliary phase MRI may avoid the tumor size overestimation, which may be related to the presence of some peri-tumor enhancement, which is often detected in neuroendocrine liver metastases as a consequence of desmoplasia, inflammation, steatosis, and vascular proliferation [45].

Nuclear Imaging

Pancreatic NETs overexpress somatostatin receptors (SSTR 2, 3, and 5) [46]: this circumstance has been exploited for somatostatin receptor scintigraphy (SRS) and more recently for PET/CT imaging, especially gallium-labeled somatostatin PET, which is considered to be more accurate than SRS. However, the physiological uptake of 68Ga-DOTANOC in the pancreas, especially in the uncinate process, compromises its specificity [47]. Furthermore, insulinomas, which are the commonest functioning pNETs, have limited SSTR expression [48, 49] thereby limiting the sensitivity of 68Ga-DOTANOC PET/CT for these tumors. According to the ENETS consensus guidelines, if basal nuclear imaging is positive, patients would have to repeat it for staging every 18–24 months [50].

Studies evaluating the accuracy of Ga-68 PET scan only in pNET patients are scanty. Kumar et al. [51] evaluated 68Ga-DOTATOC PET/CT in 20 pNET patients and found it to be better than contrast CT and 18F-FDG PET/CT for both primary tumor and metastases. In the study by Schmid-Tannwald et al. [52] including 18 patients with pNETs, 68Ga-DOTATATE PET/CT was reported to be superior to DW-MRI in terms of detection rates.

In a recent large retrospective study by Sharma et al. [53], the utility of 68Ga-DOTANOC PET/CT was assessed in 141 patients with pNETs, and 68Ga-DOTANOC PET/CT was found to be useful toward the diagnosis, staging, and restaging of patients with pNETs, even if its role is limited with regard to insulinomas. In addition, this technique may select patients for SSA (both cold and radiolabeled) therapy when needed. In the study by Haug et al. [54], 63 patients were examined with 68Ga-DOTATATE PET/CT after the primary NET curative resection. 68Ga-DOTATATE PET/CT helped correctly identify 26 out of 29 patients with recurrent NET and helped exclude NET recurrence in 28 out of 34 patients, thus indicating sensitivity at 90% and specificity at 82%, respectively, recommending its use in the follow-up of NET.

For more aggressive high-grade pNETs, fluorodeoxyglucose (FDG) as a marker of increased glucose metabolism should be preferred [55, 56]; moreover, it may be complementary to Ga68-PET scan in detecting more metastatic lesions with different histologic differentiations [57].

15.2 Conclusions

EUS has a decisive role in the setting of pNETs. It can help to correctly localize the tumor when other noninvasive procedures have failed and can provide additional useful information (i.e., distance from the pancreatic duct, Ki-67 proliferation index) toward the best therapeutic management (surgery, conservative approach, type of antitumor therapy in case of unresectable tumors). Furthermore, the possibility of EUS-guided FNA tattooing of pancreatic lesions may be extremely helpful in the preoperative setting.

Conventional radiology, including CT and MRI, plays a crucial role in staging for patients diagnosed with pNETs. The presence and extent of liver metastases as well as the presence of lymph node metastases, the extent of the lymph node metastases or the number of positive lymph nodes are among the most important prognostic factors for patients with pNETs [37]. In this setting, CT and MRI can be used as alternative modalities; however MRI has been reported to be superior, in direct comparison to CT, in the detection of liver metastases [41].

Nuclear imaging, particularly PET-Ga68 scan, aims at both identifying distant metastases – particularly bone metastases which represent a poor prognostic factor and a contraindication to surgery – and SSA receptors prior to medical therapy or radiolabeled SSAs.

Bibliography

1. Rindi G, Arnold R, Bosman F, Capella C, Kilmstra D, Kloppel G (2010) Nomenclature and classification of neuroendocrine neoplasms of the digestive system. In: Bosman FT et al (eds) WHO classification of Tumours of the digestive system. IARC Press, Lyon, pp 13–14
2. Franko J, Feng W, Yip L et al (2010) Non-functional neuroendocrine carcinoma of the pancreas: incidence, tumor biology, and outcomes in 2,158 patients. J Gastrointest Surg 14:541–548

3. Oberg K (2010) Pancreatic endocrine tumors. Semin Oncol 37:594–618
4. Sundin A, Vullierme MP, Kaltsas G et al (2009) ENETS consensus guidelines for the standards of Care in Neuroendocrine Tumors: radiological examinations. Neuroendocrinology 90:167–183
5. Metz DC, Jensen RT (2008) Gastrointestinal neuroendocrine tumors: pancreatic endocrine tumors. Gastroenterology 135:1469–1492
6. Kulke MH, Anthony LB, Bushnell DL et al (2010) NANETS treatment guidelines: well-differentiated neuroendocrine tumors of the stomach and pancreas. Pancreas 39:735–752
7. Martin-Perez E, Capdevila J, Castellano D et al (2013) Prognostic factors and long-term outcome of pancreatic neuroendocrine neoplasms: Ki-67 index shows a greater impact on survival than disease stage. The large experience of the Spanish National Tumor Registry (RGETNE). Neuroendocrinology 98:156–168
8. Massironi S, Rossi RE, Zilli A, Casazza G, Ciafardini C, Conte D (2016) A wait-and-watch approach to small pancreatic neuroendocrine tumors: prognosis and survival. Oncotarget 7:18978–18983
9. Oberg K, Kvols L, Caplin M et al (2004) Consensus report on the use of somatostatin analogs for the management of neuroendocrine tumors of the gastroenteropancreatic system. Ann Oncol 15:966–973
10. Öberg K (2012) Gallium-68 somatostatin receptor PET/CT: is it time to replace (111)indium DTPA octreotide for patients with neuroendocrine tumors? Endocrine 42:3–4
11. Kwekkeboom DJ, Kam BL, van Essen M et al (2010) Somatostatin-receptor-based imaging and therapy of gastroenteropancreatic neuroendocrine tumors. Endocr Relat Cancer 17:R53–R73
12. Panzuto F, Nasoni S, Falconi M et al (2005) Prognostic factors and survival in endocrine tumor patients: comparison between gastrointestinal and pancreatic localization. Endocr Relat Cancer 12:1083–1092
13. Klimstra DS, Modlin IR, Coppola D et al (2010) The pathologic classification of neuroendocrine tumors: a review of nomenclature, grading, and staging systems. Pancreas 39:707–712
14. Klöppel G, Couvelard A, Perren A et al (2009) ENETS consensus guidelines for the standards of Care in Neuroendocrine Tumors: towards a standardized approach to the diagnosis of gastroenteropancreatic neuroendocrine tumors and their prognostic stratification. Neuroendocrinology 90:162–166
15. Rosch T, Lightdale CJ, Botet JF et al (1992) Localization of pancreatic endocrine tumors by endoscopic ultrasonography. N Engl J Med 326:1721–1726
16. Kim MK (2012) Endoscopic ultrasound in gastroenteropancreatic neuroendocrine tumors. Gut Liver 6:405–410
17. Rustagi T, Farrell JJ (2014) Endoscopic diagnosis and treatment of pancreatic neuroendocrine tumors. J Clin Gastroenterol 48:837–844
18. Pais SA, Al-Haddad M, Mohamadnejad M et al (2010) EUS for pancreatic neuroendocrine tumors: a single-center, 11-year experience. Gastrointest Endosc 71:1185–1193
19. Pais SA, Mcgreevy K, Leblanc JK et al (2007) Utility of EUSFNA in the diagnosis of pancreatic neuroendocrine tumors: correlation with histopathology in 76 patients. Gastrointest Endosc 65:AB304
20. Atiq M, Bhutani MS, Bektas M et al (2012) EUS-FNA for pancreatic neuroendocrine tumors: a tertiary cancer center experience. Dig Dis Sci 57:791–800
21. Eloubeidi MA, Tamhane A, Varadarajulu S et al (2006) Frequency of major complications after EUS-guided FNA of solid pancreatic masses: a prospective evaluation. Gastrointest Endosc 63:622–629
22. Piani C, Franchi GM, Cappelletti C et al (2008) Cytological Ki-67 in pancreatic endocrine tumours: an opportunity for pre-operative grading. Endocr Relat Cancer 15:175–181
23. Chatzipantelis P, Konstantinou P, Kaklamanos M et al (2009) The role of cytomorphology and proliferative activity in predicting biologic behavior of pancreatic neuroendocrine tumors: a study by endoscopic ultrasound-guided fine-needle aspiration cytology. Cancer 117:211–216
24. Alexiev BA, Darwin PE, Goloubeva O, Ioffe OB (2009) Proliferative rate in endoscopic ultrasound fine-needle aspiration of pancreatic endocrine tumors: correlation with clinical behavior. Cancer 117:40–45
25. Anderson MA, Carpenter S, Thompson NW et al (2000) Endoscopic ultrasound is highly accurate and directs management in patients with neuroendocrine tumors of the pancreas. Am J Gastroenterol 95:2271–2277
26. Gouya H, Vignaux O, Augui J et al (2003) CT, endoscopic sonography, and a combined protocol for preoperative evaluation of pancreatic insulinomas. AJR Am J Roentgenol 181:987–992

27. Ardengh JC, Rosenbaum P, Ganc AJ et al (2000) Role of EUS in the preoperative localization of insulinomas compared with spiral CT. Gastrointest Endosc 51:552–555
28. Puli SR, Kalva N, Bechtold ML et al (2013) Diagnostic accuracy of endoscopic ultrasound in pancreatic neuroendocrine tumors: a systematic review and meta analysis. World J Gastroenterol 19:3678–3684
29. Sotoudehmanesh R, Hedayat A, Shirazian N et al (2007) Endoscopic ultrasonography (EUS) in the localization of insulinoma. Endocrine 31:238–241
30. Lee LC, Grant CS, Salomao DR et al (2012) Small, nonfunctioning, asymptomatic pancreatic neuroendocrine tumors (PNETs): role for non-operative management. Surgery 152:965–974
31. Gaujoux S, Partelli S, Maire F, D'Onofrio M, Larroque B, Tamburrino D, Sauvanet A, Falconi M, Ruszniewski P (2013) Observational study of natural history of small sporadic nonfunctioning pancreatic neuroendocrine tumors. J Clin Endocrinol Metab 98:4784–4789
32. Attili F, Capurso G, Vanella G, Fuccio L, Delle Fave G, Costamagna G, Larghi A (2014) Diagnostic and therapeutic role of endoscopy in gastroenteropancreatic neuroendocrine neoplasms. Dig Liver Dis 46:9–17
33. Gress FG, Barawi M, Kim D et al (2002) Preoperative localization of a neuroendocrine tumor of the pancreas with EUS-guided fine needle tattooing. Gastrointest Endosc 55:594–597
34. Zografos GN, Stathopoulou A, Mitropapas G et al (2005) Preoperative imaging and localization of small sized insulinoma with EUS guided fine needle tattooing: a case report. Hormones (Athens) 4:111–116
35. Farrell JJ, Sherrod A, Parekh D (2009) EUS guided fine needle tattooing for preoperative localization of early pancreatic adenocarcinoma. Gastrointest Endosc 69:176–177
36. Lennon AM, Newman N, Makary MA et al (2010) EUS-guided tattooing before laparoscopic distal pancreatic resection (with video). Gastrointest Endosc 72:1089–1094
37. Falconi M, Eriksson B, Kaltsas G, Bartsch DK, Capdevila J, Caplin M, Kos-Kudla B, Kwekkeboom D, Rindi G, Klöppel G, Reed N, Kianmanesh R (2016) Jensen RT; Vienna consensus conference participants. ENETS consensus guidelines update for the Management of Patients with functional pancreatic neuroendocrine tumors and non-functional pancreatic neuroendocrine tumors. Neuroendocrinology 103:153–171
38. Baur AD, Pavel M, Prasad V, Denecke T (2016) Diagnostic imaging of pancreatic neuroendocrine neoplasms (pNEN): tumor detection, staging, prognosis, and response to treatment. Acta Radiol 57:260–270
39. Kim JH, Eun HW, Kim YJ, Lee JM, Han JK, Choi BI (2016) Pancreatic neuroendocrine tumour (PNET): staging accuracy of MDCT and its diagnostic performance for the differentiation of PNET with uncommon CT findings from pancreatic adenocarcinoma. Eur Radiol 26:1338–1347
40. Farchione A, Rufini V, Brizi MG, Iacovazzo D, Larghi A, Massara RM, Petrone G, Poscia A, Treglia G, De Marinis L, Giordano A, Rindi G, Bonomo L (2016) Evaluation of the added value of diffusion-weighted imaging to conventional magnetic resonance imaging in pancreatic neuroendocrine tumors and comparison with 68Ga-DOTANOC positron emission tomography/computed tomography. Pancreas 45:345–354
41. Dromain C, de Baere T, Lumbroso J et al (2005) Detection of liver metastases from endocrine tumors: a prospective comparison of somatostatin receptor scintigraphy computed tomography, and magnetic resonance imaging. J Clin Oncol 23:70–78
42. Van Beers BE, Pastor CM, Hussain HK (2012) Primovist, Eovist: what to expect? J Hepatol 57:421–429
43. Huppertz A, Balzer T, Blakeborough A et al (2004) Improved detection of focal liver lesions at MR imaging: multicenter comparison of gadoxetic acid-enhanced MR images with intraoperative findings. Radiology 230:266–275
44. d'Assignies G, Fina P, Bruno O et al (2013) High sensitivity of diffusion-weighted MR imaging for the detection of liver metastases from neuroendocrine tumors: comparison with T2-weighted and dynamic gadolinium-enhanced MR imaging. Radiology 268:390–399
45. Semelka RC, Hussain SM, Marcos HB et al (2000) Perilesional enhancement of hepatic metastases: correlation between MR imaging and histopathologic findings-initial observations. Radiology 215:89–94
46. Oda Y, Tanaka Y, Naruse T, Sasanabe R, Tsubamoto MFH (2002) Expression of somatostatin receptor and effects of somatostatin analog on pancreatic endocrine tumors. Surg Today 32:690–694

47. Krausz Y, Rubinstein R, Appelbaum L et al (2012) Ga-68 DOTANOC uptake in the pancreas: pathological and physiological patterns. Clin Nucl Med 37:57–62
48. Grant CS (2005) Insulinoma. Best Pract Res Clin Gastroenterol 19:783–798 9
49. Zimmer T, Stölzel U, Bäder M et al (1996) Endoscopic ultrasonography and somatostatin receptor scintigraphy in the preoperative localisation of insulinomas and gastrinomas. Gut 39:562–568
50. Pavel M, Baudin E, Couvelard A et al (2012) ENETS consensus guidelines for the management of patients with liver and other distant metastases from neuroendocrine neoplasms of foregut, midgut, hindgut, and unknown primary. Neuroendocrinology 95:157–176
51. Kumar R, Sharma P, Garg P et al (2011) Role of (68)Ga DOTATOC PET-CT in the diagnosis and staging of pancreatic neuroendocrine tumours. Eur Radiol 21:2408–2416
52. Schmid-Tannwald C, Schmid-Tannwald CM, Morelli JN et al (2013) Comparison of abdominal MRI with diffusion-weighted imaging to 68Ga-DOTATATE PET/CT in detection of neuroendocrine tumors of the pancreas. Eur J Nucl Med Mol Imaging 40:897–907
53. Sharma P, Arora S, Dhull VS, Naswa N, Kumar R, Ammini AC, Bal C (2015) Evaluation of (68)Ga-DOTANOC PET/CT imaging in a large exclusive population of pancreatic neuroendocrine tumors. Abdom Imaging 40:299–309
54. Haug AR, Cindea-Drimus R, Auernhammer CJ, Reincke M, Beuschlein F, Wängler B, Uebleis C, Schmidt GP, Spitzweg C, Bartenstein P, Hacker M (2014) Neuroendocrine tumor recurrence: diagnosis with 68Ga-DOTATATE PET/CT. Radiology 270:517–525
55. Ezziddin S, Logvinski T, Yong-Hing C et al (2006) Factors predicting tracer uptake in somatostatin receptor and MIBG scintigraphy of metastatic gastroenteropancreatic neuroendocrine tumors. J Nucl Med 47:223–233
56. Kayani I, Bomanji JB, Groves A et al (2008) Functional imaging of neuroendocrine tumors with combined PET/CT using 68Ga-DOTATATE (DOTA-DPhe1,Tyr3-octreotate) and 18F-FDG. Cancer 112:2447–2455
57. Naswa N, Sharma P, Gupta SK et al (2014) Dual tracer functional imaging of Gastroenteropancreatic neuroendocrine tumours using 68 Ga-DOTANOC PET-CT and 18F-FDG PET-CT: competitive or complimentary? Clin Nucl Med 39:e27–e34§

Therapy for Locoregional Disease: Stomach/ Duodenum, Colon/ Rectum

Davide Campana, Nico Pagano, Nicole Brighi, Dario Fabbri, Maria Rinzivillo, Gianfranco Delle Fave, Guido Biasco, and Francesco Panzuto

A. Colao et al. (eds.), *Neuroendocrine Tumors in Real Life*,
https://doi.org/10.1007/978-3-319-59024-0_16

Overview

Neuroendocrine neoplasms (NENs) of the gastrointestinal (GI) tract are a heterogeneous group of tumors originating from neuroendocrine cells distributed throughout the gut and frequently presenting with correlated hypersecretory syndromes, especially in metastatic diseases. Gut-derived NENs have been classified according to their embryological origin into tumors of the foregut (bronchi, stomach, pancreas, gallbladder, duodenum), midgut (duodenum, ileum, appendix, right colon), and hindgut (left colon, rectum).

The incidence of NENs diagnosed has increased in the last years, with GI primary tumors representing the majority of diagnosis. NENs may occur as part of complex familial endocrine cancer syndromes such as multiple endocrine neoplasia type 1 (MEN 1), multiple endocrine neoplasia type 2 (MEN 2), neurofibromatosis type 1, Von Hippel–Lindau syndrome, and Carney's complex, although the majority occurs as sporadic isolated tumors.

The management of NENs of the GI tract in the setting of locoregional disease consists of different therapeutic approaches, in particular medical treatment and endoscopic procedures, and it varies greatly depending on the site of origin.

In patients with gastric NENs (gNENs), the approach depends on the clinical presentation of the tumor, classified in three types. Type 1 gNENs are associated with hypergastrinemia and chronic atrophic gastritis; the frequency of metastasis is low. Type 2 gNENs occur in patients with hypergastrinemia due to Zollinger-Ellison syndrome in combination with MEN 1. Type 3 gNENs are sporadic and have a more malignant course, frequently presenting with metastasis at the time of diagnosis.

Duodenal NENs are rare (less than 2% of all GI-NENs), and gastrinomas are the most frequent type of tumors originating in this site.

Rectal NENs are commonly small and generally low to intermediate grade (G1–2), whereas colonic NENs are often aggressive, poorly differentiated, and higher grade (G3).

Clinical Case

16

A 68-year-old woman presented to her general practitioner with a 24 months history of dyspeptic syndrome, abdominal bloating, and fasting heartburn. Blood tests revealed the presence of a microcytic iron-deficiency anemia. She underwent an upper endoscopy that showed chronic gastritis with multiple small polyps in the fundus (◘ Fig. 16.1); *Helicobacter pylori* resulted positive.

The patient was treated with clarithromycin, metronidazole, and proton pump inhibitors for *Helicobacter pylori* eradication; the urea breath test after therapy resulted negative.

The patient was then referred to our Institution of Internal Medicine because of the detection of hypergastrinemia (1450 pg/ml; normal value <50 pg/ml).

Blood tests were repeated and revealed abnormally elevated values of serum chromogranin A (CgA) (135 U/l; normal value <17 U/l) and the positivity of anti-parietal cells antibodies. Hypergastrinemia was confirmed. The biochemical markers of renal, liver, thyroid (includ-

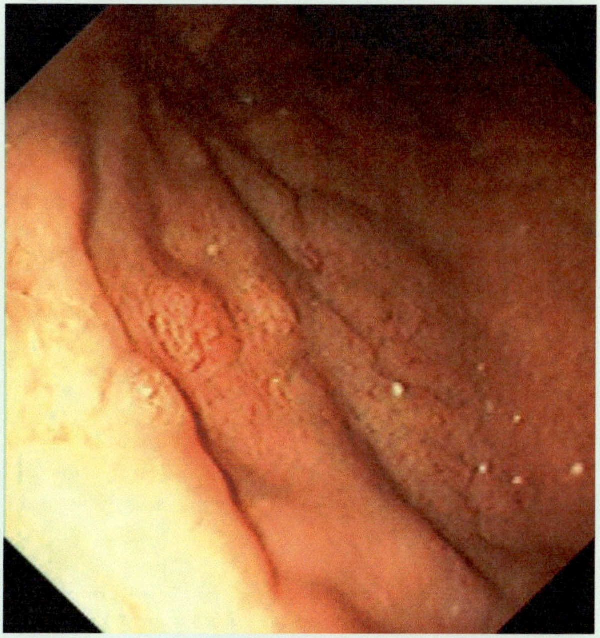

Fig. 16.1 Multiple gastric small polyps in body and fundus

ing thyroid antibodies), and parathyroid function were within normal range. Vitamin B12 was very low (90 pg/ml, nv: 195–865 pg/ml). Physical examination was negative.

Upper endoscopy was then repeated and showed a pale mucosa with multiple sessile polyps (<5 mm) in the body and fundus. Several biopsies of antrum, body, and fundus were performed.

The histological examination of body and fundus biopsies revealed multiple well-differentiated neuroendocrine neoplasms (NENs, 2010 WHO classification) on a context of moderate chronic atrophic gastritis (CAG) with widespread intestinal metaplasia; foveolar hyperplasia was present in the antrum. The Ki-67 index of the NENs was 0.8% (Fig. 16.2).

To assess the TNM stage, an endoscopic ultrasound (EUS) was performed and revealed multiple (more than 10) small hypoechoic thickenings of the mucosa of the fundus and of the gastric body (average diameter: 7 mm), with no clear signs of submucosal infiltration. No perigastric lymph nodes were detected.

The patient started treatment with long-acting somatostatin analogs (SSAs, 30 mg every 28 days, intramuscular injection).

An upper endoscopy was performed 6 months after the treatment started, showing endoscopic features of CAG with 5–6 sessile polyps (2–3 mm) in the body and fundus. The histological examination revealed micronodular hyperplasia of the neuroendocrine cells (Fig. 16.3) without evidence of NENs. Blood tests revealed a decrease in serum CgA (78 U/l vs 135 U/l) and gastrin (860 pg/ml vs 1450 pg/ml).

The patient continued the treatment with SSAs, and the upper endoscopy was repeated after 12 months from the start. The histological examination showed mild linear hyperplasia of the neuroendocrine cells. Blood tests revealed a further decrease in serum CgA (55 U/l) and gastrin (520 pg/ml).

The patient continued the treatment and repeated a gastroscopy after 24 months from the treatment start. The endoscopy showed a quiescent CAG, and the histological examination did not find any neuroendocrine cell alteration. CgA and gastrin were 45 U/L and 450 pg/ml, respectively.

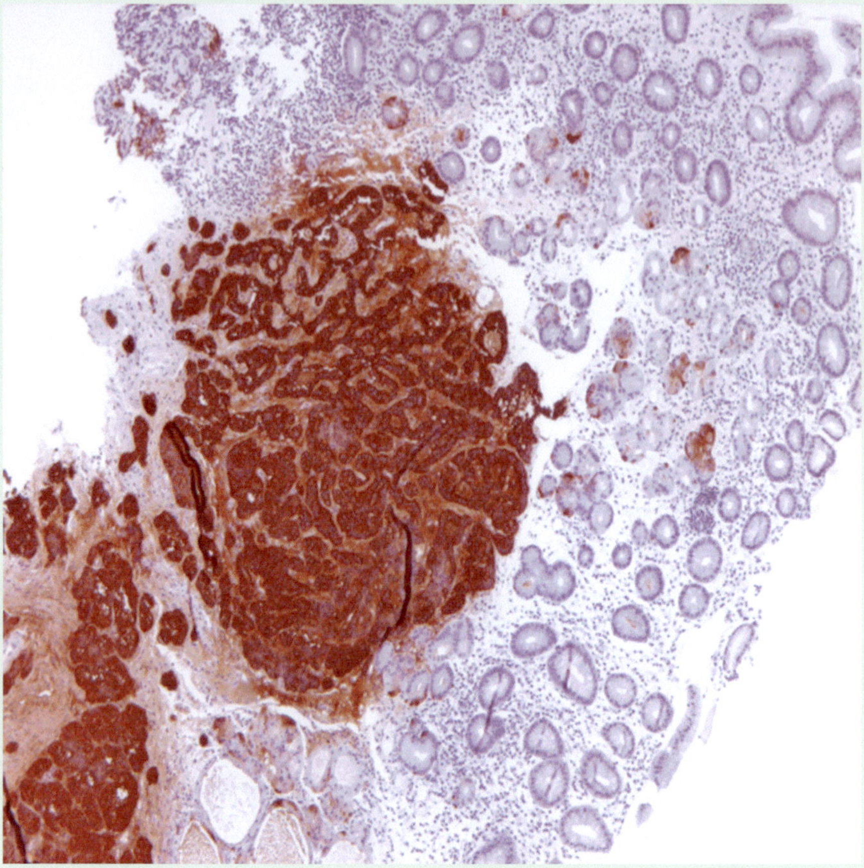

Fig. 16.2 Well-differentiated neuroendocrine neoplasm on a context of moderate chronic atrophic gastritis

The treatment was discontinued at this point, and endoscopic surveillance was established. The patient underwent a gastroscopy 12 months after treatment discontinuation, showing CAG of the fundus with intestinal metaplasia and mild linear hyperplasia of the endocrine cells at the histological examination. At this time (6 years from the end of therapy), no evidence of NEN was found.

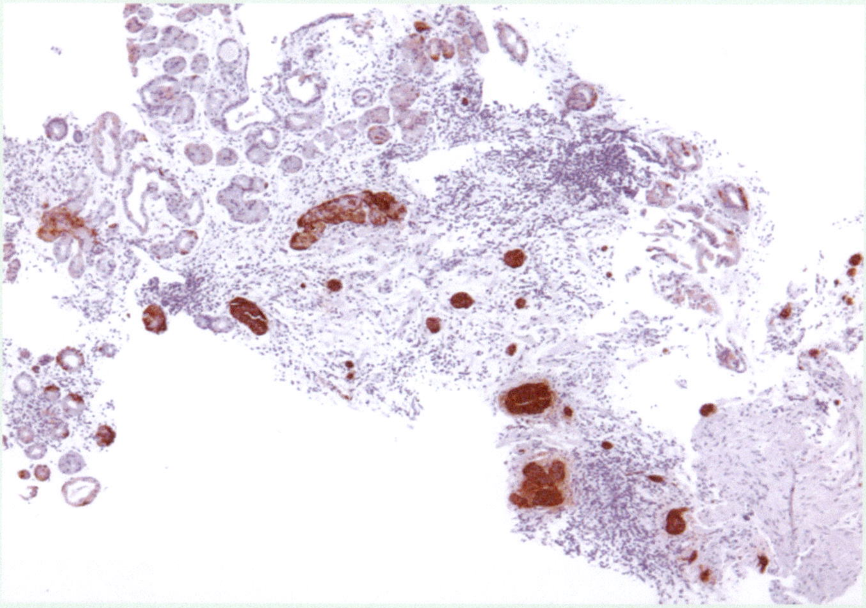

Fig. 16.3 Micronodular hyperplasia of the neuroendocrine cells without evidence of NENs

16.1 Comments to the Case

Gastric NENs (gNENs – also called «carcinoids») are tumors derived from enterochromaffin-like cells (ECL cells) localized in the gastric mucosa [1].

ECL cell tumors have been categorized into three subgroups: type 1 (70–80%) associated with CAG and hypergastrinemia, type 2 (5–8%) associated with gastrinomas in Zollinger–Ellison syndrome (ZES) and multiple endocrine neoplasia type 1 (MEN 1), and type 3 (15–20%) consisting in sporadic lesions arising in otherwise normal gastric mucosa in the absence of hypergastrinemia [2].

Neoplastic alterations in type 1 and 2 gNENs are always associated with an elevated concentration of serum gastrin [2]; gastrin exerts a trophic effect on ECL cells, leading to hyperplasia and, in some cases, to NENs [3, 4].

The majority of type 1 gNENs occurs in women and are rarely symptomatic [5]. They are nonfunctioning tumors, typically found during upper gastrointestinal (GI) endoscopy for dyspepsia or anemia [6]. Type 1 gNENs frequently present as multiple polyps, usually <1 cm in diameter, localized in the gastric corpus-fundus. They are almost exclusively benign lesions with a low risk of deep invasion of the gastric wall [7]. These tumors have a good prognosis with a 5-year survival rate quoted at 96%, comparable to the age-matched normal population [6, 8].

In the case presented, the diagnosis of CAG was suggested by the high levels of gastrin and CgA and the positivity of anti-parietal cells antibodies. Histological examination revealed a moderate CAG of corpus-fundus with multiple gNENs (type 1 gNENs). EUS examination revealed multiple lesions smaller than 1 cm, limited to the submucosa (stage I – ◘ Table 16.1). High number of the lesions (more than 10) contraindicated the endoscopic resection.

As reported in literature [10–14], the patient was treated with SSAs. After 6 months of treatment, a complete regression of the neoplastic lesions was observed. Pathological examination showed a regression from NENs to micronodular hyperplasia. Significantly

◘ Table 16.1 TNM staging of gastric neuroendocrine neoplasms

TNM			
T-primary tumor			
TX	Primary tumor cannot be assessed		
T0	No evidence of primary tumor		
Tis	In situ tumor/dysplasia (<0.5 mm)		
T1	Tumor invades lamina propria or submucosa and ≤1 cm		
T2	Tumor invades muscularis propria or subserosa or >1 cm		
T3	Tumor penetrates serosa		
T4	Tumor invades adjacent structures For any T, add (m) for multiple tumors		
N-regional lymph nodes			
NX	Regional lymph nodes cannot be assessed		
N0	No regional lymph node metastasis		
N1	Regional lymph node metastasis		
M-distant metastasis			
MX	Distant metastasis cannot be assessed		
M1	Distant metastasis		
Stage			
Stage 0	Tis	N0	M0
Stage I	T1	N0	M0
Stage IIa Stage IIb	T2 T3	N0 N0	M0 M0
Stage IIIa Stage IIIb	T4 Any T	N0 N1	M0 M0
Stage IV	Any T	Any N	M1

From Rindi et al. [9]

lower CgA levels after 6 months and after 12 months compared to baseline serum concentration were found. This decrease could be due to both an inhibitory effect produced by SSAs treatment on CgA secretion and pathological changes from neoplasia to hyperplasia [10, 15]. Finally, a significant reduction in serum gastrin levels during SSAs treatment was also found. Since hypergastrinemia plays an important role in the pathogenesis of type 1 gNENs, it is suggested that the decrease in serum gastrin levels may influence the regression of the tumors.

Questions

1. What is the role of gastrin in the aethiopathogenesis of type 1 and 2 gNENs?
2. Which parameters should be considered to guide the clinical approach in type 1 gNENs?
3. Which are the possible treatments for type 1 gNENs?

Answers

1. Neoplastic alterations in type 1 and 2 gNENs are associated with an elevated concentration of serum gastrin, which exerts a trophic effect on ECL cells, leading to hyperplasia and, in some cases, to NENs.
2. It is suggested that the decrease in serum gastrin levels due to SSAs therapy may lead to the regression of the tumors.
3. Therapeutic strategies for type 1 gNENs are based on risk stratification according to tumor size, lesion number, stage, and grade. Current ENETS guidelines suggest endoscopic management with lesion resection, while a surgical approach should be limited to cases of clearly demonstrated invasion beyond the submucosa and/or with metastasis.

Q4. Current literature points out the elevated variability existing in treatments in case of multiple, localized (mucosa or submucosa) type 1 gNENs:
   1. Careful endoscopic surveillance without any treatment [16–18]
   2. Somatostatin analogs therapy [10–14]
   3. Endoscopic resection [11, 19, 20]
   4. Surgical approach with antrectomy (to obtain a normalization of gastrin levels) [21]

Up to Date of the Topic

The choice of the clinical approach is related to the site of the NEN and to further classifications.

Stomach

The therapeutic approach of gNENs varies greatly among the three types in which they are divided.

Endoscopic surveillance without tumor resection has been proposed as a possible management option in those patients with small (<1 cm) *type 1 gNENs* [22], although recent ENETS guidelines suggest to resect all visible lesions by endoscopy when feasible [23].

Data from a retrospective multicenter Italian series included a small subgroup of patients ($n = 13$) with type 1 gNENs in which neither endoscopic resection nor antitumoral medical treatment was performed during a median follow-up time of 82 months [11]. Notably, no patient experienced tumor progression. An additional small experience in a group of 11 patients with small type 1 gNENs followed up during a median time of 54 months reported a change in endoscopic gross appearance in 4 cases (36%), without significant increase in tumor size which remained < 1 cm [18].

However, endoscopic surveillance alone may result an unsafe approach during long-term follow-up. In fact, patients with atrophic body gastritis not only have an increased risk to develop NENs but may also suffer from gastric adenocarcinoma [24]. Estimated incidence of gastric adenocarcinoma in atrophic body gastritis patients is up to 1%/year, similarly to what is observed in gastric NENs, in which the annual incidence is 0.4–2% [25]. Finally, it should be kept in mind that, although extremely rare, metastatic disease has been reported in some cases of type 1 gNENs [26].

Therefore, management of type 1 gNENs based on endoscopic surveillance without endoscopic resection cannot be recommended in the clinical practice.

For what it concerns medical therapy, long-acting SSAs (octreotide LAR and lanreotide autogel) represent the first-line therapy for GI NENs. As far as gNENs are concerned, SSAs have been proposed as effective treatment in reducing tumor burden and decreasing the risk of tumor recurrence in patients with multiple gNENs [10, 11, 13, 27–29]. Their activity is mainly based on the suppression of gastrin secretion by G cells, thus decreasing ECL cells proliferation.

Promising results have been reported by the above mentioned studies, showing a probability to obtain tumor disappearance ranging from 50% to 100%. Furthermore, circulating gastrin and CgA levels significantly decreased or even normalized in patients with type 1 gNENs receiving SSAs. As in other types of NENs, they are very well-tolerated drugs with an excellent safety profile, with mild adverse events like meteorism, bloating, diarrhea, and, rarely, cholestasis (which may cause gallbladder stones), bradycardia, and glucose intolerance [30].

Unfortunately, there are no solid data supporting their indication in the clinical setting of type 1 gNENs, since the majority of data derives from limited series analyzed retrospectively. Selection of patients to be treated, dosage and duration of treatment still remain unanswered questions. It is reasonable to consider candidates for treatment with SSAs those patients with recurrent and multiple diseases difficult to eradicate with endoscopic treatments. There are no comparative data between octreotide and lanreotide in the setting of gNENs. However, the majority of patients reported in the above mentioned small clinical series have been treated with octreotide LAR, whereas very few cases received lanreotide. Duration of treatment effective to obtain a significant tumor response is approximately 12 months, although a proposal of intermittent schedule has been recently suggested [28]. A prolonged period of Somatostatin analogs (SSAs) administration, the use of a standard full dose, and higher gastrin levels at diagnosis were suggested as predictors for a better response to the therapy during long-term follow-up [11]. However, given the high risk of tumor recurrence, occurring in almost to 2/3 of cases [14, 19, 28], the optimal timing of start and duration of therapy with SSAs in type 1 gNENs still remains unclear.

Furthermore, cost-effectiveness of the analogs has to be balanced with that of endoscopic management, which is to date considered the standard of care in type 1 gNENs. Moreover, the need to perform endoscopic follow-up also remains in patients receiving the analogs, not only to determine treatment efficacy but also to detect early neoplastic lesions (including tumors other than NENs) which may develop in patients with atrophic body gastritis [24]. There are no comparative studies on SSAs efficacy compared to endoscopic surveillance.

In conclusion, treatment with SSAs may be proposed in carefully selected patients with multiple, recurrent type 1 gNENs, in which a standard endoscopic management is not likely to efficaciously control the disease clinical course.

In the last few years, the selective gastrin/CCK-2 receptor antagonist netazepide has been proposed as an alternative medical treatment to SSAs, given its promising ability to induce regression of type 1 gNENs [31, 32]. However, such preliminary findings derived from observations in a small series of patients have not been further confirmed in randomized clinical trials. To date, netazepide remains a promising compound, but it needs further investigations to determine its role in the clinical management of type 1 gNENs.

Current ENETS guidelines for the management of patients with type 1 gNENs suggest endoscopic management as treatment of choice in case of small lesions without muscularis propria invasion [23].

Resection should be performed by experienced endoscopists in gNENs using either endoscopic mucosal resection (EMR) or endoscopic submucosal dissection (ESD). EMR is an endoscopic technique used for excision of superficial lesions of the GI tract. EMR can be performed with three modalities: injection, cap, or ligation assisted [33]. EMR can remove en bloc mucosal lesions smaller than 2 cm. When applied to NENs, only lesions smaller than 1 cm can be removed en bloc with sufficient resection margins because of the deeper location in the GI wall. ESD is a relatively new technique, developed by Japanese endoscopists in order to allow en bloc resection of lesions despite of the size. The margins (deep and lateral) of the resected specimens can be more adequately examined for lymph vascular infiltration and depth of invasion. ESD is usually performed by marking the mucosa at the edges of the lesion, providing at least 2 mm of margins, using a needle and coagulation current, then injecting fluid in the submucosal layer and cutting circumferentially the mucosa outside of the markers. The dissection of the submucosa is then performed, cutting on a plane sited at the lower third of the exposed submucosal layer. This allows to remove en bloc a lesion of virtually every size and shape. For what concerns GI-NENs, the possibility to choose the plane of dissection is a great advantage because of the major deepness of these lesions. ESD has some pitfalls though, because it requires high-level technical skills, it is time consuming, and it breeds a higher risk of complications [34–37].

Recent studies showed that endoscopic management of type 1 NENs is a safe and effective method with 100% survival rate [19, 38]. A randomized trial comparing less aggressive and more aggressive endoscopic techniques is needed.

Given the above mentioned considerations, endoscopic treatment should be considered the first-line therapy in patients with gNENs <2 cm without muscularis propria invasion (◘ Fig. 16.4).

Type 2 gNENs occur in the context of multiple endocrine neoplasia type 1 (MEN 1) with Zollinger–Ellison syndrome.

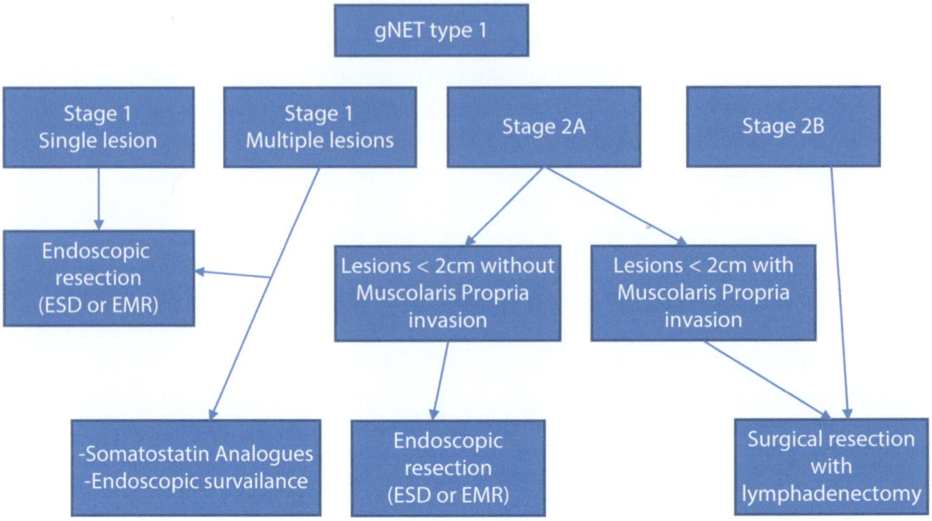

Fig. 16.4 Algorithm for type 1 gastric neuroendocrine neoplasm management

Data on SSAs in type 2 gNENs are really scarce, since no clinical trial has focused on this clinical setting so far.

Efficacy of medical treatment was initially reported in a series of three patients with type 2 gastric NENs in whom administration of octreotide induced complete tumor regression [39]. An additional report has been published in the last few years, confirming this initial observation on the efficacy of this therapy in type 2 gNENs patients [12]. However, given the limited evidence on the efficacy of SSAs to treat type 2 gNENs, their role in this particular clinical setting is not defined yet.

However, since MEN 1 syndrome patients usually present with NENs of different sites other than stomach, in particular lesions originating from the pancreas, SSAs may be used as antiproliferative therapy to inhibit the growth of other NENs. As an additional role, they may also be useful if combined with proton pump inhibitors to control ZES in those patients with MEN 1-associated gastrinomas. Reasonably, the use of SSAs in MEN 1 patients needs to be evaluated in the clinical context of each given patient, who may present several NENs rising from different endocrine sites, with or without specific tumor-related syndromes.

Type 2 gNENs can be treated by endoscopic resection with the same modalities of type 1, but deep infiltration of the gastric wall or metastatic diffusion occurs in about 12% of the cases, and the prognosis depends on the course of MEN 1 gastrinomas [40].

ENETS guidelines suggest treating patients with sporadic *type 3 gNENs* with a therapeutic approach not different from that used in non-neuroendocrine gastric carcinoma, given the potentially aggressive behavior of this NENs and the high risk of metastasis [23].

Due to the rarity of this disease, data on therapy of type 3 gNENs are usually based on anecdotic knowledge, usually deriving from single case reports or small subgroups of patients included in mixed NEN population enrolled in clinical trials.

Since no study has focused on medical treatment of this peculiar subgroup of NENs, multiple systemic treatment modalities already investigated in digestive NENs in general may be proposed in advanced type 3 gNENs. On this basis, SSAs and peptide receptor radionuclide therapy (PRRT) may have some role in somatostatin receptors expressing slow-growing tumors with low Ki67 [22]. Everolimus has been used in few patients included in the RADIANT4 trial, which showed the efficacy of this targeted agent to prolong progression-free survival in GI and lung advanced progressive NENs [41]. Platinum-based chemotherapy has been historically commonly used in advanced NENs in general (including primary gNENs) with poorly differentiated morphology and/or high proliferative index Ki67, with conflicting results [42].

Medical treatment of advanced type 3 gNENs still remains a challenge, since neither evidence-based data nor recommendations from international guidelines are available.

Duodenum

Primary duodenal NENs represent less than 2% of all GI-NENs [43]. Duodenal gastrinomas are the most common, accounting for 50–60% of all duodenal NENs. They can be either sporadic or associated with MEN 1 syndrome [44], located in the first or second portion of the duodenum. Lymph node metastasis are not uncommon at the time of diagnosis even though duodenal NENs are usually <10 mm and limited to the mucosa or submucosa [45].

Endoscopic treatment is not considered a safe option in the management of these functioning tumors. Nonfunctioning duodenal NENs metastasize only when the tumor has invaded the submucosa. They have a more favorable prognosis.

Endoscopic treatment can be considered for lesions less than 10 mm, in the absence of invasion of the muscular layer and distant metastasis [23]. Tumors located in the periampullary region tend to show a more aggressive behavior; therefore, endoscopic resection is rarely an option. Endoscopic resection with EMR has been demonstrated a safe and effective treatment for lesions of about 1 cm in diameter [46–48]. ESD in the duodenum is technically feasible and can be an option but is a very high-risk procedure, and there are only few reports from Japanese authors [49, 50].

Papillary NENs are rare. The best approach has not been established yet, but the preferred management is surgical with pancreaticoduodenectomy, given the serious consequences papillary NENs may cause by obstructing the bile and pancreatic duct [51].

Colon

Colonic NENs are most frequently located in the cecum and the ascending colon. Colonic NENs tend to present later, and at the time of diagnosis, more than two thirds are metastatic [52]. Five-year survival rate is 61.8%.

Since colonic NENs are most frequently diagnosed when they have reached dimensions >20 mm and present with regional lymph node metastasis, the treatment is commonly surgical (segmental colectomy with wide regional lymphadenectomy) [53].

An endoscopic approach can be offered for lesions <20 mm located in the mucosa and submucosa and in the absence of metastasis. Endoscopic treatment modalities are standard polypectomy and EMR, while ESD is technically more difficult in the colon, and it is associated with high risk of perforation.

Rectum

Approximately 90% of large intestinal NENs develop in the rectum [54]. Rectal NENs are usually found incidentally during screening colonoscopy. The diagnosis is often only histological, after endoscopic excision of a lesion considered to be a polyp, but sometimes, in larger lesions, the endoscopist may suspect the endocrine nature. Usually, rectal NENs are small (<10 mm) submucosal nodules or focal areas of submucosal thickening, covered with yellow-discolored mucosa. Several parameters have been suggested as predictive criteria in the assessment of the malignant potential including tumor size, histological growth patterns, muscularis propria invasion, and lymphovascular invasion. Among these parameters, size is considered the most simple and reliable parameter [55]. When tumors are smaller than 10 mm, the actual risk is extremely low. For rectal NENs measuring 10–19 mm, metastatic frequency is 5–15%, but for tumors of 20 mm or larger, the frequency rises to 80%. For all these reasons, EUS is necessary to perform a local staging (T and N) in order to decide the best treatment.

Endoscopic treatment can result in complete excision for lesions that are <10 mm, with absent invasion of the muscularis propria and no lymph node metastasis. Following local excision, patients may need to undergo further treatment according to margin status, size of the primary tumor, depth of invasion, presence of angiolymphatic invasion, and mitotic rate.

Because of the usual localization of these lesions in the submucosa, polypectomy or conventional EMR is less likely to achieve pathologically complete resection [56, 57]. Indeed, complete resection with EMR of rectal NENs varies from 28.6% to 51.7% [58].

Various techniques for endoscopic resection of rectal NENs have been reported; however, the best approach continues to be a matter of debate.

In a retrospective analysis, cap-assisted EMR was shown to be highly effective compared to EMR, and it is considered a good alternative for ESD, as this method is technically challenging. In another retrospective analysis, EMR, ESD and endoscopic mucosal resection with a ligation device were compared on therapeutic efficacy and safety. The study showed the superiority of ESD and ligation-assisted EMR in treating rectal NENs compared to EMR [59–61].

For tumors not suitable for endoscopic resection, surgery (proctectomy or transanal local excision) remains the only treatment option. In recent times, full thickness resection of the rectal wall has been proposed using the ESD technique. This approach may be useful for radicalization of a previous R1 resection, but studies are lacking. However, full thickness resection can be performed only in certain locations and requires a thorough EUS evaluation.

16.2 Conclusions

The management of NENs of the GI tract in the setting of locoregional disease consists of different therapeutic approaches, in particular medical treatment and endoscopic procedures, and it varies greatly depending on the site of origin.

Other patient-related (age, comorbidities, and performance status) and disease-related (tumor size, lesion number, stage, and grade) parameters need to be taken into account to guide the clinical management of these NENs.

Bibliography

1. Burkitt MD, Pritchard DM (2006) Review article: pathogenesis and management of gastric carcinoid tumours. Aliment Pharmacol Ther 24(9):1305–1320
2. Rindi G, Luinetti O, Cornaggia M, Capella C, Solcia E (1993) Three subtypes of gastric argyrophil carcinoid and the gastric neuroendocrine carcinoma: a clinicopathologic study. Gastroenterology 104(4):994–1006
3. Waldum HL, Sandvik AK, Idle JR (1998) Gastrin is the most important factor in ECL tumorigenesis. Gastroenterology 114(5):1113–1115
4. Lehy T, Roucayrol AM, Mignon M (2000) Histomorphological characteristics of gastric mucosa in patients with Zollinger-Ellison syndrome or autoimmune gastric atrophy: role of gastrin and atrophying gastritis. Microsc Res Tech 48(6):327–338
5. Borch K, Ahren B, Ahlman H, Falkmer S, Granerus G, Grimelius L (2005) Gastric carcinoids: biologic behavior and prognosis after differentiated treatment in relation to type. Ann Surg 242(1):64–73
6. Borch K, Renvall H, Liedberg G (1985) Gastric endocrine cell hyperplasia and carcinoid tumors in pernicious anemia. Gastroenterology 88(3):638–648
7. Rindi G, Azzoni C, La Rosa S, Klersy C, Paolotti D, Rappel S, Stolte M, Capella C, Bordi C, Solcia E (1999) ECL cell tumor and poorly differentiated endocrine carcinoma of the stomach: prognostic evaluation by pathological analysis. Gastroenterology 116(3):532–542
8. Hosokawa O, Kaizaki Y, Hattori M, Douden K, Hayashi H, Morishita M, Ohta K (2005) Long-term follow up of patients with multiple gastric carcinoids associated with type A gastritis. Gastric Cancer (Official Journal of the International Gastric Cancer Association and the Japanese Gastric Cancer Association) 8(1):42–46
9. Rindi G et al (2006) TNM staging of foregut (neuro)endocrine tumors: a consensus proposal including a grading system. Virchows Arch 449:395–401
10. Campana D, Nori F, Pezzilli R, Piscitelli L, Santini D, Brocchi E, Corinaldesi R, Tomassetti P (2008) Gastric endocrine tumors type I: treatment with long-acting somatostatin analogs. Endocr Relat Cancer 15(1):337–342
11. Campana D, Ravizza D, Ferolla P, Faggiano A, Grimaldi F, Albertelli M, Berretti D, Castellani D, Cacciari G, Fazio N, Colao A, Ferone D, Tomassetti P (2016) Clinical management of patients with gastric neuroendocrine neoplasms associated with chronic atrophic gastritis: a retrospective, multicentre study. Endocrine 51(1):131–139
12. Manfredi S, Pagenault M, de Lajarte-Thirouard AS, Bretagne JF (2007) Type 1 and 2 gastric carcinoid tumors: long-term follow-up of the efficacy of treatment with a slow-release somatostatin analogue. Eur J Gastroenterol Hepatol 19(11):1021–1025
13. Grozinsky-Glasberg S, Kaltsas G, Gur C, Gal E, Thomas D, Fichman S, Alexandraki K, Barak D, Glaser B, Shimon I, Gross DJ (2008) Long-acting somatostatin analogues are an effective treatment for type 1 gastric carcinoid tumours. European Journal of Endocrinology/European Federation of Endocrine Societies 159(4):475–482
14. Jianu CS, Fossmark R, Syversen U, Hauso O, Fykse V, Waldum HL (2011) Five-year follow-up of patients treated for 1 year with octreotide long-acting release for enterochromaffin-like cell carcinoids. Scand J Gastroenterol 46(4):456–463
15. Peracchi M, Gebbia C, Basilisco G, Quatrini M, Tarantino C, Vescarelli C, Massironi S, Conte D (2005) Plasma chromogranin A in patients with autoimmune chronic atrophic gastritis, enterochromaffin-like cell lesions and gastric carcinoids. European Journal of Endocrinology/European Federation of Endocrine Societies. 152(3):443–448
16. Rappel S, Altendorf-Hofmann A, Stolte M (1995) Prognosis of gastric carcinoid tumours. Digestion 56(6):455–462
17. Hori K, Fukui H, Imura J, Kojima T, Fujita M, Kawamata H, Chiba T, Fujimori T (2000) Benign gastric carcinoid tumor with hypergastrinemia followed up for 12 years. Gastric Cancer (Official Journal of the International Gastric Cancer Association and the Japanese Gastric Cancer Association) 3(3):161–164
18. Ravizza D, Fiori G, Trovato C, Fazio N, Bonomo G, Luca F, Bodei L, Pelosi G, Tamayo D, Crosta C (2007) Long-term endoscopic and clinical follow-up of untreated type 1 gastric neuroendocrine tumours. Dig Liver Dis 39(6):537–543

19. Merola E, Sbrozzi-Vanni A, Panzuto F, D'Ambra G, Di Giulio E, Pilozzi E, Capurso G, Lahner E, Bordi C, Annibale B, Delle FG (2012) Type I gastric carcinoids: a prospective study on endoscopic management and recurrence rate. Neuroendocrinology 95(3):207–213
20. Uygun A, Kadayifci A, Polat Z, Yilmaz K, Gunal A, Demir H, Bagci S (2014) Long-term results of endoscopic resection for type I gastric neuroendocrine tumors. J Surg Oncol 109(2):71–74
21. Ozao-Choy J, Buch K, Strauchen JA, Warner RR, Divino CM (2010) Laparoscopic antrectomy for the treatment of type I gastric carcinoid tumors. J Surg Res 162(1):22–25
22. Basuroy R, Srirajaskanthan R, Prachalias A, Quaglia A, Ramage JK (2014) Review article: the investigation and management of gastric neuroendocrine tumours. Aliment Pharmacol Ther 39(10):1071–1084
23. Delle Fave G, O'Toole D, Sundin A, Taal B, Ferolla P, Ramage JK, Ferone D, Ito T, Weber W, Zheng-Pei Z, De Herder WW, Pascher A, Ruszniewski P (2016) ENETS consensus guidelines update for Gastroduodenal neuroendocrine neoplasms. Neuroendocrinology 103(2):119–124
24. Lahner E, Esposito G, Pilozzi E, Galli G, Corleto VD, Di Giulio E, Annibale B (2015) Gastric cancer in patients with type I gastric carcinoids. Gastric Cancer (Official Journal of the International Gastric Cancer Association and the Japanese Gastric Cancer Association) 18(3):564–570
25. Vannella L, Lahner E, Annibale B (2012) Risk for gastric neoplasias in patients with chronic atrophic gastritis: a critical reappraisal. World J Gastroenterol 18(12):1279–1285
26. Grozinsky-Glasberg S, Thomas D, Strosberg JR, Pape UF, Felder S, Tsolakis AV, Alexandraki KI, Fraenkel M, Saiegh L, Reissman P, Kaltsas G, Gross DJ (2013) Metastatic type 1 gastric carcinoid: a real threat or just a myth? World J Gastroenterol 19(46):8687–8695
27. Fykse V, Sandvik AK, Qvigstad G, Falkmer SE, Syversen U, Waldum HL (2004) Treatment of ECL cell carcinoids with octreotide LAR. Scand J Gastroenterol 39(7):621–628
28. Massironi S, Zilli A, Fanetti I, Ciafardini C, Conte D, Peracchi M (2015) Intermittent treatment of recurrent type-1 gastric carcinoids with somatostatin analogues in patients with chronic autoimmune atrophic gastritis. Dig Liver Dis 47(11):978–983
29. Thomas D, Tsolakis AV, Grozinsky-Glasberg S, Fraenkel M, Alexandraki K, Sougioultzis S, Gross DJ, Kaltsas G (2013) Long-term follow-up of a large series of patients with type 1 gastric carcinoid tumors: data from a multicenter study. European Journal of Endocrinology/European Federation of Endocrine Societies 168(2):185–193
30. Oberg K (2012) Biotherapies for GEP-NETs. Best Pract Res Clin Gastroenterol 26(6):833–841
31. Moore AR, Boyce M, Steele IA, Campbell F, Varro A, Pritchard DM (2013) Netazepide, a gastrin receptor antagonist, normalises tumour biomarkers and causes regression of type 1 gastric neuroendocrine tumours in a nonrandomised trial of patients with chronic atrophic gastritis. PLoS One 8(10):e76462
32. Fossmark R, Sordal O, Jianu CS, Qvigstad G, Nordrum IS, Boyce M, Waldum HL (2012) Treatment of gastric carcinoids type 1 with the gastrin receptor antagonist netazepide (YF476) results in regression of tumours and normalisation of serum chromogranin a. Aliment Pharmacol Ther 36(11–12):1067–1075
33. Kantsevoy SV, Adler DG, Conway JD, Diehl DL, Farraye FA, Kwon R, Mamula P, Rodriguez S, Shah RJ, Wong Kee Song LM, Tierney WM (2008) Endoscopic mucosal resection and endoscopic submucosal dissection. Gastrointest Endosc 68(1):11–18
34. Yamamoto H, Kawata H, Sunada K, Sasaki A, Nakazawa K, Miyata T, Sekine Y, Yano T, Satoh K, Ido K, Sugano K (2003) Successful en-bloc resection of large superficial tumors in the stomach and colon using sodium hyaluronate and small-caliber-tip transparent hood. Endoscopy 35(8):690–694
35. Ono H, Kondo H, Gotoda T, Shirao K, Yamaguchi H, Saito D, Hosokawa K, Shimoda T, Yoshida S (2001) Endoscopic mucosal resection for treatment of early gastric cancer. Gut 48(2):225–229
36. Rosch T, Sarbia M, Schumacher B, Deinert K, Frimberger E, Toermer T, Stolte M, Neuhaus H (2004) Attempted endoscopic en bloc resection of mucosal and submucosal tumors using insulated-tip knives: a pilot series. Endoscopy 36(9):788–801
37. Gotoda T, Kondo H, Ono H, Saito Y, Yamaguchi H, Saito D, Yokota T (1999) A new endoscopic mucosal resection procedure using an insulation-tipped electrosurgical knife for rectal flat lesions: report of two cases. Gastrointest Endosc 50(4):560–563
38. Kim HH, Kim GH, Kim JH, Choi MG, Song GA, Kim SE (2014) The efficacy of endoscopic submucosal dissection of type I gastric carcinoid tumors compared with conventional endoscopic mucosal resection. Gastroenterol Res Pract 2014:253860

39. Tomassetti P, Migliori M, Caletti GC, Fusaroli P, Corinaldesi R, Gullo L (2000) Treatment of type II gastric carcinoid tumors with somatostatin analogues. N Engl J Med 343(8):551–554
40. Meko JB, Norton JA (1995) Management of patients with Zollinger-Ellison syndrome. Annu Rev Med 46:395–411
41. Yao JC, Fazio N, Singh S, Buzzoni R, Carnaghi C, Wolin E, Tomasek J, Raderer M, Lahner H, Voi M, Pacaud LB, Rouyrre N, Sachs C, Valle JW, Delle Fave G, Van Cutsem E, Tesselaar M, Shimada Y, Oh DY, Strosberg J, Kulke MH, Pavel ME (2016) Everolimus for the treatment of advanced, non-functional neuroendocrine tumours of the lung or gastrointestinal tract (RADIANT-4): a randomised, placebo-controlled, phase 3 study. Lancet 387(10022):968–977
42. Sorbye H, Welin S, Langer SW, Vestermark LW, Holt N, Osterlund P, Dueland S, Hofsli E, Guren MG, Ohrling K, Birkemeyer E, Thiis-Evensen E, Biagini M, Gronbaek H, Soveri LM, Olsen IH, Federspiel B, Assmus J, Janson ET, Knigge U (2013) Predictive and prognostic factors for treatment and survival in 305 patients with advanced gastrointestinal neuroendocrine carcinoma (WHO G3): the NORDIC NEC study. Annals of Oncology (Official Journal of the European Society for Medical Oncology/ESMO) 24(1):152–160
43. Nikou GC, Toubanakis C, Moulakakis KG, Pavlatos S, Kosmidis C, Mallas E, Safioleas P, Sakorafas GH, Safioleas MC (2011) Carcinoid tumors of the duodenum and the ampulla of Vater: current diagnostic and therapeutic approach in a series of 8 patients. Case series. Int J Surg (London, England) 9(3):248–253
44. Pipeleers-Marichal M, Donow C, Heitz PU, Kloppel G (1993) Pathologic aspects of gastrinomas in patients with Zollinger-Ellison syndrome with and without multiple endocrine neoplasia type I. World J Surg 17(4):481–488
45. Donow C, Pipeleers-Marichal M, Schroder S, Stamm B, Heitz PU, Kloppel G (1991) Surgical pathology of gastrinoma. Site, size, multicentricity, association with multiple endocrine neoplasia type 1, and malignancy. Cancer 68(6):1329–1334
46. Karagiannis S, Eshagzaiy K, Duecker C, Feyerabend B, Mozdzanowski E, Faiss S (2009) Endoscopic resection with the cap technique of a carcinoid tumor in the duodenal bulb. Endoscopy 41(Suppl 2):E288–E289
47. Dalenback J, Havel G (2004) Local endoscopic removal of duodenal carcinoid tumors. Endoscopy 36(7):651–655
48. Tai WP, Yue H (2009) Endoscopic mucosa resection of a duodenum carcinoid tumor of 1.2 cm diameter: a case report. Med Oncol (Northwood, London, England) 26(3):319–321
49. Honda T, Yamamoto H, Osawa H, Yoshizawa M, Nakano H, Sunada K, Hanatsuka K, Sugano K (2009) Endoscopic submucosal dissection for superficial duodenal neoplasms. Digestive Endoscopy (Official Journal of the Japan Gastroenterological Endoscopy Society) 21(4):270–274
50. Matsumoto S, Miyatani H, Yoshida Y, Nokubi M (2011) Duodenal carcinoid tumors: 5 cases treated by endoscopic submucosal dissection. Gastrointest Endosc 74(5):1152–1156
51. De Palma GD, Masone S, Siciliano S, Maione F, Falleti J, Mansueto G, De Rosa G, Persico G (2010) Endocrine carcinoma of the major papilla: report of two cases and review of the literature. Surg Oncol 19(4):235–242
52. Crocetti E, Paci E (2003) Malignant carcinoids in the USA, SEER 1992-1999. An epidemiological study with 6830 cases. European Journal of Cancer Prevention (The Official Journal of the European Cancer Prevention Organisation (ECP)) 12(3):191–194
53. Anthony LB, Strosberg JR, Klimstra DS, Maples WJ, O'Dorisio TM, Warner RR, Wiseman GA, Benson AB 3rd, Pommier RF (2010) The NANETS consensus guidelines for the diagnosis and management of gastrointestinal neuroendocrine tumors (nets): well-differentiated nets of the distal colon and rectum. Pancreas 39(6):767–774
54. Jetmore AB, Ray JE, Gathright JB Jr, McMullen KM, Hicks TC, Timmcke AE (1992) Rectal carcinoids: the most frequent carcinoid tumor. Dis Colon Rectum 35(8):717–725
55. Soga J (1997) Carcinoids of the rectum: an evaluation of 1271 reported cases. Surg Today 27(2):112–119
56. Son HJ, Sohn DK, Hong CW, Han KS, Kim BC, Park JW, Choi HS, Chang HJ, Oh JH (2013) Factors associated with complete local excision of small rectal carcinoid tumor. Int J Color Dis 28(1):57–61

57. Park CH, Cheon JH, Kim JO, Shin JE, Jang BI, Shin SJ, Jeen YT, Lee SH, Ji JS, Han DS, Jung SA, Park DI, Baek IH, Kim SH, Chang DK (2011) Criteria for decision making after endoscopic resection of well-differentiated rectal carcinoids with regard to potential lymphatic spread. Endoscopy 43(9):790–795
58. Iishi H, Tatsuta M, Yano H, Narahara H, Iseki K, Ishiguro S (1996) More effective endoscopic resection with a two-channel colonoscope for carcinoid tumors of the rectum. Dis Colon Rectum 39(12):1438–1439
59. Boskoski I, Volkanovska A, Tringali A, Bove V, Familiari P, Perri V, Costamagna G (2013) Endoscopic resection for gastrointestinal neuroendocrine tumors. Expert Rev Gastroenterol Hepatol 7(6):559–569
60. Zhao ZF, Zhang N, Ma SR, Yang Z, Han X, Zhao YF, Gao F, Gong ZJ, Yang L (2012) A comparative study on endoscopy treatment in rectal carcinoid tumors. Surg Laparosc Endosc Percutan Tech 22(3):260–263
61. Kim KM, Eo SJ, Shim SG, Choi JH, Min BH, Lee JH, Chang DK, Kim YH, Rhee PL, Kim JJ, Rhee JC, Kim JY (2013) Treatment outcomes according to endoscopic treatment modalities for rectal carcinoid tumors. Clin Res Hepatol Gastroenterol 37(3):275–282

Therapy for Locoregional Disease: Pancreas

Francesca Muffatti, Mauro Cives, Stefano Partelli, Franco Silvestris, and Massimo Falconi

A. Colao et al. (eds.), *Neuroendocrine Tumors in Real Life*,
https://doi.org/10.1007/978-3-319-59024-0_17

Overview

Surgery is the mainstay for the treatment of localized pancreatic neuroendocrine neoplasm tumors (PanNENs). Either formal or limited pancreatic resections are commonly used for large (>2 cm), sporadic PanNENs and for functioning neoplasms. However, given the high rate of perioperative morbidity and mortality after pancreatic surgery and the indolent behavior of PanNETs, a conservative approach consisting of active surveillance has been proposed for small, nonfunctioning, low-to-intermediate-grade tumors. Treatment of locally advanced PanNENs appears particularly challenging. Although surgery can be proposed in the presence of tumor invasion of nearby organs, it is currently unclear whether an aggressive surgical approach is associated with improved survival outcomes. On the other hand, it has been suggested that chemotherapy or peptide receptor radionuclide therapy (PRRT) is effective in the neoadjuvant setting and may lead to increased rates of curative resections in patients with locally advanced disease. Studies investigating the molecular underpinnings of PanNENs in relation to their clinical behavior are needed for optimal treatment tailoring.

Clinical Case

A 58-year-old woman presented at our attention for persistent meteorism. At physical examination, a large mass in the epigastric region was found, with no other related symptoms. An ultrasound confirmed the presence of a 20 cm abdominal lesion. The patient performed an abdominal computed tomography (MDCT) and an abdominal magnetic resonance (MRI) which demonstrated a 20 cm neoplasm with areas of necrosis and defined margins, probably originating from the head of the pancreas and close to the left hepatic lobe as well as to the stomach (◘ Fig. 17.1). Two hypervascularized hepatic lesions (segment V and segment VIII) suspicious for metastases were present as well. Serum carbohydrate (CA) 19.9 and carcinoembryonic antigen (CEA) were within the normal range. Patient underwent percutaneous fine needle aspiration (FNA) of the primitive tumor

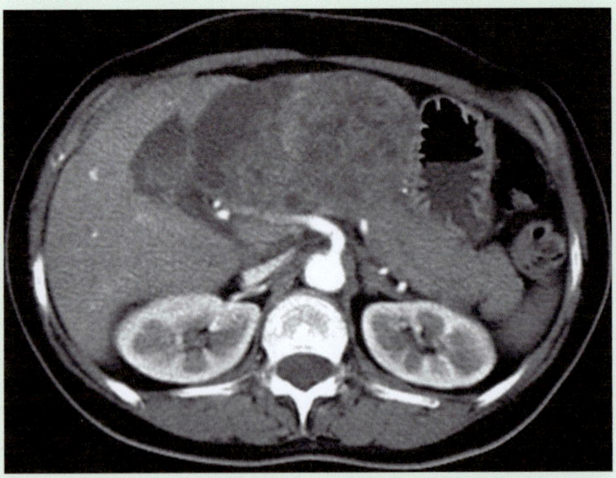

◘ **Fig. 17.1** Abdominal computed tomography at initial diagnosis with a 20 cm partially necrotic mass with defined margins, originating from the head of the pancreas and close to the left hepatic lobe as well as to the stomach (July 2014)

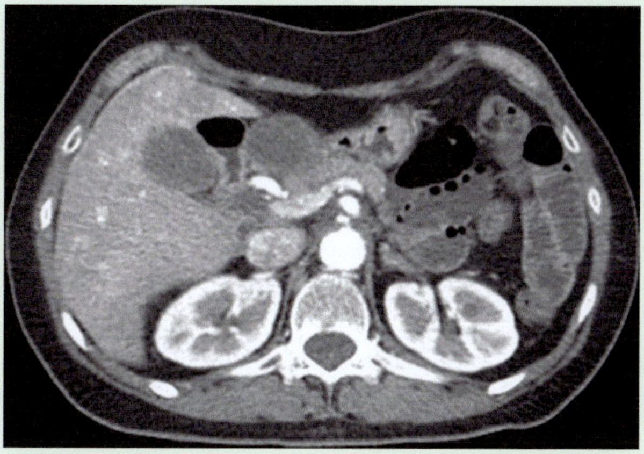

Fig. 17.2 Abdominal computed tomography after neoadjuvant treatment with 5 cycles of PRRT with 90Y–DOTATOC associated with octreotide® LAR 30 mg/28 days i.m. MDCT performed in September 2015 showed a reduction of the pancreatic mass (maximum diameter: 3.5 cm)

that revealed a well-differentiated neuroendocrine tumor (NET) with a Ki-67 = 3%. Combined ^{18}FDG- and ^{68}Ga-PET/CT were both positive in the pancreatic head and in the liver (segment V and segment VIII).

After a multidisciplinary tumor board meeting discussion, a neoadjuvant treatment based on peptide receptor radionuclide therapy (PRRT) with ^{90}Y-DOTATOC associated with octreotide® LAR 30 mg/28 days i.m. was offered to the patient. Overall, five cycles of PRRT were administered between December 2014 and June 2015. Treatment was well tolerated without significant side effects.

In September 2015 patient underwent a restaging with MDCT scan and ^{68}Ga-PET/CT, which showed a dramatic reduction of the pancreatic mass (maximum diameter, 3.5 cm) (Fig. 17.2). Hepatic lesion localized in segment VIII was no longer visible, whereas the metastasis in segment V was decreased in size. An abdominal MRI with liver-specific enhancement failed to reveal the segment V hepatic metastasis.

Patient underwent surgery in November 2015, and after laparotomy a 3 cm pancreatic mass was enucleated. Prophylactic cholecystectomy was performed as well. The tumor was exophytic with a small and thin peduncle originating from the posterior aspect of the pancreatic neck. An intraoperative ultrasound failed to reveal nodules in the liver. Postoperative course was uneventful and patient was discharged on postoperative day 6. Octreotide®-LAR administration was not discontinued.

Pathological examination revealed the presence of a well-differentiated nonfunctioning neuroendocrine neoplasm with a Ki-67 of 1% (NET G1 according to 2010 WHO classification [1]). The neoplasm measured 3 cm in size, and all the six harvested nodes were negative for metastasis (stage II according to ENETS staging system [2]). Diffuse areas of necrosis and fibrosis were observed. Eighteen months after surgery, the patient is still free of disease with no symptoms.

17.1 Comments to the Case

Pancreatic neuroendocrine neoplasms (PanNENs) are biologically heterogeneous tumors that can be categorized by hormone secretion, differentiation, grade, pace of disease, pattern of metastatic spread, and somatostatin receptor expression [3]. Recent advances in our understanding of the pathobiology of these neoplasms have expanded the therapeutic landscape for patients with PanNENs. Also, as frequently occurs, they concurrently generated a multitude of new questions, particularly regarding selection, timing, and sequence of treatments. The case presented above illuminates some of these aspects and suggests that (i) uniform criteria for the definition of locally advanced or oligometastatic PanNETs need to be incorporated in clinical trials and clinical practice; (ii) new therapeutic approaches should be systematically investigated in patients with locally advanced/oligometastatic PanNETs; and (iii) predictors of response are needed to better select treatment choices and improve outcomes.

17.1.1 Criteria for the Definition of Locally Advanced or Oligometastatic PanNETs

Until recently, the ability to stratify patients with PanNETs into prognostic groups has been limited by the absence of a commonly accepted staging classification. In fact, different staging systems have been adopted by the European Neuroendocrine Tumor Society (ENETS) [2] and the American Joint Committee on Cancer (AJCC) [4], thus generating some confusion (◘ Table 17.1). Although their prognostic ability has been

◘ **Table 17.1** TNM staging definitions by ENETS and AJCC for PanNENs. The ENETS staging system [5] maintains the ENETS T, N, and M definitions [2] while adopting the AJCC stage definitions [4]

	ENETS staging system	AJCC staging system	
TNM			
T1	Tumor limited to the pancreas, <2 cm	Tumor limited to the pancreas, ≤2 cm	
T2	Tumor limited to the pancreas, 2–4 cm	Limited to the pancreas, >2 cm	
T3	Tumor limited to the pancreas, >4 cm, or invading the duodenum or common bile duct	Beyond the pancreas but without involvement of the superior mesenteric artery	
T4	Tumor invades adjacent structures	Involvement of the celiac axis or superior mesenteric artery (unresectable tumor)	
N0	No regional lymph node metastasis	No regional lymph node metastasis	
N1	Regional lymph node metastasis	Regional lymph node metastasis	
M0	No distant metastasis	No distant metastasis	
M1	Distant metastasis	Distant metastasis	
Stage			
I	T1, N0, M0	I	T1, N0, M0
IIA	T2, N0, M0	IB	T2, N0, M0
IIB	T3, N0, M0	IIA	T3, N0, M0
IIIA	T4, N0, M0	IIB	T1–3, N1, M0
IIIB	Any T, N1, M0	III	T4, any N, M0
IV	Any T, any N, M1	IV	Any T, any N, M1

validated by large series studies [6, 7], both classifications have shown some drawbacks. In fact, while in the ENETS staging system patients with stage IIIA disease (invasion of peripancreatic structures) showed worse prognosis than patients with stage IIIB cancer (nodal metastases), in the AJCC classification only 4–5% of patients had tumor involvement of the celiac axis or the superior mesenteric artery (stage III). To overcome the shortcomings of both ENETS and AJCC classifications, a new staging system, the so-called modified ENETS (mENETS) classification, has been recently proposed and revealed improved prognostic capability [5]. Based on the mENETS staging system, stage III disease is defined by invasion of peripancreatic structures, regardless of nodal metastatic involvement. Similarly to the ENETS classification, in the mENETS staging system, patients with stage III disease have worse outcomes as compared to those with intrapancreatic tumors and nodal metastases (stage IIB), thus confirming that invasion of adjacent organs per se exerts an influence on survival greater than node metastases. Whether this is related to a more aggressive intrinsic tumor biology of larger tumors or to surgical issues leading to decreased rates of radical resections in the presence of peripancreatic invasion still needs to be elucidated.

Criteria for the surgical resection of PanNENs do not exclude the presence of nearby organ invasion nor the invasion of vascular structures. Whenever feasible, a formal resection combined with lymphadenectomy and nearby organ resection is currently the treatment of choice for patients with locally advanced disease. While the presence of celiac trunk invasion is not an absolute limitation for distal pancreatectomy, circumferential invasion of the portal vein and/or of the superior mesenteric artery contraindicates extended pancreatic surgery [8].

Surgery is curative only when a complete resection of the tumor is achieved. Although potentially resectable, large PanNENs invading adjacent structures may be less likely to undergo R0/R1 surgery, with obviously limited patients' outcomes. Over the last few decades, neoadjuvant treatments have been extensively used for a variety of cancers, leading to remarkable clinical results [9–11]. This kind of approach may be potentially useful for the downstaging/downsizing of PanNETs, but high-level evidence in this context may derive only from trials accruing very homogeneous patient populations. To this aim, uniform, universally accepted criteria for the definition of locally advanced disease need to be adopted. The possibility of identifying patients with locally advanced disease as those falling in the stage III group of the mENETS classification may currently represent the most convenient approach to select patients who potentially benefit from neoadjuvant treatments.

Similarly to patients with locally advanced disease, patients with PanNEN metastatic to the liver may still be cured by surgery, if adequately preselected. Because of the high incidence of multifocal and bilateral hepatic metastases, R0/R1 resections are usually feasible in less than 20% of patients with liver metastatic PanNENs [12]. However, in contrast with other cancers [13], there are no criteria to univocally define PanNENs as oligometastatic. Technical resectability and prognostic aspects related to the number and size of hepatic metastases should be taken into account in the elaboration of such criteria. In the absence of data showing that the outcomes of oligometastatic PanNENs are comparable with those of patients with locally advanced disease, inclusion of both patient categories in studies investigating either neoadjuvant or adjuvant therapies could be performed only if subset analyses are adequately powered.

17.1.2 New Therapeutic Approaches for Locally Advanced/Oligometastatic PanNETs

Patients with locally advanced or metastatic PanNENs have a 5-year overall survival (OS) of 85% and 60%, respectively [6]. However, 80% of patients who undergo radical resection of their liver metastases survive at least 5 years [14], thus suggesting that surgery has a major influence on disease's outcomes. Tumor burden reduction by neoadjuvant treatment facilitates surgery and may have a positive impact on the rates of curative resections. Although induction therapy is currently not considered standard of care for the treatment of locally advanced/oligometastatic PanNETs, evidence of its potential utility in selected clinical scenarios is presently growing [15].

Chemotherapy, external beam radiotherapy, and PRRT have been used as neoadjuvant treatments for advanced PanNENs (Table 17.2). Chemotherapeutic regimens including etoposide/cisplatin, capecitabine/temozolomide, streptozocin, doxorubicin, and the oral fluoropyrimidine S-1 have shown variable efficacy in the neoadjuvant setting. In a seminal study, Sorbye et al. described a single patient with pancreatic neuroendocrine carcinoma (PanNEC) and liver metastases treated with etoposide and cisplatin as neoadjuvant therapy. Following disease downsizing, the patient underwent curative surgery, remaining free of disease after 5 years of follow-up [16]. In a subsequent series of five patients with advanced PanNEC treated with the same neoadjuvant combination, radical surgery was reported as feasible in four patients [18]. In a recent retrospective series of 42 patients with low-to-intermediate-grade, advanced PanNENs treated with different neoadjuvant chemotherapy protocols, the rate of R0 and R1 resections was 46% and 21%, respectively. Although generally safe, pancreatic surgery following neoadjuvant chemotherapy was associated with one perioperative death and severe complications in five patients [19].

The preoperative use of external beam radiotherapy has been recently reported by Lee et al. In a single patient with locally advanced PanNET who underwent surgical resection after neoadjuvant radiotherapy, a R0 resection was achieved, and a disease-free status was documented after 5 years of follow-up [22]. The neoadjuvant use of PRRT in patients with unresectable PanNETs appears very promising. Several case reports and case series have already highlighted the potential for downstaging of preoperative radionuclide therapy with ^{177}Lu-DOTATATE, with or without concurrent 5-FU [23–26]. Recently, in a cohort of 29 patients with borderline unresectable or oligometastatic disease (≤3 liver metastases) who received neoadjuvant lutetium, a 31% rate of successful surgery was reported. The median PFS was 69 months for patients who underwent successful surgery and 49 months for the others [27].

Although intriguing in their results, case reports and retrospective series do not allow to draw any firm conclusions on the efficacy of neoadjuvant therapy in PanNETs. Future research is therefore needed to define the role of neoadjuvant chemotherapy and/or PRRT in patients with locally advanced or oligometastatic PanNETs. Prospective, controlled, randomized clinical trials preselecting patients based on their likelihood of response to treatment will certainly provide new insightful information to advance the field.

Prevention of tumor growth after spread owing to tumor manipulation during surgery or eradication of preexisting micrometastases may be achieved through adjuvant therapy. At present, adjuvant therapy has not been formally investigated in patients with

Table 17.2 Efficacy of neoadjuvant treatment for PanNENs: current evidence

Neoadjuvant regimen	*N*. of cycles	Disease features	*N*. of patients[b]	Outcome	Comments	References
Etoposide/cisplatin	4	PanNEC, pancreatic head, 14 mm Single liver metastasis, 20 cm Enlarged regional lymph nodes, 10 cm	1	Free of disease after 60 months of follow-up	A partial response was obtained after 4 cycles of neoadjuvant chemotherapy. Liver resection, regional lymph node dissection, Billroth I gastric resection, and enucleation of the pancreatic lesion were followed by 4 cycles of adjuvant etoposide/cisplatin	[16]
Etoposide/cisplatin	Pt. #1: 6 Pt. #2: 4	Pt. #1 PanNEC, pancreatic head, invading the duodenum Enlarged regional lymph nodes encasing the superior mesenteric artery and portal vein Pt. #2 PanNEC, pancreatic head, 10 cm, invading the duodenum, colon and stomach Enlarged regional and mesenteric lymph nodes	2	Pt. #1: Free of disease after 18 months of follow-up Pt. #2: Postoperative recurrence, patient died 5 months after surgery	Pt. #1 After tumor downstaging, complete separation from the superior mesenteric artery and portal vein was achieved. The patient underwent radical pancreaticoduodenectomy. Pathology examination showed fibrous replacement of the tumor tissue. Pt. #2 After a partial response to neoadjuvant chemotherapy, the patient underwent pancreaticoduodenectomy with en bloc resection of the right colon	[17]
Etoposide/cisplatin	NR	Locally advanced NEC and/or presence of hepatic metastases	5	NR	After neoadjuvant chemotherapy, 3 pancreatoduodenectomies, 1 distal pancreatectomy, and 1 distal pancreatectomy with tumor debulking of liver metastases were performed	[18]

(continued)

Table 17.2 (continued)

Neoadjuvant regimen	*N*. of cycles	Disease features	*N*. of patients[b]	Outcome	Comments	References
5-FU (*n* = 31) Streptozocin (*n* = 21) Doxorubicin (*n* = 21) Platinum salts (*n* = 10) Etoposide (*n* = 7)		Stage IV PanNETs (*n*: 34) Stage IIIA[a] PanNETs (*n*: 6) Stage IIIB[a] PanNETs (*n*: 2)	42	A complete tumor macroscopic resection was performed in 19 patients (45%)	One patient (4%) died postoperatively because of septic shock. Five patients (20%) experienced severe complications (III–IV)	[19]
5-FU (*n* = 31) Streptozocin (*n* = 21) Doxorubicin (*n* = 21) Platinum salts (*n* = 10) Etoposide (*n* = 7)		Stage IV PanNETs (*n*: 34) Stage IIIA[a] PanNETs (*n*: 6) Stage IIIB[a] PanNETs (*n*: 2)	42	A complete tumor macroscopic resection was performed in 19 patients (45%)	One patient (4%) died postoperatively because of septic shock. Five patients (20%) experienced severe complications (III–IV)	[19]
CAPTEM	8	PanNET, pancreatic head, 6 cm encasing the superior mesenteric vein and superior mesenteric artery Borderline enlarged regional lymph nodes	1	Free of disease after 3 months of follow-up	After a partial response to CAPTEM, the patient underwent R0 pancreatic surgery	[20]
S-1	4	PanNET, pancreatic body Multiple liver metastases	1	Free of disease after 6 months of follow-up	After a partial response to neoadjuvant chemotherapy, the patient underwent distal pancreatectomy	[21]
IMRT + Etoposide/carboplatin/5-FU	Total dose: 55.7 Gy	Locally advanced PanNET	1	Free of disease after 60 months of follow-up	After neoadjuvant radiotherapy, the patient underwent R0 tumor resection	[22]

PRRT (^{90}Y–DOTATATE)	2	PanNEC, pancreatic head encasing the mesenteric vessels Enlarged para-aortic lymph nodes	1	Free of disease after 18 months of follow-up	Following partial response to PRRT, the patient underwent Traverso-Longmire pancreaticoduodenectomy, with R0 resection	[23]
PRRT (90Y–DOTATATE)	NR	PanNET, pancreatic body Multiple liver metastases	1	NR	Neoadjuvant PRRT induced complete response of the hepatic lesions and partial response of the pancreatic primary, thus enabling surgery	[24]
PRRT (^{177}Lu-octreotate)						[25]
PRRT (^{177}Lu-octreotate) + 5-FU	4	Locally advanced PanNET	1	Free of disease after 12 months of follow-up	Following achievement of partial response after 6 months of PRRT completion, a R0 was performed. Ki-67% decreased following neoadjuvant PRRT	[26]
PRRT (^{177}Lu-octreotate)	4	Patient group 1: Borderline or unresectable PanNET ($n = 15$) Patient group 2: Oligometastatic ($\leq$3 liver metastases) PanNET ($n = 14$)	29	Successful surgery was performed in 31% of patients	No perioperative mortality was noted. All resection specimens showed fibrosis or necrosis as consequence of the neoadjuvant treatment. Of the nine operated patients, four remained disease-free after a median follow-up of 59 months	[27]

NR not reported, *IMRT* intensity-modulated radiotherapy
[a]According to ENETS staging system
[b]Only patients with PanNETs are reported

PanNENs following curative surgery. In an animal model, treatment with ^{177}Lu-octreotate prevented or significantly reduced the growth of tumors in the liver after injection of NET cells via the portal vein [28]. Large, multicenter trials with very long follow-up would be needed to detect difference in recurrence rates or survival in NET patients treated with or without adjuvant protocols.

17.1.3 Predictors of Treatment Response for Patient Preselection

The identification of response predictors may be particularly important for the management of patients with locally advanced or oligometastatic PanNENs. In fact, while bringing the hope of tumor shrinkage and consequent improved rates of curative surgery, neoadjuvant therapies (when ineffective or limitedly effective) also expose the patient to the risk of further disease progression. Moreover, since both chemotherapy and PRRT are associated with high rates of objective responses and may be effective in the neoadjuvant setting, allocation of the right patient to the right treatment becomes essential.

Currently available biomarkers for PanNENs have poor sensitivity, specificity, and predictive ability [29]. Secretory peptides including insulin, glucagon, gastrin, etc. are effective serum indicators of tumor activity, but their utility is limited to functioning tumors, which constitute less than 25% of PanNENs [30]. Chromogranin A (CgA) is a constitutive product of the neuroendocrine cell secretory granule and is widely used as prognostic factor. However, its clinical limitations have become increasingly evident [31], and novel biomarkers with improved predictive capability are currently in advanced clinical development. Among them, there are circulating tumor cells (CTCs) and a multianalyte whole blood RNA signature (NETest). Changes in CTC count have been recently associated with treatment response and survival [32], but treatment individualization based on CTCs is currently not feasible for PanNENs. On the other hand, the NETest has shown impressive results in terms of sensitivity and specificity [33], and its posttreatment changes seem to accurately predict response to operative resection and PRRT [34, 35]. However, similarly to CTCs, treatment personalization based on NETest baseline value has never been evaluated so far. Both CTCs and NETest might be useful for follow-up in the adjuvant setting, although clinical validation is still needed.

Differentiation, grade, methylguanine methyltransferase (MGMT) status, and alternative lengthening of telomere (ALT) pathway activation have been assessed as potential predictors of response to chemotherapy in PanNENs, but inconclusive results have been achieved so far. Several studies [36, 37] have demonstrated the activity of platinum-based doublets in poorly differentiated PanNECs, and higher rates of response were reported in tumors with very high Ki-67 proliferation index (>55%) [38]. However, although tumor responses to chemotherapy seem to increase in parallel with Ki-67 index [39], the predictive value of grade by WHO 2010 is considered quite low, particularly with temozolomide-based combinations [40]. MGMT is a DNA repair enzyme that counteracts the genotoxic damage induced by alkylating agents, and its overexpression is theoretically associated with resistance to temozolomide [41]. Nevertheless, contrasting results have been reported so far concerning the predictive role of MGMT loss in PanNENs, and its systematic determination in daily clinical practice cannot be recommended at this time [40, 42–45]. Similarly, activation of the ALT pathway, which correlates with chromosomal instability and tumor clinical aggressiveness, has failed to predict response to chemotherapy [40].

In contrast with chemotherapy, PRRT has a clear predictive biomarker, namely, the somatostatin receptor (SSTR) expression [46]. Increased response rates have been demonstrated in patients with higher degree of radiotracer uptake on SSTR scintigraphy (Octreoscan®), and an overall response rate (ORR) of ~60% has been reported for patients with grade 4 uptake by Krenning score (tumor uptake greater than that of the spleen or kidneys) [47]. By ^{68}Ga-DOTATOC-PET/CT scan, a maximum standard uptake value (SUV) higher than 16 predicts tumor response with a sensitivity and specificity of 95% and 60%, respectively [48]. Overall, while patients with poorly differentiated, highly proliferating, SSTR-negative, locally advanced PanNENs may potentially benefit of chemotherapy in the neoadjuvant setting, upfront PRRT could be more active in low-grade PanNETs overexpressing SSTRs. Other genetic and epigenetic biomarkers are currently under intensive investigation. In the precision medicine era, treatment tailoring based on disease's mutatomic, epigenomic, metabolomic, transcriptomic, and proteomic profiling is necessary, although clinical applicability and economic sustainability must be always taken into account.

Assessment of the location and extent of PanNENs is crucial for their management. Radiographically, PanNENs often appear as infiltrative masses homogenously enhancing during arterial and pancreatic or portal venous phases of imaging. Occasionally they can be cystic, and this can lead to diagnostic delay [49]. Given their high degree of vascularization, PanNENs may be successfully imaged by 3-phase MDCT scans with iodinated contrast. In patients with gastrointestinal NENs, MRI scans were shown to be superior to MDCT imaging for the detection of liver metastases. The optimal MRI sequences were T2-weighted images or arterial phase-enhanced T1-weighted images [50]. To rule out stage IV, Eovist contrast may be used to optimize the detection of subcentimeter hepatic metastases [51]. Somatostatin receptor scintigraphy (SRS, Octreoscan®) is the most established functional imaging for NENs. The sensitivity of SRS for PanNENs is 60–90% [52, 53]. However, SRS may be inadequate for the detection of metastases smaller than 1.5 cm, with a sensitivity less than 35% [50]. Imaging with ^{68}Ga-PET/CT has the highest sensitivity (86–100%) and specificity (79–100%) for localizing PanNENs [8]. Given their low expression of SSTRs, insulinomas are not adequately imaged by either Octreoscan® or ^{68}Ga-PET/CT scans [54]. The use of ^{68}Ga-PET/CT has been shown to modify the surgical or medical management of PanNEN patients in 20–55% of cases [55, 56]. Radiotracer uptake levels of SRS or ^{68}Ga-PET/CT have prognostic value and can be also used to predict response to PRRT, whereas the predictive value for response to somatostatin analogs (SSAs) is still debated. ^{18}FDG-PET/CT scans may be useful in rapidly progressing patients, in particular if harboring high-grade tumors [8].

At diagnosis of locally advanced PanNEN, cross-sectional imaging should be performed to assess resectability, while prognostic/predictive information should be acquired by SSTR imaging. The same conventional imaging technique used at diagnosis should be employed during follow-up. The role of functional imaging during PanNEN follow-up is currently unclear.

Questions

1. What is the best management of small, incidentally detected PanNENs?
2. Should open surgery be preferred over the laparoscopic approach for PanNENs?
3. Should lymphadenectomy be always performed in patients with PanNENs?
4. Should neoadjuvant or adjuvant strategies be used for locally advanced PanNENs?
5. Which criteria should drive the treatment choice in patients with PanNENs?

Answers

1. Because of the widespread use of high-quality cross-sectional imaging and endoscopy, up to 60% of PanNENs are currently diagnosed when their diameter is inferior to 2 cm [57, 58]. Incidentally discovered, hormonally nonfunctioning, well-differentiated PanNENs smaller than 2 cm often have a very indolent behavior and patients harboring these tumors carry a 5-year survival of 100% [58]. Although surgery is considered the mainstay for the management of local PanNENs [59], its role in patients with G1, asymptomatic PanNETs smaller than 2 cm has been recently questioned, and, because of the substantial morbidity and mortality associated with both conventional and parenchyma-sparing pancreatectomy [60, 61], a «wait and see» policy has been formally advocated by ENETS for this selected group of patients. A conservative approach seems also appropriate for PanNET patients with multiple endocrine neoplasia type 1 (MEN1) [8]. In this setting, a treatment with SSA has been proposed [62]. Nevertheless, further studies should evaluate the real efficacy as well as the cost-effectiveness of this treatment before considering it as a valid option in patients with small PanNETs.

   Curative resection of PanNECs is associated with improved survival, and surgery plays a key role in the localized, resectable setting. At present, it is very difficult to define the specific indications for pancreatic resection in patients with locally advanced disease, in particular when a radical intervention cannot be guarantee. Although several retrospective studies suggest a potential benefit of primary tumor resection in the context of advanced G1/G2 PanNENs [63, 64], palliative resection of primary PanNEC should not be performed in the presence of metastatic or unresectable disease [18].
2. Laparoscopic procedures are increasingly used for the surgical treatment of PanNENs, particularly insulinomas. Although there is evidence that laparoscopic distal pancreatectomy or tumor enucleation are safe and feasible in PanNEN patients [65], resection of large tumors infiltrating the adjacent structures may require an open approach. If an adequate tumor shrinkage is achieved by preoperative induction therapy, there is no formal contraindication to use minimally invasive approaches. Laparoscopic pancreatic surgery is associated with a lower rate of complications and a shorter hospitalization [66].
3. Given the weak association between lymph node metastasis and survival [67, 68], the role of lymphadenectomy for patients with PanNENs has been long debated. However, recent evidence suggests that nodal involvement per se, number of metastatic lymph nodes, and lymph node ratio (positive lymph nodes/total examined lymph nodes) are important predictors of recurrence after surgery [69, 70]. As result, systematic removal of lymph nodes in the peritumoral area has been recently recommended by ENETS [8], irrespective of the operation performed.

4. At present, neoadjuvant or adjuvant strategies are not recommended as standard therapies for locally advanced PanNENs. While data on adjuvant treatment of PanNEN patients are very limited, evidence of the efficacy of neoadjuvant therapies is based only on case reports or small case series, as discussed above. Future clinical trials of induction therapy in locally advanced PanNENs should focus on chemotherapy or PRRT, as these agents are most likely to induce objective responses as compared with other treatment options (i.e., SSAs, everolimus, sunitinib, etc.). The possibility to preselect patients putatively responding to PRRT through functional imaging renders neoadjuvant PRRT particularly attractive. Given its longer tissue penetration as compared with ^{177}Lu [71], ^{90}Y appears a good candidate in the setting of large, primarily inoperable tumors. Whether low-to-intermediate (G1–G2) tumors may benefit from neoadjuvant treatments more than high-grade PanNECs is largely unclear.
5. Treatment decisions for PanNEN patients may be particularly challenging, particularly in the presence of locally advanced disease. Patients with sporadic PanNENs larger than 2 cm should undergo surgery, if feasible. Patients with locally advanced disease should be treated according to operability and resectability criteria. Inoperable patients should be treated similarly to those with stage IV tumors. Operable patients with primarily unresectable PanNEN may undergo downstaging/downsizing with upfront chemotherapy or PRRT, provided that a sufficient degree of tumor shrinkage can be achieved to enable subsequent surgery. SSAs, everolimus, and sunitinib are usually associated with response rates in the range of 5–10% in PanNETs [59] and should therefore be used in locally advanced patients only if the goal of treatment is disease stability. Patients with functioning PanNETs may benefit from surgery even when disease cure is not feasible anymore. Given that emerging evidence suggests that mixed grades can occur in well-differentiated NETs and that well-differentiated tumors with high-grade component (NET G3) are genotypically different from poorly differentiated tumors (NEC G3) [72], both grade and tumor differentiation should always inform treatment decisions. For locally advanced PanNENs in the setting of hereditary syndromes such as MEN1 or von Hippel-Lindau (VHL) disease, the goals of therapy should be palliation of symptoms and tumor control. Management of hereditary PanNENs is however influenced by other comorbidities at presentation [8].

Up to Date of the Topic

Patients with locoregional PanNENs are usually treated with surgery upfront. The surgical approach primarily depends on the primary tumor size and localization and can vary from conservative procedures to extended surgical resections [73]. As discussed above, there is increasing awareness that a «watchful waiting» policy is indicated for small, incidentally discovered, nonfunctioning PanNETs. However, this approach should be considered only in the presence of low-grade tumors, thus rendering mandatory the fine needle aspiration (FNA) or the tumor biopsy [8]. Relative concern remains on the accuracy of a preoperative FNA, especially for small lesions; however, a high concordance between tumor grading as per preoperative FNA and that defined by the final histological report has been recently shown [74]. Although a surveillance protocol has not been formally adopted for incidentally detected PanNETs, follow-up visits with cross-sectional imaging and tumor markers every 6–12 months seem reasonable.

For patients with PanNENs >2 cm and/or symptomatic tumors, surgery still represents the treatment of choice. Either formal or limited pancreatic resections can be used and differ according to the tumor site. While pancreatoduodenectomies are usually performed for tumors of the pancreatic head, lesions of the body or tail are treated with distal pancreatectomy. When performed in high-volume centers, pancreatic formal resections have a mortality rate of less than 5%, with perioperative complications in up to 50% of patients [75, 76]. Both endocrine and exocrine insufficiency have been described in patients subjected to formal pancreatic resections [77], so that parenchyma-sparing techniques have been developed and are currently employed in selected cases. In particular, tumor enucleation or middle pancreatectomy may be indicated for small (<2 cm) functioning PanNETs, particularly insulinomas. In fact, insulinomas usually present as small, well-demarcated, solitary nodule and are associated with favorable outcomes [78]. Minimally invasive techniques including laparoscopy or robotic surgery can be also used for these neoplasms. Although they are associated with a reduced rate of exocrine and endocrine pancreatic insufficiency, parenchyma-sparing approaches increase the risk of pancreatic fistulas [61]. The role of prophylactic cholecystectomy in patients with locoregional PanNENs is currently under debate. Indeed, although there is a clear association between long-term SSA use and development of biliary gallstones, the incidence of cholecystitis is apparently low. Moreover, given recent advances in the selectivity of «embolotherapies», cholecystitis by reflux of microspheres after liver embolization is currently extremely rare [73].

Patients with G1/G2, locally advanced PanNENs may benefit of an aggressive surgical approach only in selected cases. In a recent retrospective analysis of patients who underwent «en bloc» resection of PanNENs and nearby organs, the 5-year disease-free survival (DFS) was 42%, and did not differ from that of patients undergoing pancreatic resection alone [79]. Of note, palliation of symptoms may be achieved by debulking surgery, mostly as part of multistep or multimodal treatment [80]. As in pancreatic adenocarcinoma, no survival gain has been observed in locally advanced, G3 PanNENs undergoing resection [81], so that surgery is currently not considered an option in this group of patients. Neoadjuvant strategies may be used to facilitate curative surgery in selected patients, as discussed above. As a rule of thumb, while PRRT appears more effective for tumor expressing high levels of SSTRs, chemotherapy may be appropriate for highly proliferating tumors.

The management of MEN1-associated PanNENs is similar to that of sporadic PanNENs. Up to 80% of patients with MEN1 develop synchronous or metachronous PanNENs or duodenal NENs [82]. While surgery is usually performed in patients with functioning tumors or symptoms caused by the tumor mass, a conservative management is indicated in patients with nonfunctioning tumors or gastrinomas smaller than 2 cm and with a yearly increased size below 0.5 cm [8]. Due to the high rate of multicentric lesions, intraoperative ultrasonography is mandatory in case of surgery for patients with MEN1 syndrome [73]. Up to 17% of patients with VHL develop PanNETs, which are almost always nonfunctioning [83]. As for MEN1 patients, VHL-associated PanNENs should be resected when symptomatic. However, mass-related symptoms occur in less than 5% of patients [83]. Currently, VHL-associated PanNENs are conservatively managed when their size is under 1.5 cm [8]. However, since PanNENs in patients with VHL syndrome may demonstrate a nonlinear growth pattern, special attention should be paid during their follow-up [84]. Tumor diameter > 3 cm, mutations in the exon 3 of the VHL gene, and high tumor doubling time (>500 days) have been shown to predict poor outcomes in VHL-associated PanNENs [85]. Patients with neurofibromatosis type 1 (NF1) present with periampullary somatostatin immunostaining neoplasms in up to 10% of cases. Because of their relatively high tumor malignancy, standard resections or local resections are commonly performed for NF1-associated PanNENs, irrespective of tumor size [86].

Approved medical therapies for patients with inoperable or unresectable locoregional PanNENs span from SSAs (octreotide and lanreotide) to the mammalian target of rapamycin (mTOR) inhibitor everolimus and the antiangiogenic agent sunitinib. It is still not clear if PRRT with lutetium will gain formal acceptance by regulatory authorities for patients with PanNETs, based on the results of the NETTER-1 trial [3]. However, there is wealth of low-level evidence indicating that PRRT is effective across a broad spectrum of NETs, and the highest rates of responses are observed in PanNETs [71]. Cytotoxic drugs including alkylating agents (streptozocin, temozolomide, platinum, dacarbazine) as well as fluoropyrimidines induce high rates of objective responses and are therefore commonly used in PanNET/C patients [59]. Currently, there are no data to drive treatment selection or sequencing.

17.2 Conclusions

At present time, surgery represents the only curative treatment for PanNETs. However, given the significant morbidity and mortality associated with pancreatic surgery even in high-volume centers, adequate patient selection is mandatory. While patients with small, nonfunctioning PanNETs may undergo active surveillance, subjects with tumors larger than 2 cm must be treated surgically. In the presence of nearby organ invasion, neoadjuvant strategies may be used to obtain tumor shrinkage. Recently, the combination of ^{177}Lu-DOTATATE, capecitabine, and temozolomide has been investigated in patients with advanced NETs and was associated with an overall response rate of 80% [87]. Although a higher percentage of objective responses should not be necessarily interpreted as an indicator of improved survival outcomes in the metastatic setting, the tandem association of preoperative chemo radionuclide therapy and surgery may be potentially curative for locally advanced patients, if R0 tumor resections are achieved. Protocols combining both ^{90}Y and ^{177}Lu have been evaluated in several nonrandomized trials of advanced NETs, resulting in ~40% of objective responses [88, 89]. Whether combinations of the two radioisotopes, that preferentially target large and small lesions respectively, may result in preoperative macroscopic tumor shrinkage and concurrent microscopic disease eradication is currently unknown. Since PRRT induces a large fraction of single-strand DNA breaks, inhibition of the machinery devoted to DNA repair may increase its efficacy. Of note, the poly-ADP-ribose-polymerase-1 (PARP-1) inhibitor olaparib has been recently shown to synergistically sensitize NET cells to PRRT, at least in vitro [90]. If associated with adequate objective response rates in PanNET patients, this treatment combination should be tested in the locally advanced setting.

While delay of tumor progression is the main treatment goal for patients with metastatic PanNENs, disease eradication via surgery or combinations of surgery and systemic/local treatments may be considered the ultimate objective in patients with locoregional disease. Multimodal or multistep therapies are thus requested for optimal treatment of locoregional PanNENs, and multidisciplinary team integration is key in this context, particularly in experienced, high-volume centers. Future research is needed to move the field of NENs to one dominated by empirical clinical judgment to one relying on molecularly tailored treatment choices.

Bibliography

1. Rindi G, Arnold R (2010) Nomenclature and classification of neuroendocrine neoplasms of the digestive system. In: Bosman F, Carneiro F, Hruban R, Theise N (eds) World Health Organization classification of tumours of the digestive system. IARC Press, Lyon, 13–14
2. Rindi G, Klöppel G, Alhman H, Caplin M, Couvelard A, de Herder WW, Erikssson B, Falchetti A, Falconi M, Komminoth P, Körner M, Lopes JM, McNicol AM, Nilsson O, Perren A, Scarpa A, Scoazec JY, Wiedenmann B, all other Frascati consensus conference participants; European Neuroendocrine tumor society (ENETS) (2006) TNM staging of foregut (neuro)endocrine tumors: a consensus proposal including a grading system. Virchows Arch 449(4):395–401
3. Cives M, Soares HP, Strosberg J (2016 Jul) Will clinical heterogeneity of neuroendocrine tumors impact their management in the future? Lessons from recent trials. Curr Opin Oncol 28(4):359–366
4. Bilimoria KY, Bentrem DJ, Merkow RP et al (2007) Application of the pancreatic adenocarcinoma staging system to pancreatic neuroendocrine tumors. J Am Coll Surg 205:558–563
5. Luo, G., et al (2017) Modified staging classification for pancreatic neuroendocrine tumors on the basis of the American Joint Committee on cancer and european neuroendocrine tumor society systems. J Clin Oncol 35(3):274–280
6. Strosberg JR, Cheema A, Weber J et al (2011) Prognostic validity of a novel American Joint Committee on Cancer Staging Classification for pancreatic neuroendocrine tumors. J Clin Oncol 29:3044–3049
7. Rindi G, Falconi M, Klersy C et al (2012) TNM staging of neoplasms of the endocrine pancreas: results from a large international cohort study. J Natl Cancer Inst 104:764–777
8. Falconi M, Eriksson B, Kaltsas G et al (2016) ENETS consensus guidelines update for the management of patients with functional pancreatic neuroendocrine tumors and non-functional pancreatic neuroendocrine tumors. Neuroendocrinology 103(2):153–171
9. Heestand GM, Murphy JD, Lowy AM (2015) Approach to patients with pancreatic cancer without detectable metastases. J Clin Oncol 33(16):1770–1778
10. Smith JJ, Garcia-Aguilar J (2015) Advances and challenges in treatment of locally advanced rectal cancer. J Clin Oncol 33(16):1797–1808
11. Wright AA, Bohlke K, Armstrong DK et al (2016) Neoadjuvant chemotherapy for newly diagnosed, advanced ovarian cancer: Society of Gynecologic Oncology and American Society of Clinical Oncology Clinical Practice Guideline. J Clin Oncol 34(28):3460–3473
12. Steinmuller T, Kianmanesh R, Falconi M et al (2008) Consensus guidelines for the management of patients with liver metastases from digestive (neuro)endocrine tumors: foregut, midgut, hindgut, and unknown primary. Neuroendocrinology 87(1):47–62
13. Reyes DK, Pienta KJ (2015) The biology and treatment of oligometastatic cancer. Oncotarget 6(11):8491–8524
14. Scigliano S, Lebtahi R, Maire F et al (2009) Clinical and imaging follow-up after exhaustive liver resection of endocrine metastases: a 15-year monocentric experience. Endocr Relat Cancer 16(3):977–990

15. Perysinakis I, Aggeli C, Kaltsas G, Zografos GN (2016) Neoadjuvant therapy for advanced pancreatic neuroendocrine tumors: an emerging treatment modality? Hormones (Athens) 15(1):15–22
16. Sorbye H, Westre B, Horn A et al (2007) Curative surgery after neoadjuvant chemotherapy in metastatic poorly differentiated neuroendocrine carcinoma. Eur J Surg Oncol 33:1209–1210
17. Lessing Y, Ben-Haim M, Lahat G et al (2011) Surgery after neoadjuvant chemotherapy for locally advanced extrapulmonary poorly differentiated neuroendocrine cancer. Am Surg 77(8):1102–1104
18. Crippa S, Partelli S, Bassi, Berardi R, Capelli P, Scarpa A, Zamboni G, Falconi M (2016) Long-term outcomes and prognostic factors in neuroendocrine carcinomas of the pancreas: morphology matters. Surgery 159(3):862–871
19. Dumont F, Goudard Y, Caramella C et al (2015) Therapeutic strategies for advanced pancreatic neuroendocrine tumors with segmental portal hypertension. World J Surg 39:1974–1980
20. Devata S, Kim EJ (2012) Neoadjuvant chemotherapy with capecitabine and temozolomide for unresectable pancreatic neuroendocrine tumor. Case Rep Oncol 5(3):622–626
21. Sato I, Ueda N, Kinoshita E et al (2010) Curatively resected case of non-functioning pancreatic neuroendocrine carcinoma with multiple liver metastases after downstaging with S-1 monotherapy. Gan To Kagaku Ryoho 37(7):1341–1344
22. Lee J, Choi J, Choi C, Seong J (2013) Role of radiotherapy for pancreatobiliary neuroendocrine tumors. Radiat Oncol J 31:125–130
23. Kaemmerer D, Prasad V, Daffner W et al (2009) Neoadjuvant peptide receptor radionuclide therapy for an inoperable neuroendocrine pancreatic tumor. World J Gastroenterol 15(46):5867–5870
24. Sowa-Staszczak A, Pach D, Chrzan R et al (2011) Peptide receptor radionuclide therapy as a potential tool for neoadjuvant therapy in patients with inoperable neuroendocrine tumours (NETs). Eur J Nucl Med Mol Imaging 38(9):1669–1674
25. Ezziddin S, Lauschke H, Schaefers M et al (2012) Neoadjuvant downsizing by internal radiation: a case for preoperative peptide receptor radionuclide therapy in patients with pancreatic neuroendocrine tumors. Clin Nucl Med 37(1):102–104
26. Barber TW, Hofman MS, Thomson BN, Hicks RJ (2012) The potential for induction peptide receptor chemoradionuclide therapy to render inoperable pancreatic and duodenal neuroendocrine tumours resectable. Eur J Surg Oncol 38(1):64–71
27. van Vliet EI, van Eijck CH, de Krijger RR et al (2015) Neoadjuvant treatment of nonfunctioning pancreatic neuroendocrine tumors with [177Lu-DOTA0,Tyr3]Octreotate. J Nucl Med 56(11):1647–1653
28. Breeman WA, Mearadji A, Capello A et al (2003) Anti-tumor effect and increased survival after treatment with [177Lu-DOTA0,Tyr3]octreotate in a rat liver micrometastases model. Int J Cancer 104(3):376–379
29. Oberg K, Krenning E, Sundin A et al (2016) A Delphic consensus assessment: imaging and biomarkers in gastroenteropancreatic neuroendocrine tumor disease management. Endocr Connect 5(5):174–187
30. Halfdanarson TR, Rubin J, Farnell MB et al (2008) Pancreatic endocrine neoplasms: epidemiology and prognosis of pancreatic endocrine tumors. Endocr Relat Cancer 15(2):409–427
31. Kidd M, Bodei L, Modlin IM (2016) Chromogranin a: any relevance in neuroendocrine tumors? Curr Opin Endocrinol Diabetes Obes 23(1):28–37
32. Khan MS, Kirkwood AA, Tsigani T et al (2016) Early changes in circulating tumor cells are associated with response and survival following treatment of metastatic neuroendocrine neoplasms. Clin Cancer Res 22(1):79–85
33. Modlin IM, Kidd M, Bodei L et al (2015) The clinical utility of a novel blood-based multi-transcriptome assay for the diagnosis of neuroendocrine tumors of the gastrointestinal tract. Am J Gastroenterol 110(8):1223–1232
34. Modlin IM, Frilling A, Salem RR et al (2016) Blood measurement of neuroendocrine gene transcripts defines the effectiveness of operative resection and ablation strategies. Surgery 159(1):336–347
35. Bodei L, Kidd M, Modlin IM et al (2016) Measurement of circulating transcripts and gene cluster analysis predicts and defines therapeutic efficacy of peptide receptor radionuclide therapy (PRRT) in neuroendocrine tumors. Eur J Nucl Med Mol Imaging 43(5):839–851
36. Moertel CG, Kvols LK, O'Connell MJ, Rubin J (1991) Treatment of neuroendocrine carcinomas with combined etoposide and cisplatin. Evidence of major therapeutic activity in the anaplastic variants of these neoplasms. Cancer 68:227–232

37. Mitry E, Baudin E, Ducreux M et al (1999) Treatment of poorly differentiated neuroendocrine tumours with etoposide and cisplatin. Br J Cancer 81:1351–1355
38. Sorbye H, Welin S, Langer SW et al (2013) Predictive and prognostic factors for treatment and survival in 305 patients with advanced gastrointestinal neuroendocrine carcinoma (WHO G3): the NORDIC NEC study. Ann Oncol 24:152–160
39. Childs A, Kirkwood A, Edeline J et al (2016) Ki-67 index and response to chemotherapy in patients with neuroendocrine tumours. Endocr Relat Cancer 23(7):563–570
40. Cives M, Ghayouri M, Morse B et al (2016) Analysis of potential response predictors to capecitabine/temozolomide in metastatic pancreatic neuroendocrine tumors. Endocr Relat Cancer 23(9):759–767
41. Gerson SL (2004) MGMT: its role in cancer aetiology and cancer therapeutics. Nat Rev Cancer 4:296–307
42. Ekeblad S, Sundin A, Janson ET et al (2007) Temozolomide as monotherapy is effective in treatment of advanced malignant neuroendocrine tumors. Clin Cancer Res 13:2986–2991
43. Kulke MH, Hornick JL, Frauenhoffer C et al (2009) O6-methylguanine DNA methyltransferase deficiency and response to temozolomide-based therapy in patients with neuroendocrine tumors. Clin Cancer Res 15:338–345
44. Schmitt AM, Pavel M, Rudolph T et al (2014) Prognostic and predictive roles of MGMT protein expression and promoter methylation in sporadic pancreatic neuroendocrine neoplasms. Neuroendocrinology 100:35–44
45. Walter T, van Brakel B, Vercherat C et al (2015) O6-Methylguanine-DNA methyltransferase status in neuroendocrine tumours: prognostic relevance and association with response to alkylating agents. Br J Cancer 112:523–531
46. Van Essen M, Krenning EP, De Jong M et al (2007) Peptide receptor radionuclide therapy with radiolabelled somatostatin analogues in patients with somatostatin receptor positive tumours. Acta Oncol 46(6):723–734
47. Kwekkeboom DJ, Kam BL, van Essen M et al (2010) Somatostatin-receptor-based imaging and therapy of gastroenteropancreatic neuroendocrine tumors. Endocr Relat Cancer 17(1):R53–R73
48. Kratochwil C, Stefanova M, Mavriopoulou E et al (2015) SUV of [68Ga]DOTATOC-PET/CT predicts response probability of PRRT in neuroendocrine tumors. Mol Imaging Biol 17(3):313–318
49. Legmann P, Vignaux O, Dousset B et al (1998) Pancreatic tumors: comparison of dual-phase helical CT and endoscopic sonography. AJR Am J Roentgenol 170:1315–1322
50. Dromain C, de Baere T, Lumbroso J et al (2005) Detection of liver metastases from endocrine tumors: a prospective comparison of somatostatin receptor scintigraphy, computed tomography, and magnetic resonance imaging. J Clin Oncol 23:70–78
51. Kim YK, Lee MW, Lee WJ et al (2012) Diagnostic accuracy and sensitivity of diffusion-weighted and of gadoxetic acid-enhanced 3-T MR imaging alone or in combination in the detection of small liver metastasis (≤ 1.5 cm in diameter). Investig Radiol 47(3):159–166
52. Sundin A, Garske U, Orlefors H (2007) Nuclear imaging of neuroendocrine tumours. Best Pract Res Clin Endocrinol Metab 21(1):69–85
53. Binderup T, Knigge U, Loft A et al (2010) Functional imaging of neuroendocrine tumors: a head-to-head comparison of somatostatin receptor scintigraphy, 123I-MIBG scintigraphy, and 18F-FDG PET. J Nucl Med 51(5):704–712
54. Sharma P, Arora S, Karunanithi S et al (2016) Somatostatin receptor based PET/CT imaging with 68Ga-DOTA-Nal3-octreotide for localization of clinically and biochemically suspected insulinoma. Q J Nucl Med Mol Imaging 60(1):69–76
55. Ambrosini V, Campana D, Bodei L et al (2010) 68Ga-DOTANOC PET/CT clinical impact in patients with neuroendocrine tumors. J Nucl Med 51(5):669–673
56. Wild D, Bomanji JB, Benkert P et al (2013) Comparison of 68Ga-DOTANOC and 68Ga-DOTATATE PET/CT within patients with gastroenteropancreatic neuroendocrine tumors. J Nucl Med 54(3):364–372
57. Cheema A, Weber J, Strosberg JR (2012) Incidental detection of pancreatic neuroendocrine tumors: an analysis of incidence and outcomes. Ann Surg Oncol 19:2932–2936
58. Bettini R, Partelli S, Boninsegna L et al (2011) Tumor size correlates with malignancy in nonfunctioning pancreatic endocrine tumor. Surgery 150:75–82

59. Cives M, Strosberg J (2014) An update on gastroenteropancreatic neuroendocrine tumors. Oncology (Williston Park) 28(9):749–756. 758
60. Cherif R, Gaujoux S, Couvelard A et al (2012) Parenchyma-sparing resections for pancreatic neuroendocrine tumors. J Gastrointest Surg 16:2045–2055
61. Falconi M, Mantovani W, Crippa S et al (2008) Pancreatic insufficiency after different resections for benign tumours. Br J Surg 95(1):85–91
62. Ramundo V, Del Prete M, Marotta V et al (2014) Impact of long-acting octreotide in patients with early-stage MEN1-related duodeno-pancreatic neuroendocrine tumours. Clin Endocrinol 80(6):850–855
63. Capurso G, Bettini R, Rinzivillo M et al (2011) Role of resection of the primary pancreatic neuroendocrine tumour only in patients with unresectable metastatic liver disease: a systematic review. Neuroendocrinology 93(4):223–229
64. Frilling A, Modlin IM, Kidd M et al (2014) Recommendations for management of patients with neuroendocrine liver metastases. Lancet Oncol 15(1):e8–21
65. Fernández-Cruz L, Blanco L, Cosa R, Rendón H (2008) Is laparoscopic resection adequate in patients with neuroendocrine pancreatic tumors? World J Surg 32(5):904–917
66. Drymousis P, Raptis DA, Spalding D et al (2014) Laparoscopic versus open pancreas resection for pancreatic neuroendocrine tumours: a systematic review and meta-analysis. HPB (Oxford) 16(5):397–406
67. Conrad C et al (2016) Prognostic value of lymph node status and extent of lymphadenectomy in pancreatic neuroendocrine tumors confined to and extending beyond the pancreas. J Gastrointest Surg 20(12):1966–1974
68. Bilimoria KY, Talamonti MS, Tomlinson JS et al (2008) Prognostic score predicting survival after resection of pancreatic neuroendocrine tumors: analysis of 3851 patients. Ann Surg 247(3):490–500
69. Boninsegna L, Panzuto F, Partelli S et al (2012) Malignant pancreatic neuroendocrine tumour: lymph node ratio and Ki67 are predictors of recurrence after curative resections. Eur J Cancer 48(11):1608–1615
70. Hashim YM, Trinkaus KM, Linehan DC et al (2014) Regional lymphadenectomy is indicated in the surgical treatment of pancreatic neuroendocrine tumors (PNETs). Ann Surg 259(2):197–203
71. Bodei L, Kwekkeboom DJ, Kidd M et al (2016) Radiolabeled somatostatin analogue therapy of gastroenteropancreatic cancer. Semin Nucl Med 46(3):225–238
72. Tang LH, Untch BR, Reidy DL et al (2015) Well differentiated neuroendocrine tumors with a morphologically apparent high-grade component: a pathway distinct from poorly differentiated neuroendocrine carcinomas. Clin Cancer Res 22:1011–1017
73. Partelli S, Maurizi A, Tamburrino D et al (2014) Surgical management of pancreatic neuroendocrine neoplasms. Ann Saudi Med 34(1):1–5
74. Larghi A, Capurso G, Carnuccio A et al (2012) Ki-67 grading of nonfunctioning pancreatic neuroendocrine tumors on histologic samples obtained by EUS-guided fine-needle tissue acquisition: a prospective study. Gastrointest Endosc 76(3):570–577
75. Büchler MW, Wagner M, Schmied BM et al (2003) Changes in morbidity after pancreatic resection: toward the end of completion pancreatectomy. Arch Surg 138(12):1310–1314
76. Yeo CJ, Cameron JL, Sohn TA et al (1997) Six hundred fifty consecutive pancreaticoduodenectomies in the 1990s: pathology, complications, and outcomes. Ann Surg 226(3):248–257
77. Smith JK, Ng SC, Hill JS et al (2010) Complications after pancreatectomy for neuroendocrine tumors: a national study. J Surg Res 163(1):63–68
78. de Herder WW, Niederle B, Scoazec JY et al (2006) Well-differentiated pancreatic tumor/carcinoma: insulinoma. Neuroendocrinology 84(3):183–188
79. Birnbaum DJ, Turrini O, Vigano L et al (2015) Surgical management of advanced pancreatic neuroendocrine tumors: short-term and long-term results from an international multi-institutional study. Ann Surg Oncol 22(3):1000–1007
80. Partelli S, Inama M, Rinke A et al (2015) Long-term outcomes of surgical management of pancreatic neuroendocrine tumors with synchronous liver metastases. Neuroendocrinology 102(1–2):68–76
81. Fischer L, Kleeff J, Esposito I et al (2008) Clinical outcome and long-term survival in 118 consecutive patients with neuroendocrine tumours of the pancreas. Br J Surg 95(5):627–635

82. Triponez F, Cadiot G (2007) Non-functioning tumours of the pancreas in MEN1 patients. J Gastrointestin Liver Dis 16(3):295–296
83. Jensen RT, Berna MJ, Bingham DB, Norton JA (2008) Inherited pancreatic endocrine tumor syndromes: advances in molecular pathogenesis, diagnosis, management, and controversies. Cancer 113(7 Suppl):1807–1843
84. Gaujoux S, Gonen M, Tang L et al (2012) Synchronous resection of primary and liver metastases for neuroendocrine tumors. Ann Surg Oncol 19(13):4270–4277
85. Blansfield JA, Choyke L, Morita SY et al (2007) Clinical, genetic and radiographic analysis of 108 patients with von Hippel-Lindau disease (VHL) manifested by pancreatic neuroendocrine neoplasms (PNETs). Surgery 142(6):814–818
86. Hartel M, Wente MN, Sido B et al (2005) Carcinoid of the ampulla of Vater. J Gastroenterol Hepatol 20(5):676–681
87. Claringbold PG, Turner JH (2016) Pancreatic neuroendocrine tumor control: durable objective response to combination 177Lu-octreotate-capecitabine-temozolomide radiopeptide chemotherapy. Neuroendocrinology 103(5):432–439
88. Seregni E, Maccauro M, Chiesa C et al (2014) Treatment with tandem [90Y]DOTA-TATE and [177Lu] DOTA-TATE of neuroendocrine tumours refractory to conventional therapy. Eur J Nucl Med Mol Imaging 41(2):223–230
89. Villard L, Romer A, Marincek N et al (2012) Cohort study of somatostatin-based radiopeptide therapy with [(90)Y-DOTA]-TOC versus [(90)Y-DOTA]-TOC plus [(177)Lu-DOTA]-TOC in neuroendocrine cancers. J Clin Oncol 30(10):1100–1106
90. Nonnekens J, van Kranenburg M, Beerens CE et al (2016) Potentiation of peptide receptor radionuclide therapy by the PARP inhibitor olaparib. Theranostics 6(11):1821–1832

Therapy for Locoregional Disease: Ileum

Olov Norlen, Peter Stålberg, and Per Hellman

A. Colao et al. (eds.), *Neuroendocrine Tumors in Real Life*,
https://doi.org/10.1007/978-3-319-59024-0_18

Overview

SI-NET is one of the most common neuroendocrine tumours, as well as the most common malignant tumour found in the small bowel. The majority of cases are diagnosed when liver metastases, peritoneal carcinomatosis or other distant metastases are present, while others present in with only lymph node metastases, whereas tumours without any metastases at diagnosis are uncommon. In some of these patients, the locoregional disease is asymptomatic, while in others abdominal symptoms such as pain or small bowel obstruction are present. This chapter focuses on the primary surgical approach in these patients, where the prognosis is very good with correct treatment.

Clinical Case

A 67-year-old man presents in the emergency department with colicky abdominal pain, distension and vomiting. The medical history does not reveal any prior diseases nor any heredity for malignant diseases. He is a non-smoker and does not use any medications. Prior to the last 2 days of abdominal pain and absence of passing of flatus and stools, there is history of loose stools/diarrhoea for several months. He also complains of flushing, and on specific questioning, he admits it happens after the use of red wine and chocolate. General physical examination reveals metallic abdominal sounds, a distended abdomen but no peritonitis.

After prescribing 1000 ml of Ringer's solution, 5 mg of morphine i.v. for the abdominal pain, a nasogastric tube and routine bloods and an abdominal computed tomography (CT) scan are ordered. The CT scan reveals distended small bowel loops with gas-fluid levels. There are signs of small bowel obstruction before the most distal part of the ileum, as this segment of the ileum and the colon is not distended. In the mesentery, lymph node metastases, with for small intestinal neuroendocrine tumour (SI-NET) typically associated desmoplastic reaction presenting as a spoke-wheel sign, is seen (◘ Fig. 18.1). In coronary sections, the mesenteric mass is seen not to involve the central mesenteric root (◘ Fig. 18.1). The CT scan reveals a few liver metastases located in both lobes of the liver. The patient is, after initial resuscitation, subjected to an emergency laparotomy, and the abdominal cavity is explored. Before anaesthesiological induction, an infusion of a somatostatin analogue at 50 ug/h is started in order to prevent a carcinoid crisis during surgery.

On the surface of the liver, more than 20 small metastases are palpated. There are no signs of peritoneal carcinomatosis in the abdominal cavity. The small bowel is palpated from the ligament of Treitz to the ileocecal valve, and the obstructive mechanism is found approximately 50 cm before the ileocecal valve. The small intestine is here incorporated in a fibrotic mass and is kinked by adherences around an obvious primary tumour of about 1.5 cm in size in the intestinal wall. In addition, between 20 and 70 cm from the ileocecal valve, eight small intraluminal small bowel tumours are also found. In the mesentery the lymph node metastases are palpated extending up to and surrounding the ileocolic artery as it branches off the superior mesenteric artery. To achieve a macroscopically radical operation in the mesentery, the right side of the colon including the hepatic flexure is mobilized, and an extended right-sided haemicolectomy, also removing the last 70 cm of the ileum with all tumours palpable in the intestinal wall, as well as clearance of the mesentery to the origin of the ileocolic artery, with a primary anastomosis is performed. The postoperative course is uneventful and the patient is discharged after 4 days.

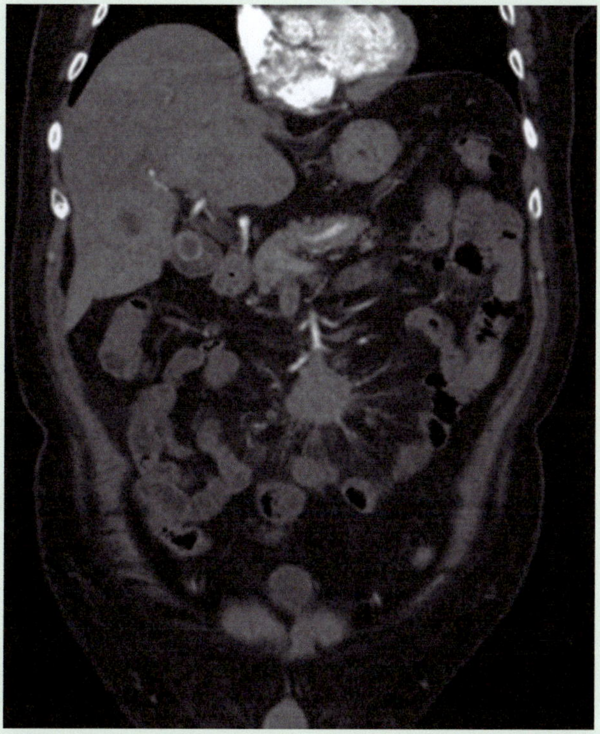

Fig. 18.1 Coronary section of a CT scan of a patient with SI-NET. The typical spoke-wheel appearance of the desmoplastic reaction surrounding the mesenteric metastasis is clearly seen

18.1 Comments to the Case

A spoke-wheel sign is pathognomonic to SI-NETs. Somatostatin analogues should always be given preoperatively if a metastatic SI-NET is suspected. Often radical surgery can be achieved; however, if enough jejunal branches cannot be spared, it may be better to leave lymph node metastases and not risk a short bowel syndrome.

Questions

1. Is laparoscopic resection an option when operating on these tumours?
2. What is the prognosis after resection of the primary in a patient in SI-NET and what influences it?

Answers

1. Laparoscopy makes palpation of the small bowel impossible, and as 35% of all SI-NET are multiple, the risk of missing multiple bowel tumours is high. Therefore, we recommend laparotomy or at least handport-assisted surgery to facilitate palpation of the entire small bowel.
2. The prognosis is generally very good with a median survival that surpasses 10 years. The most negative prognostic factors are increasing age, remaining peritoneal carcinomatosis, extra-abdominal disease, para-aortal metastases and an increasing degree of comorbidity.

Up to Date of the Topic

Introduction and Treatment Options for Locoregional Disease

SI-NET are in the majority of cases diagnosed in stage IV, when liver metastases or other distant metastases are present, while others present in stage IIIb, but rarely in earlier stages [1, 2]. In some of these patients, the locoregional disease is asymptomatic, while in others abdominal symptoms such as pain or small bowel obstruction are present [2]. However, some cases are found incidentally by radiology performed either due to an unrelated cause or as a work-up for long-standing diffuse abdominal pain (Fig. 18.2). Patients in stage I–IIIa, thus without even locoregional dissemination to the lymph nodes, are usually only found during laparotomy for an unrelated cause [2]. Each of these situations calls for a strategy for work-up, treatment and follow-up.

The only treatment shown to reduce tumour burden in locoregional disease is surgery, although biotherapy by somatostatin analogues or interferon alpha may exhibit «stabilization» of the disease, leading to hampered continuous growth and in some cases also marginal reduction of the tumour sizes. In locally advanced cases, novel therapies including mTOR or tyrosine kinase inhibitors may be used, and if the fibrotic reaction impairs the ureters or mesenteric vessels, stenting may alleviate symptoms.

Work-Up Before Surgery

In the elective setting, patients with suspected SI-NET should, initially, be diagnosed, most preferably by a biopsy, usually from a liver lesion, but confirmatory findings of high U-5-HIAA levels are supportive. It is wise, also in the emergency situation if preoperative diagnostics is not possible, to collect blood for later measurements of biomarkers, such as chromogranin A. If not in emergency, an abdominal CT scan with arterial and venous contrast phases should be obtained to assess for metastatic disease and the extent of locoregional disease. Coronary sections of the contrast phases are often helpful to display the relationship of the vessels in the mesenteric root in relationship with the mesenteric mass (Fig. 18.1). The extent of lymph node involvement may be classified according to Ohrvall et al., where lymph node stage IV represents inoperable disease [3].

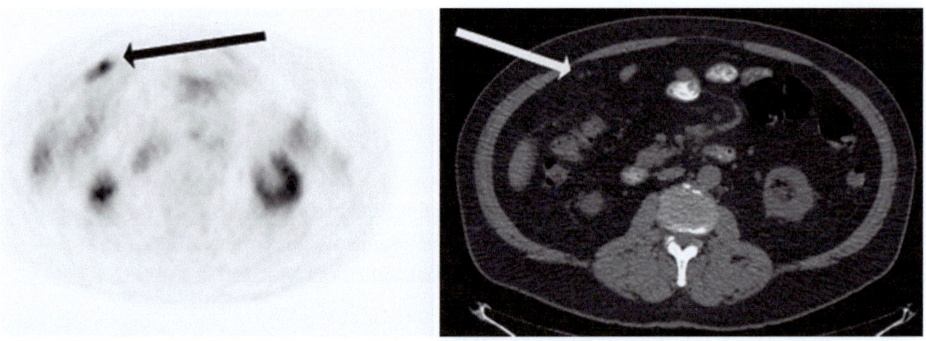

Fig. 18.2 68Ga-DOTATOC PET and corresponding CT image of a patient with SI-NET, revealing peritoneal carcinomatosis (*arrows*)

In equivocal cases, when biochemistry or radiology is not definitive of the diagnosis, a somatostatin analogue receptor scintigraphy or rather a 68Ga-DOTATOC/DOTATATE/DOTANOC PET may be obtained. These functional scans will also sometimes upstage the tumour as they are more sensitive than abdominal CT, and they are indicated prior to surgery in some cases, especially in asymptomatic patients where accurate preoperative staging may alter the decision of surgery (◘ Fig. 18.2).

Patients with advanced stage IV disease and/or signs of cardiac incompensation should undergo an echocardiography to exclude carcinoid heart disease. If present, the cardiac heart disease should be assessed and operated on if necessary before abdominal surgery.

Indications for Surgery for Locoregional Disease

In TNM stage I–III, all patients fit for surgery should undergo radical resection of the locoregional disease if technically feasible, with the aim to perform radical surgery. Likewise in technically operable TNM stage IV, all patients with symptoms related to the abdominal disease have a clear indication for surgery, as surgery often relieves symptoms and may inhibit pending bowel obstruction. In asymptomatic stage IV patients, the evidence for locoregional surgery is more equivocal. A paradigm has been that all these patients eventually progress also in the mesentery and therefore the locoregional tumour should be resected prophylactically before it causes any problems [2, 4, 5]. However, there are no randomized trials to support this, although most retrospective series show a possible survival benefit of locoregional surgery also in these patients [2, 4, 5].However, these series are, even though attempting to adjust for confounders, probably influenced by bias. As always, the morbidity and mortality associated with locoregional surgery must be weighed against the potential benefit.

In asymptomatic TNM stage IV disease, the age and comorbidity of the patient, the size and location of the mesenteric tumour and the general tumour load may aid the surgeon to decide if surgery is indicated. The ENETS guideline promotes prophylactic locoregional resection of asymptomatic stage IV patients, whereas NCNN most recent guidelines recommend against it [6, 7].

Peroperative Considerations and Surgical Technique

All patients undergoing surgery for SI-NET should receive antibiotics and thrombosis prophylaxis according to local hospital routine. Moreover, somatostatin analogues should be administered peroperatively in all patients with stage III–IV disease or, if unknown stage, with symptoms of the carcinoid syndrome to avoid peroperative carcinoid crisis. Carcinoid crisis presents as hypotension, flushing and tachycardia, and if it occurs, one or several bolus doses of somatostatin analogue may be administered or the rate of the infusion may be increased.

Surgery is often performed as a laparotomy, although laparoscopic resections have been reported. However, laparoscopy makes palpation of the entire small bowel virtually impossible, and as this is an important step of the operation since one third of all SI-NETs are multiple, laparoscopy is not recommended. A hybrid solution to facilitate palpation of the small bowel may be a handport-assisted laparoscopy. The first step after entering the abdominal cavity is to explore the abdominal cavity for signs of metastatic disease, either peritoneal carcinomatosis or in the liver.

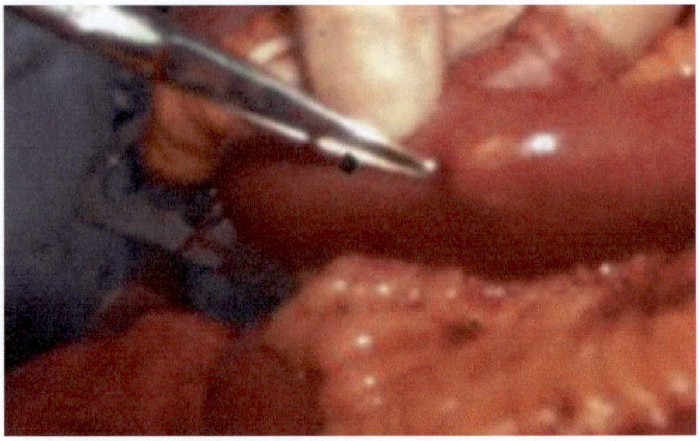

Fig. 18.3 Small incidental tumour found in the ileum at operation due to intestinal obstruction. The primary tumour per se, later confirmed as an SI-NET, did not cause any obstruction

In women, the ovaries contain metastases in up to 20% of all cases [2]. In patients with no or only single liver metastases, an intraoperative ultrasound may be performed to assess the liver for additional metastases to determine if resection of the liver metastasis is possible and to stage the patient to accurately be able to determine future adjuvant therapy.

After this the ligament of Treitz is found, and the small bowel palpated from the proximal jejunum to the distal ileum. Most primary tumours are located in the distal 100 cm of the ileum (Fig. 18.3). When the small bowel tumours are localized, the mesentery is palpated, and the relationship between the superior mesenteric artery and its branches is assessed. Depending on the location and extent of the mesenteric mass, a small bowel resection with or without a right-sided haemicolectomy is performed, including a wedge-shaped resection of the mesentery and the mesenteric mass. Meticulous dissection is done to avoid injury to jejunal branches of the superior mesenteric artery. If in doubt if the tumour is resectable due to a close relationship to these branches, a vascular haemostat may be applied at the thought line of the resection, and if the proximal bowel does not become ischaemic, the resection may continue. The surgeon should always weigh the benefit of a radical resection in the mesentery against the risk of small bowel infarction and subsequent short bowel syndrome.

After the resection is complete, a primary anastomose is made, with either a handsewn or stapled technique. The abdomen is then closed according to the surgeon's preference.

Short- and Long-Term Complications After Locoregional Surgery

Morbidity of locoregional surgery ranges from 5.8% to 7.8%, probably depending on case-mix and definition of morbidity [2]. Short-term complications may include fascia dehiscence, bleeding, anastomotic leak, infection and deep vein thrombosis. Long-term complications include small bowel obstruction and abdominal wall hernias. Thirty-day mortality has been reported to be 1.6% [2].

Prognosis and Follow-Up After Locoregional Surgery

Overall 5-year survival after locoregional resection in stage I–III patients is reported to be 84–100%, and for stage IV patients, the 5-year survival ranges from 57 to 74% [2, 4, 5] (Fig. 18.4).

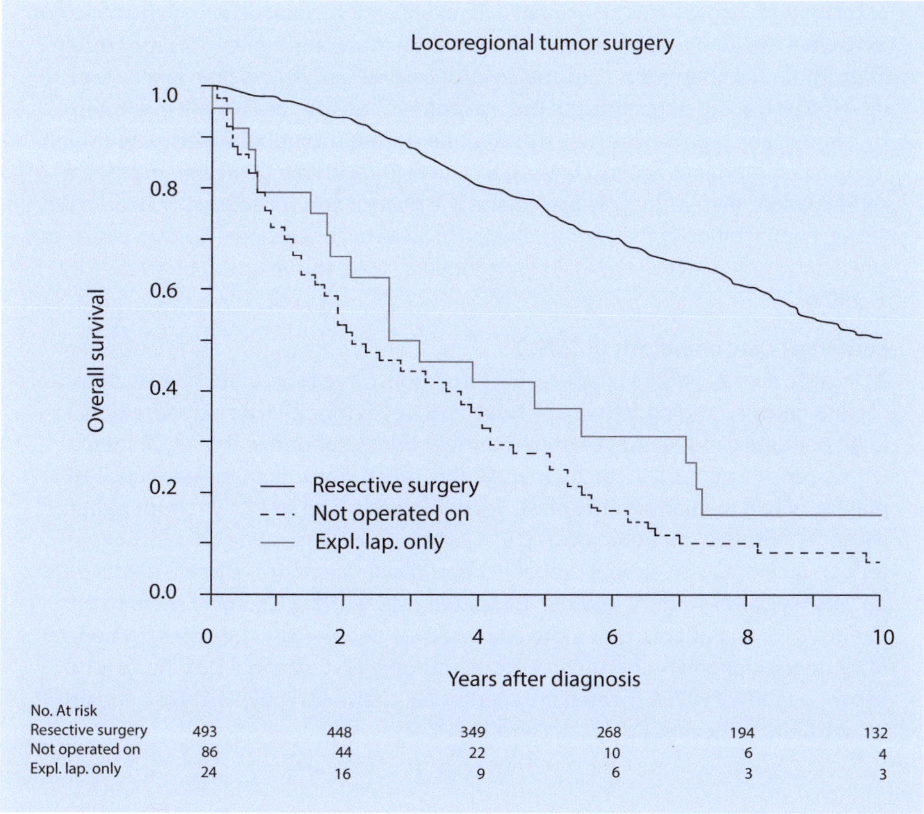

Fig. 18.4 Kaplan-Meier survival curve of patients with SI-NET, due to type of surgery performed, in a retrospective material [2]

All grade 1–2 tumours that have undergone radical surgery should be followed up every 6–12 months. G3 tumours should be followed more often, every 3 months according to current ENETS guidelines [7]. For patients with residual disease after surgery, the interval is initially 3–6 months for G1/G2 tumours and 3 months for G3 tumours, although this interval can be increased in slow progressing tumours. Triphasic computed tomography, measurement of urinary 5-HIAA and serum CgA are mandatory. In the case of a suspected recurrence, somatostatin receptor scintigraphy or rather somatostatin analogue PET/CT should be performed [7]. The follow-up should be life-long, considering that after 25 years only approximately 20% of all patients are free of disease [7].

Treatment for Patients with Locally Advanced Mesenteric or Retroperitoneal Disease

Some patients have an advanced locoregional disease with a mesenteric mass surrounding the mesenteric root and are generally deemed inoperable as the risk of surgery exceeds the potential benefit. However, in some SI-NET patients, the mesenteric metastases and accompanying fibrosis may cause venous stasis, development of tortuous varicose veins associated with eventual intestinal bleeding and incipient ischaemia due to direct pressure of the proximal mesenteric veins. This may result in postprandial abdominal pain, malabsorption and weight loss or in some cases develop into acute ischaemia [8]. The mesenteric veins are usually not infiltrated by tumour, and a guidewire may therefore be passed through the obstructed vein using a percutaneous access via the portal vein [9]. With the guidewire in place, a self-expandable stent may be placed and the obstruction subsequently cleared [9]. Other manifestations of advanced disease include retroperitoneal fibrosis, which can cause obstruction of the ureter. In symptomatic cases, this may also be treated by stenting.

Peritoneal Carcinomatosis in SI-NET

At least 20% of all patients undergoing laparotomy due to an SI-NET have peritoneal carcinomatosis, ranging from a few small nodules in the small bowel mesentery to large peritoneal metastases scattered throughout the abdominal cavity. Patients with extensive peritoneal carcinomatosis fare much worse than the general SI-NET patient, with a median survival of 4.0 years in comparison to 11.1 years for patients without peritoneal carcinomatosis [10]. Easily resected moderate amounts of peritoneal carcinomatosis should probably be surgically treated, as these patients often do very well after surgery, and the associated risks with such surgery seem to be minimal [10]. In patients with more advanced carcinomatosis, the potential benefit of surgery is unknown, and the risk of such surgery is substantial [11]. There is no known benefit of HIPEC (heated intraperitoneal chemotherapy) in SI-NET, and ENETS most recent guidelines do not support HIPEC [7].

Bibliography

1. Yao JC, Hassan M, Phan A, Dagohoy C, Leary C, Mares JE et al (2008) One hundred years after "carcinoid": epidemiology of and prognostic factors for neuroendocrine tumors in 35,825 cases in the United States. J Clin Oncol 26(18):3063–3072
2. Norlen O, Stalberg P, Oberg K, Eriksson J, Hedberg J, Hessman O et al (2012) Long-term results of surgery for small intestinal neuroendocrine tumors at a tertiary referral center. World J Surg 36(6):1419–1431
3. Ohrvall U, Eriksson B, Juhlin C, Karacagil S, Rastad J, Hellman P et al (2000) Method for dissection of mesenteric metastases in mid-gut carcinoid tumors. World J Surg 24(11):1402–1408
4. Ahmed A, Turner G, King B, Jones L, Culliford D, McCance D et al (2009) Midgut neuroendocrine tumours with liver metastases: results of the UKINETS study. Endocr Relat Cancer 16(3):885–894
5. Strosberg J, Gardner N, Kvols L (2009) Survival and prognostic factor analysis of 146 metastatic neuroendocrine tumors of the mid-gut. Neuroendocrinology 89(4):471–476
6. Kulke MH, Shah MH, Benson AB 3rd, Bergsland E, Berlin JD, Blaszkowsky LS et al (2015) Neuroendocrine tumors, version 1. 2015. J Natl Compr Cancer Netw 13(1):78–108
7. Niederle B, Pape UF, Costa F, Gross D, Kelestimur F, Knigge U et al (2016) ENETS consensus guidelines update for neuroendocrine neoplasms of the jejunum and ileum. Neuroendocrinology 103(2):125–138
8. Åkerstrom G, Hellman P, Hessman O (2005) Midgut carcinoid tumours: surgical treatment and prognosis. Best Pract Res Clin Gastroenterol 19(5):717–728
9. Hellman P, Hessman O, Akerstrom G, Stalberg P, Hennings J, Bjorck M et al (2010) Stenting of the superior mesenteric vein in midgut carcinoid disease with large mesenteric masses. World J Surg 34(6):1373–1379

10. Norlen O, Edfeldt K, Akerstrom G, Westin G, Hellman P, Bjorklund P et al (2014) Peritoneal carcinomatosis from small intestinal neuroendocrine tumors: clinical course and genetic profiling. Surgery 156(6):1512–1521; discussion 21–22
11. Elias D, Sideris L, Liberale G, Ducreux M, Malka D, Lasser P et al (2005) Surgical treatment of peritoneal carcinomatosis from well-differentiated digestive endocrine carcinomas. Surgery 137(4): 411–416

Therapy for Locoregional Disease: Bronchi

Niccolò Daddi, Valentina Tassi, Marco Lupattelli, Vincenzo Minotti, Francesco Puma, and Piero Ferolla

A. Colao et al. (eds.), *Neuroendocrine Tumors in Real Life*,
https://doi.org/10.1007/978-3-319-59024-0_19

Overview

Central endobronchial carcinoid represents often the subtype characterised by the least aggressive behaviour in the entire spectrum of differentiation of neuroendocrine tumours of the lung. Being central, they became generally early symptomatic and therefore is not unfrequent, an early diagnosis when their diffusion is still locoregional. As is well known, WHO Classification [1] subdivides carcinoid on the basis of the mitotic count and the presence or lack of necrosis in typical (TC) and atypical (AC). It should be remarked that these tumours, although may have an indolent biological behaviour, are not benign and even the lower-grade TC may be associated with a haematogenous and lymphatic spread. Therefore the therapeutic approach, either surgical, interventional endoscopic or medical, requires always a careful multidisciplinary planning at the light of the distinctive peculiarities of these subcategories. Finally, an accurate and extensive follow-up plays a crucial role even in the cases apparently radically cured. This chapter will review, starting from the clinics of two evidence-based practice cases, the therapeutic options available for locoregional bronchial carcinoids in a multidisciplinary setting.

Clinical Case 1

A 21-year-old male (C.D.) was hospitalised for progressive episodes of dyspnoea on exertion and the persistence, in the past 6 months, of recurrent episodes of inspiratory siblings and concomitant cough with haemoptoic sputum. A CT scan showed the presence of a 11 mm diameter left endobronchial polypoid lesion. Fibrebronchoscopy evidenced a pedunculated lesion partially occluding the main left bronchus (◘ Fig. 19.1a). Under general anaesthesia, a rigid bronchoscopy with endobronchialneodymium:yttrium-aluminium-garnet (Nd:YAG) laser disobliteration was performed. The residual tissue scar was spotted at the mucosal area of the segmental bronchi for the apical segment (B6) of the lower lobe.

The final pathology report described an atypical carcinoid (AC) due to the presence of necrosis. Despite that the excision was apparently radical at bronchoscopy and CT, after discussion with the patients, we convene, for a curative intent, to proceed

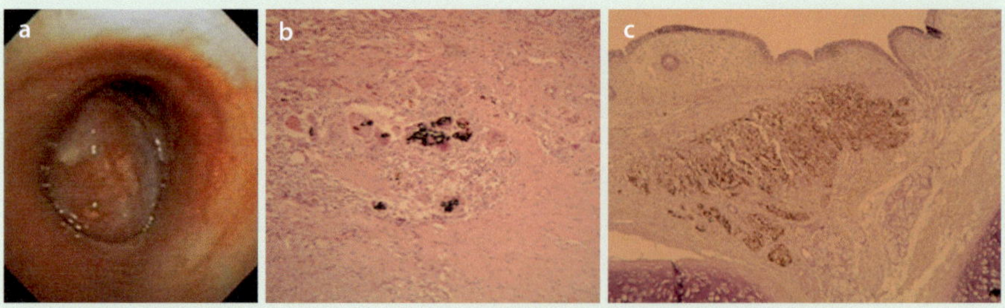

◘ **Fig. 19.1** Endoscopic appearance **a** of the typical carcinoid tumour resected with neodymium:yttrium-aluminium-garnet (Nd:YAG) laser. At the final pathology report on the lung specimen, in the submucosal space, under the area treated endoscopically [**b**; black spots of photocoagulation], a 0.7 cm area of disease was detected [**c**; highlighted brownish area obtained with Chromogranin A staining]

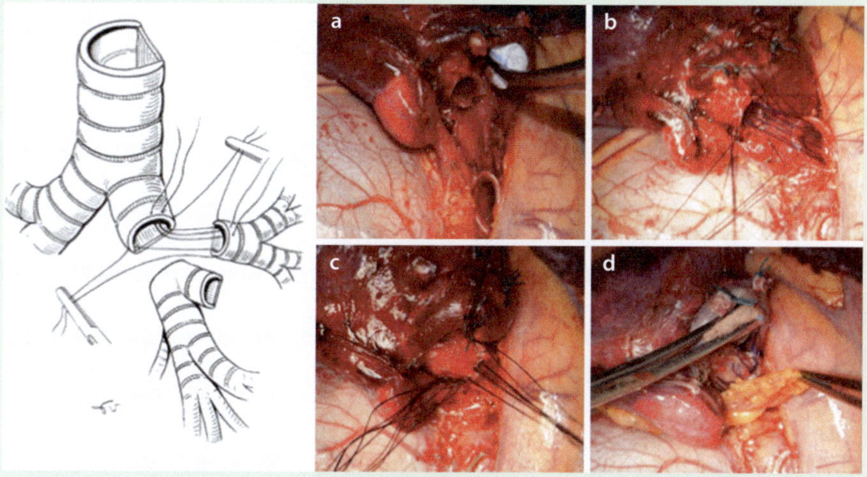

Fig. 19.2 Left lower lobe sleeve resection [drawing] of the endobronchial submucosal remnant of typical carcinoid. The two sides of the bronchi without the disease **a** were attached **b** with separate 3-0 Vicryl stitches. Final result of the procedure **c** and suture coverage with a pedunculated fat pad **d** from the mediastinum

for surgery. The patient underwent therefore to a left lower sleeve lobectomy (Fig. 19.2) with systematic lymph node dissection for a pathological stage IA (T1b N0 M0, AJCC 8th Edition [2]) low-grade typical carcinoid (TC) detected under the scar tissue of the previous laser treatment site (Fig. 19.1a, c). The patient started post-surgical follow-up according to the current ENETS and ESMO Guidelines 8 [3]. At 7 years no recurrence has been detected, but the patient will continue the follow-up at least till 15 years postsurgery.

19.1 Comments to the Case

This case is an emblematic example of how the locoregional treatment with only Nd:YAG laser disobliteration for an endobronchial TC cannot sufficiently eradicate the disease. Indeed, despite an apparent radical endobronchial excision, under the scar, a persistence of disease was demonstrated by surgery (Fig. 19.1b, c). Furthermore endobronchial resection does not allow the lymph-nodal resection and is now well known how lymph-nodal metastases may be present at diagnosis up to 20% of TC and in more than 50% of AC [4]. In these cases endobronchial treatment may result incomplete in a significant percentage of patients, while surgical treatment may offer the definitive cure to the patient if done with a proper lymph nodal dissection [4, 5]. The young age, like in this case, may be crucial to choose a treatment that offers a higher possibility of cure, while in elderly patients, with a lower performance status and/or co-morbidity, an endoscopic treatment with palliative intent may be justified [4].

Pathology report, such as in this patient, may be misleading [5] if the multiple samples are collected after laser treatment, due to the fact that the presence of artificial coagulative necrosis, induced by the treatment, may lead to a diagnosis of AC rather than TC. In the postsurgical histological diagnosis, the mitotic rate less than 2 mitoses per 10 HPF and the absence of necrosis (Ki-67 was less than 2%) were consistent with the definitive diagnosis of TC according to the WHO criteria [1].

Questions

1. May endoscopic treatment (i.e. laser or brachytherapy) be considered a valid alternative to surgery in bronchial carcinoids?
2. May carcinoid have metastatic spread? How is the cancer specific survival rate? Is recurrence more frequently locoregional or at distance?
3. Besides CT scan, are there other diagnostic tools to evaluate metastatic diffusion?
4. Is lung parenchyma-sparing resection a valid substitute of major lung resection (i.e. lobectomy or pneumonectomy) for endobronchial lesions?

Answers

1. Endobronchial disobliteration using neodymium:yttrium-aluminium-garnet (Nd:YAG) laser or other local treatments such as photodynamic therapy, cryotherapy and mechanical removal has been described in some series in literature [6, 7], in a cohort of highly selected patients, associated with good outcome after short-term follow-up in an interval time ranging from 1 to a maximum of 5 years. It should be however remarked that an accurate and protracted follow-up is always necessary [8] to consider the patient cured. The peak of recurrence is generally located within 5 years in AC and over 10 years in TC [4, 8, 9]. Furthermore the impossibility to evaluate and remove lymph node candidates an high percentage of patients (around 20% of the total in TC and more than 50% in AC) to a persistence of disease, while in most of the patients surgery may obtain an R0 resection [4, 9, 10] with distant metastases detected during the follow-up [4, 5].

   Surgery should therefore still be considered the treatment of choice. However endobronchial resections may play an important role in a multidisciplinary setting to allow presurgical disobliteration or in the palliative setting in the elderly patients with/without relevant co-morbidities who cannot be candidates for surgery [3, 4, 11].
2. Histological distinction between TC and AC represents the most important prognostic factor [1, 3, 4]. Haematogenous and lymphatic metastatic spread may be possible in both subtype but more common in AC [1, 4]. In older series, overall cancer-specific survival for resectable tumours, after the Travis Classification [12, 13], was reported to be for TC 95% (range 87–100%) at 5 years, 91% (range 82–87%) at 10 years and 85% (range 83–87%) at 15 years and for AC 72% (range 56–78%) at 5 years, 55% (range 73–98%) at 10 years and 53% at 15 years [4].

   In a recent meta-analyses study done by Detterbeck [4], most of the patient had the disease distally recurred (74% TC and 82% AC). A 13% of local or local + distant metastases were described in TC, while a 7% of local and 11% local + distant recurrences were evident in AC patients. Bone metastases have been reported in the only prospective study in around 70% of the cases (Ferolla et al. LUNA Trial NCT01563354 presented at ESMO 2016 in submission).

3. A careful preoperative, surgical and postoperative diagnostic workup is of crucial importance [3, 8, 9, 11, 13]. Recently new endoscopic tools such as endobronchial ultrasound probes or fibre optic narrowband images and 3-D navigation system guidance may add some value [14]. Nuclear medicine techniques like SRS and Ga^{68}-DOTA PET may play a relevant role in the staging, and MR of the spine may be associated to evaluate bone metastatic spread in the symptomatic patients [3].
4. Data from the literature highlight how lobectomies are the predominant operations [4, 5, 7, 9, 10]. Among the other available techniques, there is a tendency towards conservative surgery (sublobar resections and sleeve lobectomies), although a considerable number of pneumonectomies are still reported (up to 27%) [4]. The main concern in surgical treatment of carcinoids is to avoid unnecessary removal of functioning pulmonary tissue [3, 8–11]. However, while parenchyma-sparing operations such as sleeve lobectomies or tracheo-bronchoplasties represent the procedure of choice for centrally located carcinoid tumours in experienced centres [4, 5, 9, 10], the outcome might be questionable if the lymphadenectomy is not properly performed and the endoscopic follow-up not periodically done [4, 9].

Clinical Case 2

A 39-year-old male was referred to our hospital for metastatic typical bronchial carcinoid. When he was 25, he underwent in another hospital bilobectomy of the lower and middle lobe without lymphadenectomy for a typical carcinoid. He then developed multiple recurrences after 8 years with metastatic diffusion to the liver, lungs, lymph nodes and bones (spine, sternum, iliac). Subsequent treatments, including locoregional procedures for metachronous liver metastases and for a single lesion of the lower part of the sternum, were performed. After radiological progression of the metastatic spread at the liver, bone and lymph nodes, the patients were treated with long-acting somatostatin analogues obtaining a stable disease according to RECIST 1.0 criteria for 36 months. After a new RECIST progression of the patient at lymph node and liver level, the patient was enrolled in a phase III trial with a combination of octreotide LAR 30 mg every 28 days and everolimus 10 mg/day obtaining a stable disease for the following 30 months.

In March 2010, the patient was admitted at our institution complaining with cough, dyspnoea and fever. Chest-abdomen CT scan revealed partial atelectasis of the residual right lung, multiple pulmonary nodules in the left lung (◘ Fig. 19.3, panel 1a) and increasing in size and number of liver and lymph-nodal metastasis. Fibrebronchoscopy showed a centimetric red polypoid neoplasm originating from the stump of the intermediate bronchus and partially obliterating the upper lobar bronchus (◘ Fig. 19.3, panel 1b). Furthermore, three lesions on the vertebral body of T2, sternum and the right sacrum ala were detected at MR imaging. Multimodality therapy was indicated. External radiation therapy was delivered to sternum, right sacral ala and vertebral body. The patient received also palliative endobronchial high-dose rate BT (*Iridium*^{192}) with a total dose of *20 Gy* in four weekly fractions over 1 month (◘ Fig. 19.3, panel 2a and 2b). Although a complete change in the vascularization of the endobronchial lesion was observed (◘ Fig. 19.3, panel 3b), no changes in the

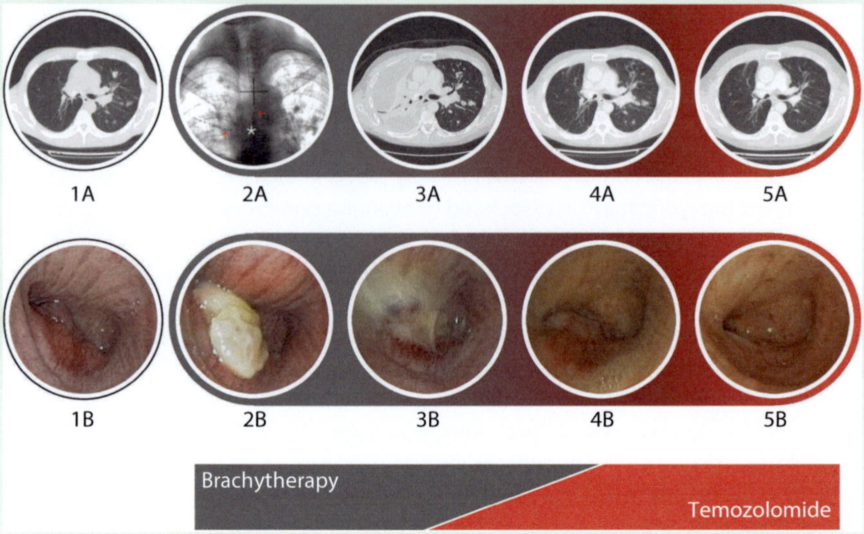

Fig. 19.3 The CT scan initial appearance of the carcinoid tumour (Fig. 19.1 panel **1a**) shows a metastatic spread in both lungs and an endobronchial recurrence of the typical carcinoid in the stump of the bronchus intermedius (Fig. 19.1 panel **1b**). Furthermore the endoscopic view of the carcinoid tumour (Fig. 19.1 panel **1b**) was surrounded by capillary web particularly on the cartilaginous part of the main right bronchus mucosa (*arrow*). After the first fraction of brachytherapy (Fig. 19.1 panel **2a**, *arrows* on the two beads of the centring intraluminal guide probe, *asterisk*, whereas the HDR field was performed), the endobronchial lesion increased in volume due to the necrotic tissue (Fig. 19.1 panel **2b**). At the third fraction of BT, the right lung was completely atelectasic (Fig. 19.1 panel **3a**) with fibrous tissue occluding completely the lumen of the bronchus for the right upper lobe at the endoscopic view (Fig. 19.1 panel **3b**). Furthermore decreased extension of the capillary web, covered by white induitus of fibrin, was fairly present (Fig. 19.1 panel **3b** *arrow*). During this period chemotherapy with TMZ was started (red fading field). At the 6-month period after the initial TMZ treatment, the endobronchial lesion shrinks 20% (Fig. 19.1 panel **4b**) with a slight decrease of the previously described capillary area (*arrow*). At the CT scan was clearly evident the re-expansion of the right upper lobe (Fig. 19.1 panel **4a**). Control after 1 year of treatment shows a reduction in size and numbers of the lung metastatic lesions (Fig. 19.1 panel **5a**) and a complete disappearance of the endobronchial lesion as well as the capillary web on the cartilaginous part of the main right bronchus (Fig. 19.1 panel **5b** *arrow*)

tumour volume were noted in this phase. Furthermore the residual right lung was completely atelectasic (Fig. 19.3, panel 3a). Adjuvant temozolomide (TMZ) 200 mg/m^2 per os for 5 days associated with octreotide LAR 30 mg in every 28 days was administered. After 1 month from the start of the therapy with TMZ, a partial reduction in the tumour volume was observed (Fig. 19.3, panel 4b) that allowed the re-expansion of the residual right lung parenchyma (Fig. 19.3, panel 4a). Eighteen months later, clinical and radiological workup with CT scan and MRI demonstrated partial remission of disease in the liver, bone, lymph nodes and bilateral pulmonary parenchyma; fibrebronchoscopy revealed complete disappearance of the bronchial polypoid lesion (Fig. 19.3, panel 5b). No relevant side effects were observed. Three years later, with stable disease, the patient passed away for other causes not related to his disease (traumatic death).

19.2 Comments to the Case

This case leads to some considerations:

1. The multimodal approach to an endobronchial carcinoid has been associated in this case with a significant efficacy and low toxicity, probably superior to an only systemic medical approach. Although the timing of the clinical response does not indicate a sure direct correlation, TMZ is a drug that is well known to increase radio sensitivity; therefore a synergistic late addictive effect [15] of the BT may be suspected.
2. Being associated with a major rate of objective response when compared to everolimus utilised in the previous case, TMZ may be of choice when a tumour shrinkage is the main aim of the treatment.
3. Disobliteration may be an important aim in bronchial carcinoid, which is generally associated with a long-time survival also in the metastatic phase. In this case the disobliteration allowed the resolution of the obstructive pneumonitis and the re-expansion of the collapsed lung.
4. The patients several years before underwent in another hospital surgical resection without lymphadenectomy. The brief time between surgery and recurrence raises reasonable doubt on the radicality of the intervention. Again it should in fact be remembered that also in TC the percentage of lymph-nodal metastatic spread may reach 20% of the cases. We recommend therefore always the systematic lymph nodal dissection, particularly in young patient like this.

Questions

1. Is TMZ alone or in combination with BT an option in metastatic bronchial carcinoids?

Answers

1. Temozolomide (TMZ) [15, 16] is an alkylating drug inserted as a possible therapeutic option both in ESMO and ENETS Guidelines [3, 11]. The activity of this drug has been showed in retrospective NET phase II clinical trials [16], while the first prospective trial in lung NET is actually ongoing (Ferolla et al. ATLANT study NCT02698410 enrolling). Brachytherapy (BT) has been used so far as a palliative treatment of NSCLC but not clearly codified for the treatment of well-differentiated neuroendocrine tumours of the lung [17], and further evidences are needed for a routinely use in these tumours.

Up to Date of the Topic

The bronchial tree represents one of the most frequent sites of origin of neuroendocrine tumours (NET) with a prevalence ranging between 25% and 30% of all NET [1, 3, 4, 20]. Approximately 70% of carcinoid tumours present as an endoscopically visible tumour, usually located in a segmental bronchus, less often in main bronchi, rarely in the carina or trachea [4].

When feasible, surgery represents the treatment of choice in well-differentiated lung NET (TC and AC) and the only procedure that can cure the patients [4, 5, 9, 10]. It should always be remarked however that the definitive cure should be established in these tumours only after an accurate and protracted follow-up, reaching more than 15 years till in the case associated with a radical resection [8]. Since the advent of the minimally invasive surgery in the early 1990s and recently the robotic surgery as well as the renaissance of sublobar resections as a possible alternative tool for the low-grade neuroendocrine tumours of the lung, the best surgical treatment for primary lung carcinoid tumours represents a benchmark for the surgeon [10]. Minimally invasive surgery is based upon limited access (from one to three centimetric incisions) to the thoracic cavity achieved through video-assisted or pure videothoracoscopic techniques. In both cases standard lobectomies or sublobar resections may be performed. The main controversy concerning the minimally invasive approach with sublobar or bronchoplastic resections lies in the possibility of performing a true systematic lymph node dissection. Several authors claim their results with this technique are equal to those obtained with thoracotomies [4, 10]. However, until randomised trials will prove or disprove this assertion, we believe that an open access, with a small muscle-sparing thoracotomy particularly in young patients, for bronchoplastic procedures represents the safest approach for centrally located tumours. Furthermore limited resection or bronchoplastic procedures might be applicable in the TC or patient with limited lung function and/or cardiovascular impairment [21]; AC carcinoid should be treated with more oncological aggressiveness with a mandatory lymph nodal dissection. Considering the frequent occurrence of metastatic lymph nodes even in TC, a lymph node sampling cannot be accepted, and a systematic mediastinal dissection should always be done [5]. In our experience, this technique yielded over 13% of metastatic lymph nodes in patients affected by TC [9, 21].

Endobronchial laser treatment and cryotherapy or photodynamic clearance of the affected site are justified as palliative management in patients not fit for operative treatment and as a useful adjunct to surgery since preoperative removal of obstructing lesions allows clearing of the bronchial tree from secretions [4, 9, 11, 21]. These techniques should not be used with a curative intent because, according to our experience, residual nests of tumour cells can be detected in the submucosa after an apparent radical removal. However in the rare cases of primary multiple endobronchial lesions, laser treatment might allow a more limited resection and a systematic oncological treatment.

Moreover lymphatic spread cannot be assessed unless proven by mediastinoscopy or with the recent endobronchial ultrasound technique [14].

A particular word needs to be spent on multiple neuroendocrine forms such as diffuse idiopathic pulmonary neuroendocrine cell hyperplasia (DIPNECH) and tumourlets detected in the lung parenchyma around the primary resected tumour: should it be considered neoplasm? The pathologist should always be aware about these possible findings and always search carefully in the lung parenchyma. In our experience [9], 25% of patients had the presence of these lesions when the parenchyma was carefully analysed by our pathologist. The final answer will be obtained from molecular biology studies. Conversely, multiple endobronchial carcinoids, as primitive lesions, are rare and should always beware of the possibility that they might represent just a sign of submucosal lymphatic spread.

At the moment there are no prospective studies evaluating the role of an adjuvant medical therapy after a radical surgery, and no indication is actually expressed in the main international guidelines [3, 11]. The design of specific randomised prospective trials, particularly in the AC associated with nodal involvement, employing low-toxicity drugs like long-acting somatostatin analogues would be of interest but will require a prolonged time of observation to be significant.

Medical therapy may play a role in the palliative setting till in the locoregional disease, whenever surgical treatment may be not feasible both for the extension of the disease both for the performance status and co-morbidity of the patients [18, 19].

The choice of the therapy should be evaluated in the course of a multidisciplinary tumour board. The options start with the control of the hormonal hypersecretions when present to the anti-proliferative intent. The main aim of the medical treatment is generally a stabilisation of the tumour growth rather than an objective response. The first-line therapy in TC and AC with locoregional disease is generally based on long-acting somatostatin. Their use is generally extrapolated from the results of two phase III studies performed in GEP NET (the PROMID study using octreotide LAR and CLARINET study using lanreotide) [22]. However at the time of publication of this chapter, a phase III study with lanreotide dedicated to lung NET (the SPINET study) is ongoing and enrolling. Another study exploring the efficacy and safety of the combination of lanreotide and temozolomide in TC and AC with progressive disease (ATLANT study) is ongoing and enrolling. Another somatostatin analogue, pasireotide, has shown activity in TC and AC alone or in combination with everolimus (LUNA study presented at ESMO 2016, in submission).

As second line, the drug everolimus has shown activity in TC and AC in the phase III trial RADIANT IV and in the cited LUNA study alone or in combination with pasireotide [23, 24]. Retrospective series report efficacy of temozolomide in retrospective series, and the first prospective study in this context is ongoing. PRRT has been evaluated in small retrospective series [25].

In conclusion every decision in the palliative setting, particularly when facing with locoregional disease, should be evaluated in a multidisciplinary setting weighing the balance between toxicities and benefit, and the therapeutic approach should be always tailored on the single patients in centre with high level of expertise.

Bibliography

1. Beasley MB, Brambilla E, Chirieac LR, Austin JHM, Devesa SS, Hasleton P, Jett J, Marchevsky AM, Nicholson S, Papotti M, Pelosi G, Rami-Porta R, Scagliotti G, Thunnissen E, Travis WD, van Schil P, Yang P (2015) Carcinoid tumour. In: Travis WD, Brambilla E, Burke AP, Marx A, Nicholson AG (eds) WHO classification of tumours of lung, pleura, thymus and heart, 4th edn. IARC, Lyon, pp 73–77
2. Rami-Porta R, Asamura H, Travis WD, Rusch VW (2017) Chapter 36: Lung. In: American Joint Committee on Cancer (AJCC) staging manual, 8th edn. Springer, pp 431–457
3. Öberg K, Hellman P, Ferolla P, Papotti M, ESMO Guidelines Working Group (2012) Neuroendocrine bronchial and thymic tumors: ESMO Clinical Practice Guidelines for diagnosis, treatment and follow-up. Ann Oncol 23 Suppl 7:vii120–vii123
4. Escalon JC, Detterbeck FC (2009) Chapter 122: Carcinoid tumors. In: Shields TW, Locicero III J, Reed CE, Feins RH (eds) General thoracic surgery, 7th edn. Wolters Kluwer and Lippincott Williams & Wilkins, pp 1539–1554

5. Daddi N, Schiavon M, Filosso PL, Cardillo G, Ambrogi MC, De Palma A, Luzzi L, Bandiera A, Casali C, Ruffato A, De Angelis V, Andriolo LG, Guerrera F, Carleo F, Davini F, Urbani M, Mattioli S, Morandi U, Zannini P, Gotti G, Loizzi M, Puma F, Mussi A, Ricci A, Oliaro A, Rea F, Multi-Institutional Italian Pathology Group (2014) Prognostic factors in a multicentre study of 247 atypical pulmonary carcinoids. Eur J Cardiothorac Surg 45(4):677–686
6. Boxxen study and Neyman K, Sundset A, Naalsund A, Espinoza A, Solberg S, Kongerud J, Fosse E (2012) Endoscopic treatment of bronchial carcinoids in comparison to surgical resection: a retrospective study. J Bronchology Interv Pulmonol 19(1):29–34
7. Raz DJ, Nelson RA, Grannis FW, Kim JY (2015) Natural history of typical pulmonary carcinoid tumors: a comparison of nonsurgical and surgical treatment. Chest 147(4):1111–1117
8. Ferolla P, Daddi N, Puma F, Crinò L (2014) Postsurgical follow-up is always necessary in bronchial carcinoid. Ann Thorac Surg 98(3):1143–1144
9. Ferolla P, Daddi N, Urbani M, Semeraro A, Ribacchi R, Giovenali P, Ascani S, De Angelis V, Crinò L, Puma F, Daddi G (2009) Tumorlets, multicentric carcinoids, lymph-nodal metastases, and long-term behavior in bronchial carcinoids. J Thorac Oncol 4(3):383–387
10. Fox M, Van Berkel V, Bousamra M 2nd, Sloan S, Martin RC 2nd (2013) Surgical management of pulmonary carcinoid tumors: sublobar resection versus lobectomy. Am J Surg 205(2):200–208
11. Caplin ME, Baudin E, Ferolla P, Filosso P, Garcia-Yuste M, Lim E, Oberg K, Pelosi G, Perren A, Rossi RE, Travis WD, ENETS consensus conference participants (2015) Pulmonary neuroendocrine (carcinoid) tumors: European Neuroendocrine Tumor Society expert consensus and recommendations for best practice for typical and atypical pulmonary carcinoids. Ann Oncol 26(8):1604–1620
12. Travis WD, Rush W, Flieder DB, Falk R, Fleming MV, Gal AA, Koss MN (1998) Survival analysis of 200 pulmonary neuroendocrine tumors with clarification of criteria for atypical carcinoid and its separation from typical carcinoid. Am J Surg Pathol 22(8):934–944
13. Faggiano A, Ferolla P, Grimaldi F, Campana D, Manzoni M, Davì MV, Bianchi A, Valcavi R, Papini E, Giuffrida D, Ferone D, Fanciulli G, Arnaldi G, Franchi GM, Francia G, Fasola G, Crinò L, Pontecorvi A, Tomassetti P, Colao A (2012) Natural history of gastro-entero-pancreatic and thoracic neuroendocrine tumors. Data from a large prospective and retrospective Italian epidemiological study: the NET management study. J Endocrinol Investig 35(9):817–823
14. Lee P, Colt HG (2010) Bronchoscopy in lung cancer: appraisal of current technology and for the future. J Thorac Oncol 5(8):1290–1300
15. Stupp R, Mason WP, van den Bent MJ et al (2005) Radiotherapy plus concomitant and adjuvant temozolomide for glioblastoma. N Engl J Med 352:987–996
16. Ekeblad S, Sundin A, Janson ET, Welin S, Granberg D, Kindmark H, Dunder K, Kozlovacki G, Orlefors H, Sigurd M, Oberg K, Eriksson B, Skogseid B (2007) Temozolomide as monotherapy is effective in treatment of advanced malignant neuroendocrine tumors. Clin Cancer Res 13(10):2986–2991
17. Chalmers AJ, Ruff EM, Martindale C, Lovegrove N, Short SC (2009) Cytotoxic effects of temozolomide and radiation are additive- and schedule-dependent. Int J Radiat Oncol Biol Phys 75(5):1511–1519
18. Ferolla P (2014) Medical treatment of advanced thoracic neuroendocrine tumors. Thorac Surg Clin 24(3):351–355
19. Ferolla P (2015) Medical therapy of pulmonary neuroendocrine neoplasms: targeted, symptomatic and chemotherapy. Front Horm Res 44:193–197
20. Ferolla P, Faggiano A, Avenia N, Milone F, Masone S, Giampaglia F, Puma F, Daddi G, Angeletti G, Lombardi G, Santeusanio F, Colao A (2007) Epidemiology of non-gastroenteropancreatic (neuro) endocrine tumours. Clin Endocrinol 66(1):1–6
21. Daddi N, Ferolla P, Urbani M, Semeraro A, Avenia N, Ribacchi R, Puma F, Daddi G (2004 Oct) Surgical treatment of neuroendocrine tumors of the lung. Eur J Cardiothorac Surg 26(4):813–817
22. Caplin ME, Pavel M, Ćwikła JB, Phan AT, Raderer M, Sedláčková E, Cadiot G, Wolin EM, Capdevila J, Wall L, Rindi G, Langley A, Martinez S, Blumberg J, Ruszniewski P, CLARINET Investigators (2014) Lanreotide in metastatic enteropancreatic neuroendocrine tumors. N Engl J Med 371(3):224–233

23. Yao JC, Fazio N, Singh S, Buzzoni R, Carnaghi C, Wolin E, Tomasek J, Raderer M, Lahner H, Voi M, Pacaud LB, Rouyrre N, Sachs C, Valle JW, Delle Fave G, Van Cutsem E, Tesselaar M, Shimada Y, Oh DY, Strosberg J, Kulke MH, Pavel ME, RAD001 in Advanced Neuroendocrine Tumours, Fourth Trial (RADIANT-4) Study Group (2016) Everolimus for the treatment of advanced, non-functional neuroendocrine tumours of the lung or gastrointestinal tract (RADIANT-4): a randomised, placebo-controlled, phase 3 study. Lancet 387(10022):968–977
24. Yao J, Fazio N, Buzzoni R, Delle Fave G, Tesselaar M, Wolin E, Van Cutsem E, Tomassetti P, Strosberg J, Voi M, Pacaud L, Ridolfi A, Singh S, Pavel M, Kulke M (2016) ORAL02.02: efficacy and safety of everolimus in advanced, progressive, nonfunctional neuroendocrine tumors (NET) of the lung: RADIANT-4 Subgroup Analysis: Topic: Medical Oncology. J Thorac Oncol 11(11S):S253
25. Parghane RV, Talole S, Prabhash K, Basu S (2017) Clinical Response Profile of Metastatic/Advanced Pulmonary Neuroendocrine Tumors to Peptide Receptor Radionuclide Therapy with 177Lu-DOTATATE. Clin Nucl Med 42(6):428–435

Therapy for Metastatic Disease: Stomach/Duodenum, Colon/Rectum

Salvatore Tafuto, Chiara De Divitiis, Antonella Bianco, Monica Capozzi, Francesco Lassandro, Fabiana Tatangelo, Nicolina De Rosa, Alessandro Ottaiano, Carlo Bergaminelli, Antonella Petrillo, Elena Di Girolamo, and Antonella Di Sarno

On behalf of the ENETS Center of Excellence Multidisciplinary Group for Neuroendocrine Tumors in Naples, Italy

A. Colao et al. (eds.), *Neuroendocrine Tumors in Real Life*,
https://doi.org/10.1007/978-3-319-59024-0_20

Overview

Neuroendocrine tumors (NET), especially those of the pancreas and gastrointestinal tract, are frequently metastatic at the time of initial diagnosis. Because of a better knowledge of the molecular and cell-biological aspects as well as the clear pathological characterization of this tumor entity, a worldwide overall increase of these neuroendocrine tumors is reported. Therapeutic approaches for management of metastatic disease include surgical, medical, radiological, and nuclear medicine strategies. We present our experiences of management of three clinical cases of ileum, rectum, and gastric metastatic neuroendocrine tumors treated at the ENETS Center for Neuroendocrine Tumors of Naples, Italy. In the case of ileum-NET, we demonstrate the potent antiproliferative effect of SSA and the decisive role of the multidisciplinary approach which is able by itself to impact on survival. Then, in the case of gastric NET, we stress such awful consequences; a late and misunderstood diagnosis may have on prognosis and on the quality of life of a young patient. The role of a center of excellence devoted to NETs becomes crucial in these situations. Regarding the last case, it is a patient with G2 rectum NET. His clinical history, characterized by successive progressions of disease, is a paradigm of the G2 metastatic neuroendocrine tumors treatment. Three lines of therapy (SSA, chemotherapy, and PRRT) have followed ensuring a prolongation of survival of the patient and a good quality of life. The patient is in follow-up and maintains additional therapeutic chance.

Clinical Case 1

Gastric Neuroendocrine Tumor

In July 2015 the case of a 57-year-old man who is unable to walk independently because of myelopathy which is a suffering not better diagnosed, with a history of chronic atrophic gastropathy known for about 2 years, comes to our attention. Such patient is subjected to endoscopic examination of the stomach, which confirms the diagnosis of atrophic gastropathy and detects the presence of multiple polypoid formations localized to the body of the stomach, some with superficial ulcerations and with variable ranging from a few millimeters to approximately 2 cm (◘ Fig. 20.1). Some polyps are removed for histology with biopsy forceps. Histological examination diagnosed the presence of a spectrum of lesions of the neuroendocrine system (chromogranin +, synaptophysin +, CD56 +, Ki-67 6%) variables from hyperplasia areas of the diffuse type, linear (chain-forming), micronodular, and adenomatoid until the formation of dysplastic foci (enlarged micronodules) (◘ Fig. 20.2). Elevated levels of gastrin and very low levels of cyanocobalamin were found. A CT scan total body with contrast performed in August 2015 shows the presence of 3 mm hypervascular liver lesions, visible only in the arterial phase, at the VII segment (7 × 7 mm, 9 × 6 mm) and at the II segment (8 × 7 mm), suspicious for disease localization (◘ Fig. 20.3). A scintigraphy with octreoscan shows pathological areas of uptake at the body of the stomach.

In July 2015, the case of this patient is brought to the attention of the members of our multidisciplinary group for neuroendocrine tumors. The board suggests that patient for vitamin supports with additional B12, medical therapy with somatostatin analogue, and a program of clinical and instrumental follow-up. After 3 months of vitamin B12 supplementation and somatostatin analogue therapy, the patient resumes a normal and independent deambulation, and serum gastrin levels were normal. A CT scan total body shows stable disease.

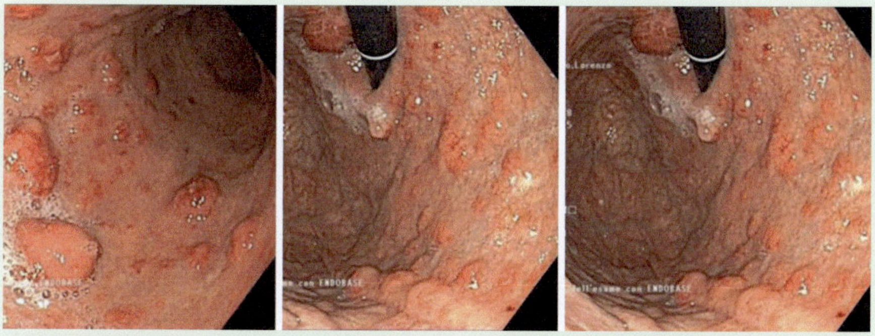

Fig. 20.1 At gastric body the endoscopy shows multiple sessile polypoid formations, with certain superficial ulcerations. The diameter varies from a few mm to about 2 cm (polyp localized on the small curve)

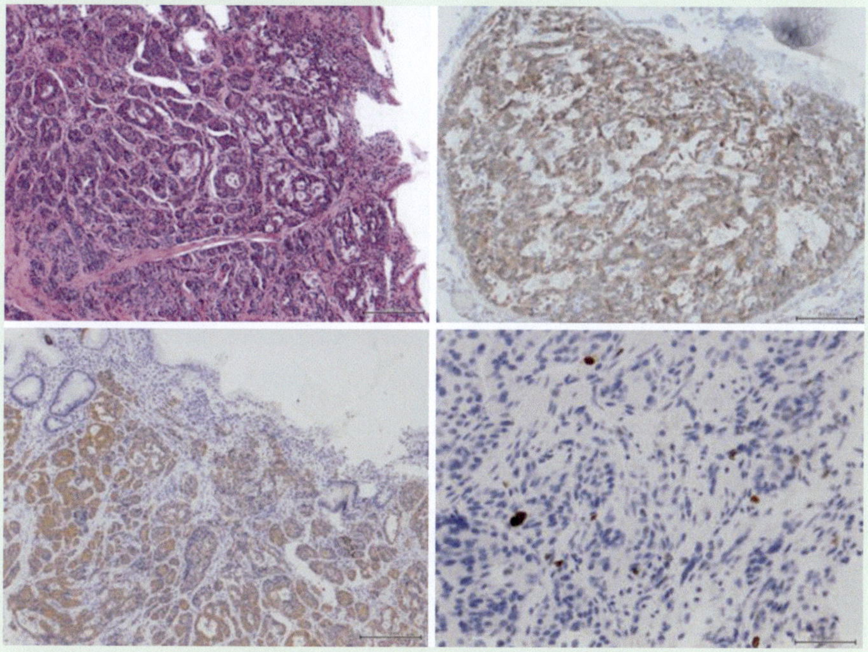

Fig. 20.2 These figures show the presence of a spectrum of lesions of the neuroendocrine system (chromogranin +, Syn +, CD56 +, Ki-67% 6) variables from hyperplasia areas of the diffuse type, linear (chain-forming), micronodular, and adenomatoid until the formation of dysplastic foci (enlarged micronodules)

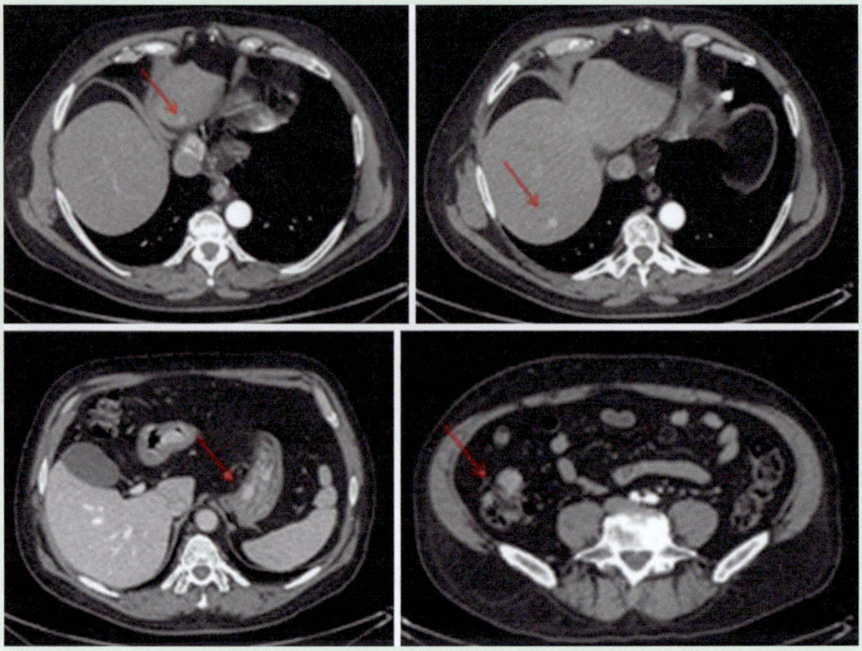

Fig. 20.3 CT scan total body with contrast performed that shows the presence of 3 mm hypervascular liver lesions, visible only in the arterial phase, at the VII segment (7 × 7 mm, 9 × 6 mm) and at the II segment (8 × 7 mm), suspicious for disease localization

20.1 Comments to the Case

Gastric neuroendocrine tumors (G-NET) are increasingly recognized due to expanding indications of upper gastrointestinal (UGI) endoscopy. We showed a case of a gastric neuroendocrine tumor which is defined as «type 1» (Table 20.1), small, multiple, polypoid well-differentiated G1 neuroendocrine tumors, associated with chronic atrophic gastritis, a serum gastrin levels elevated, and suspected liver metastases, too small to be further characterized. In patients with type 1 gastric carcinoids, in accordance to ENETS guidelines of G-NET, conservative management based on endoscopic follow-up and lesion resection should be preferred. Indications to treatment by somatostatin analogues (SSA) or surgical antrectomy to suppress hypergastrinemia and limit ECL growth are still debated. SSA proved good antiproliferative properties, but their role in patients with type 1 G-NET should be proposed only according to expert opinion. In this case we chose to start with SSA because of liver metastasis suspected. For metastatic disease today, we have many different options for the medical treatment of gastric neuroendocrine tumors, from somatostatin analogues to the biological treatment with everolimus.

Table 20.1 Summary of the main characteristics of G-NENs

	Type 1	Type 2	Type 3
Proportion among g-NENs, %	70–80	5–6	14–25
Tumor characteristics	Often small (<1–2 cm), multiple in 65% of cases, polypoid in 78% of cases	Often small (<1–2 cm) and multiple, polypoid	Unique, often large (>2 cm) polypoid and ulcerated
Associated conditions	Chronic atrophic gastritis	Gastrinoma/MEN1	None
Pathology	Often NET G1	NET G1-G2	NEC G3
Serum gastrin levels	↑	↑	Normal
Gastric pH	↑↑	↓↓	Normal
Metastases, %	2–5	10–30	50–100
Tumor-related deaths, %	0	<10	25–30

Modified by Delle Fave et al. [15]

Questions

1. Indications to treatment with SSA in gastric neuroendocrine tumors are still debated. What about in clinical practice?
2. Is it correct to associate the ultrasound examination to the standard EGDS in gastric NET?

Answers

1. SSA proved good antiproliferative properties in metastatic disease, but their role in patients with gastric neuroendocrine tumor should be proposed only according to expert opinion.
2. Gastric endoscopic ultrasonography is strongly advised at least in the process of staging for the study of the gastric wall and infiltration levels.

Clinical Case 2

Ileal Neuroendocrine Tumor

A 63-year-old female patient was admitted in May 2012 for recurrent abdominal pain (numeric analogue scale = 6–7), weight loss (7 kg over 5 months), diarrhea (4–5 stools per day), and alternating subocclusive symptoms, anorexia, asthenia, and facial and neck flush (4 times per day) lasting for 6 months; she also had an Eastern Cooperative Oncology Group (ECOG) performance status (ECOG PS) of 2. Physical examination revealed diffuse abdominal sensitivity at palpation and hepatomegaly.

An abdominal computed tomography (CT) scan, performed in May 2012, showed multiple nodular liver lesions, of which the largest were in the fourth segment (S) (about 37 × 35 mm), which were extended in part to the fifth S and into the right lobe (seventh S and eighth S of about 23 × 16 mm and 13 mm, respectively). The hypervascular pattern of secondary lesions was compatible with a neuroendocrine tumor (NET); an oval area of 3.2 cm (maximum diameter) with sharp margins compressing the ileal loops and with an expansive aspect was found in the anterior hypogastrium. An abdominal magnetic resonance imaging (MRI) scan confirmed the presence of liver metastases.

In July 2012, a liver biopsy was performed. Histological examination revealed the presence of neoplastic proliferation in the solid growth patterns of insular cells; immunohistochemistry (pan-cytokeratin-positive, chromogranin-positive, synaptophysin-positive, CD56-negative/positive, and Ki-67,20%) was consistent with the diagnosis of NET (◘ Fig. 20.4). Urinary excretion of 5-hydroxyindoleacetic showed a little increase of values. Chromogranin was high (131.6 U/L; range, 2–18 U/L) in the absence of proton pump inhibitors or kidney failure. In accordance with the European Neuroendocrine Tumor Society (ENETS) consensus guidelines, the radiological methods for staging are MRI, CT scan total body, and octreoscan scintigraphy.

An octreoscan scintigraphy, performed in September 2012, showed two areas of uptake of the radiotracer in correspondence of the hepatic parenchyma at the level of the fourth S and fifth S and of the mesogastric region; MRI revealed two nodular areas consistent with neoplastic tissue. In October 2012, the case was discussed by the tumor board of our institution, and the board suggested surgery for this patient. So in October 2012, the patient underwent surgery. We must remember that the palliative surgery for patients with endocrine tumors of the jejunum-ileum has the objective to make liver metastases the only persisting problem. Patients

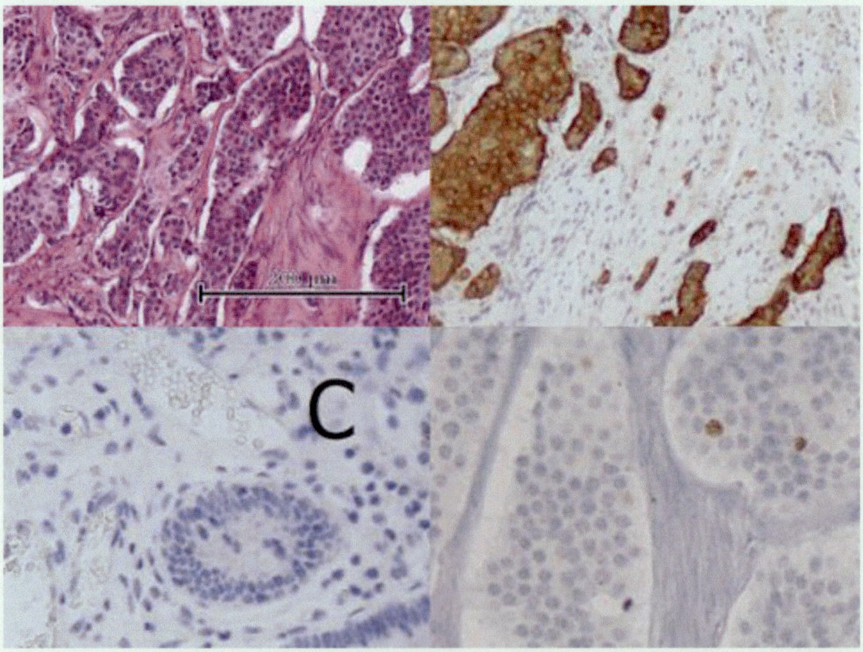

◘ **Fig. 20.4** Histological examination with immunohistochemistry and hematoxylin-eosin staining (e/e). Notes: **a** e/e 20× magnification, **b** chromogranin 20× magnification, **c** synaptophysin 20× magnification, and **d** Ki-67 40× magnification

suitable for palliative procedures are those presumed to benefit from tumor reduction performed in accordance with given guidelines.

A stenosing tumor was found in the terminal ileum. Lymph nodes that had increased in size were identified along the right colonic artery, ileum, and cecum. An ileotransversal terminolateral anastomosis was performed. Histopathologic examination revealed a malignant intestinal NET with lymph node metastases: NET G1;22 and pT3 pN1 pv1 pR0 G2 (AJCC 2010). Postsurgical recovery was favorable, and the patient started therapy with OCT-LAR 30 mg intramuscularly every 28 days.

At 1-month follow-up, the patient had marked improvement in her clinical conditions, with a significant weight increase. After 3 months of medical treatment, a complete clinical response with regression of symptoms, normalization of chromogranin levels, and PS recovery from ECOG PS 2 to ECOG PS 0 was obtained. A total body CT scan showed a single secondary nodular lesion in the liver of about 34 × 30 mm (versus 37 × 34 mm) (◘ Fig. 20.5a versus 20.5b), with a slight decrease in its density. The other secondary lesions (present at the previous exam)

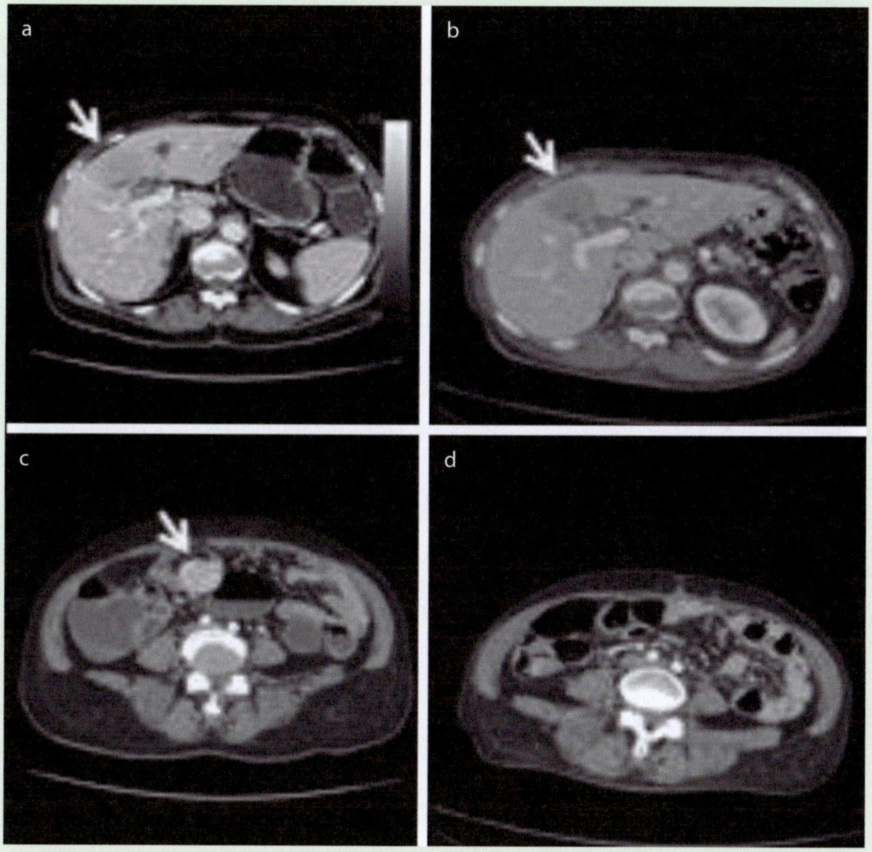

◘ **Fig. 20.5** Liver metastatic NET: **a**–**d** Contrast-enhanced CT. **a** and **c** Double-contrast study of the stomach. The difference between the abdominal parenchyma visualized in the two examinations lies in the different degree of filling of the stomach and in the patient's different breaths. Before treatment, the hepatic lesions of the seventh and eighth segments appear as soft hypodense inhomogeneous lesions (*white arrow*). **b** and **d** After treatment, the lesions are not more appreciable. *Abbreviations*: *LVR* liver, *ST* stomach, *SPL* spleen, *LKD* left kidney, *NET* neuroendocrine tumor, *CT* computed tomography were not clearly identified (▪ Fig. 20.5a versus 20.5b; ▪ Fig. 20.5c versus 20.5d).

We submitted the case to the attention of our tumor board. We decided to reevaluate the patient with a new total body CT scan after 2 months in order to confirm the clinical response in the liver to determine between performing hepatic surgery or a locoregional treatment (i.e., transarterial embolization).

In November 2014 a CT scan confirmed the clinical response, and in November 2014 the patient underwent hepatic surgery. Currently, after 26 months, the patient continues with the instrumental and clinical follow-up program which shows complete response (R0).

20.2 Comments to the Case

This case report shows that OCT-based therapy is able to produce an objective response and clinical benefit in NET, whereas cytotoxic chemotherapy is rarely effective. SSAs are typically used to treat the symptoms caused by NET, but they are not used as a primary treatment to induce tumor shrinkage. In this case report, symptom control was clearly obtained, resulting in an improvement in the patient's ECOG PS (0 versus 2) (ECOG). After the surgery approach and after 1 month of OCT treatment, the patient, once again in the presence of smaller liver metastasis, showed a complete regression of symptoms.

In addition, it is paramount to underline that an objective response in the liver, with the disappearance of secondary lesions during CT scan, was observed after just 3 months of treatment. These clinical, objective responses are commonly observed in metastatic colorectal cancer in patients treated with chemotherapy. The shrinkage obtained can lead the patient to liver resection or locoregional treatment, with a strong impact on survival time. In midgut metastatic NETs, this opportunity is rarely found using the SSAs alone and, of course, when it occurs, it can be due only to the proven antiproliferative activity of SSAs in NET.

This case also shows that a multidisciplinary approach improves the choice of the best and most appropriate treatment strategy. In fact, the presence of liver metastases largely influences the prognosis in all types of NET, and surgical resection with curative intent remains the gold standard in the treatment of liver metastases, achieving a survival rate of 60–80% at 5 years with low mortality (0–5%) and acceptable morbidity (close to 30%).

The use of SSA and surgery, as well as future targeted drugs, may increase the long-term control of some patients with advanced NET. An early multidisciplinary approach remains fundamental for the selection of the most appropriate treatments to adopt.

? Questions

1. Unlike other solid tumors typically considered inoperable in the presence of metastatic disease, in well or moderately differentiated NETs, the surgical approach would have a considerable role.

✓ Answers

1. In accordance with the European Neuroendocrine Tumor Society (ENETS) consensus guidelines, the indications for surgery in this case were:
   The presence of symptomatic disease
   The risk of occlusion
   The presence of liver metastases alone

Clinical Case 3

Rectal Neuroendocrine Tumor

The patient initially presented in January 2014 at the age of 70 with recurrent abdominal pain, weight loss (5% in a 3-month time), and diarrhea (3–4 movements a day). Abdominal conventional ultrasound, visualized multiple hypoechoic liver lesions suspicious for a metastases, and contrast-enhanced ultrasound (CEUS) showed the characteristics early and homogenous hypervascular pattern in the arterial phase typical for the majority of metastases (80%) of neuroendocrine tumors (NET). Abdomen CT scan confirmed the diagnosis of multiple liver metastases from neuroendocrine tumor. Blood levels of chromogranin A and 24-hour urine 5-hydroxyindoleacetic acid were in the normal range. ^{18}F-FDG PET/CT scan reported low focal uptake in the liver and no other pathological uptake within the body. Colonoscopy visualized a distal rectum polyp (>2 cm) with a superficial ulcer area; pathology showed a well-differentiated NET (◘ Fig. 20.6) G2 (Ki-67 5%) (◘ Fig. 20.7a) chromogranin A, synaptophysin (◘ Fig. 20.7b), and CD 56 positive. Fine-needle liver lesion aspiration biopsy confirmed diagnosis of well-differentiated NET G2 (Ki-67 10% more elevated than primary tumor) metastasis chromogranin A, synaptophysin, and CD 56 positive. Endoscopic ultrasound was also performed. Somatostatin-receptor scintigraphy showed increased tracer uptake in the liver (as grade 3) and in the pelvic area (score 1). The patient did not agree with anterior resection of primary tumor, chemotherapy, and locoregional therapies for liver metastases. In February 2014 treatment with somatostatin analogues (SSAs) administered every 4 weeks (OCT-LAR 30 mg/28 days) was commenced. Response to the SSA treatment was satisfactory with resolution of abdominal pain and diarrhea after 1–3 months, respectively, and stability of the disease (SD) at CT scan. The patient continued on 4-weekly SSA treatment and a regular follow-up. In November 2014 CT scan showed a disease progression with new multiple liver lesions based on RECIST criteria. So, the patient received

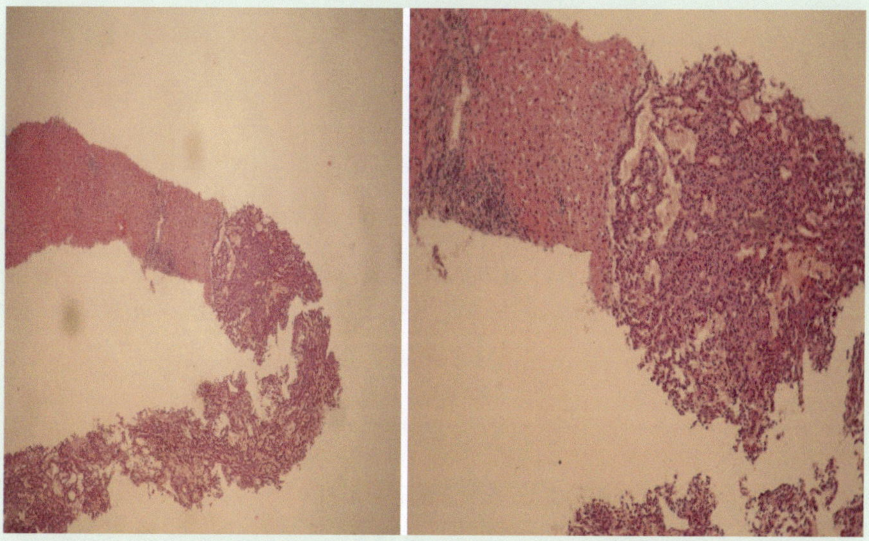

◘ **Fig. 20.6** Liver biopsy. Histology (EE)

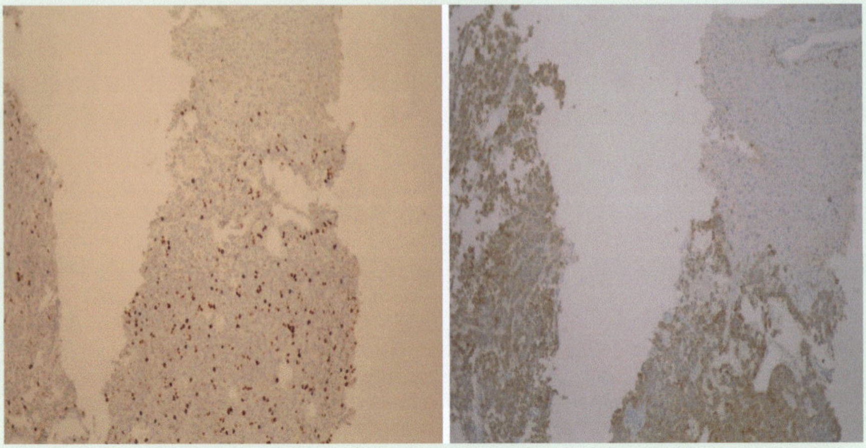

Fig. 20.7 Liver biopsy immunochemistry. **a** ki-67 index (Mib1 immunostaning). **b** Synaptophysin immunostaining

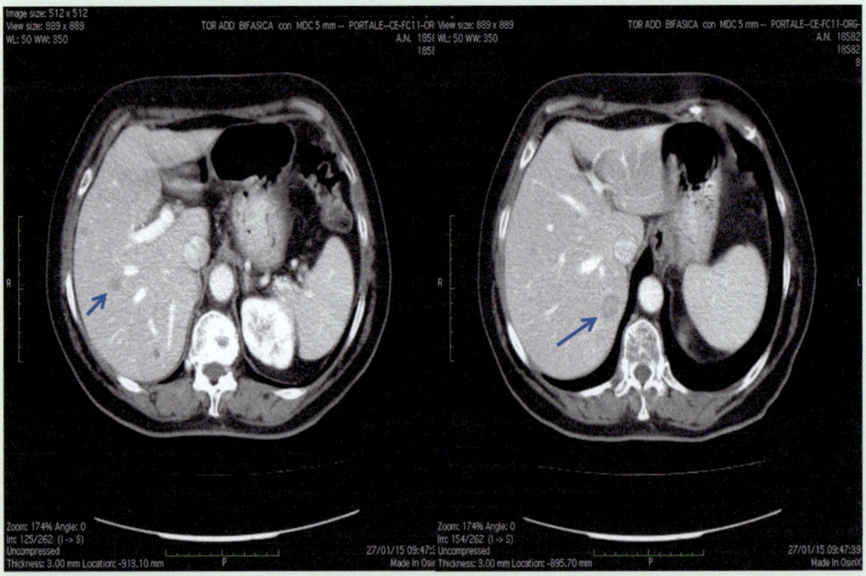

Fig. 20.8 CT scan (January 2015): multiple liver metastases (*blue arrows*)

high dose of SSA between November 2014 and February 2015 (Fig. 20.8). Dose escalation was performed by shortening the injection interval from 3 to 4 weeks (OCT-LAR 30 mg/21 days). Treatment was well tolerated. In February 2015 the patient presented with a severe lumbar pain; a CT scan revealed for the first time spine lesions. ^{18}F–FDG PET/CT and MRI scan were consistent with the CT scan findings and confirmed a new metastatic bone lesions (D12, L1-L4). CgA was above the normal range. Due to progressive disease between March 2015 and

October 2015, the patient commenced chemotherapy with capecitabine (2000 mg for 2/day every 14 days, q21 for 8 cycles) combined with high dose of SSA (OCT-LAR 30 mg every 3 weeks). No toxicity was observed. In October 2015, bone and liver metastases were stable at MRI and CT scan, respectively; however, CT scan revealed a new metastatic bilateral pulmonary lesions. Capecitabine and high dose of SSA were discontinued. Between November 2015 and April 2016, the patient commenced treatment with temozolomide (120 mg/day for 7 days per week on alternate weeks for 7 cycles). Treatment was well tolerated and the disease maintained stable at radiological imaging. In June 2016 new metastatic bone lesions (ischium) (◘ Fig. 20.9) and new metastatic abdominal lymph nodes were visualized. In July 2016 ^{68}Ga-DOTA-TATE PET/CT scan confirmed as metastatic all liver (◘ Fig. 20.10), bone, pulmonary, and mesenteric lymph nodes lesions CgA was progressively raised. The patient reported the persistence of abdominal and lumbar pain. Based on high expression of SSTR in the metastatic lesions on ^{68}Ga-DOTA-TATE PET/CT scan, advanced, and progressive disease, the patient was qualified for peptide receptor radioisotope therapy. Between July 2016 and January 2017, the patient received four cycles of ^{90}Y/^{177}Lu DOTATOC treatment (cumulative activity of 79 and 193 mCi of ^{90}Yttrio-DOTATOC and 177Lu-DOTATOC, respectively). Three cycles of PRRT resulted in normalization of serum CgA and satisfactory control of abdominal and lumbar pain. Since then, treatment was well tolerated, and the disease was stable at radiological imaging. At present the patient stays under a regular follow-up.

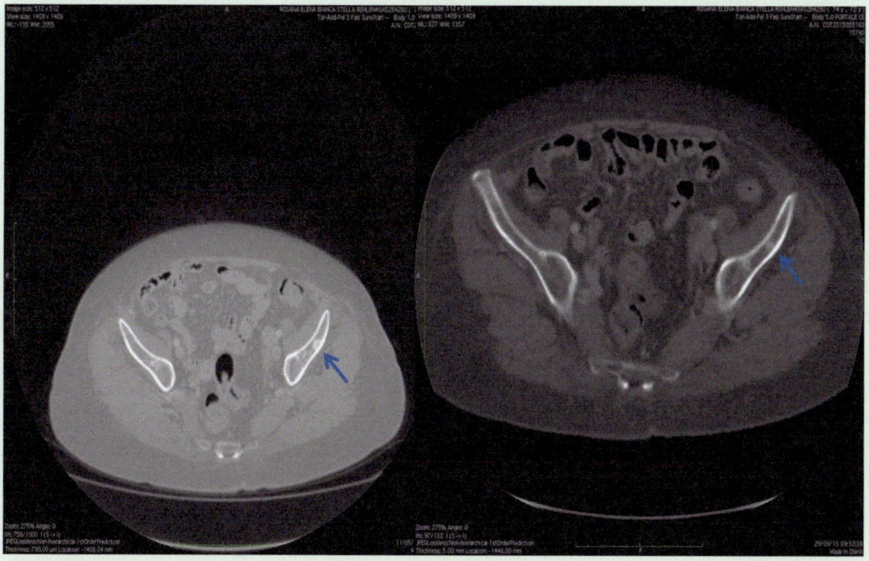

◘ **Fig. 20.9** CT scan (June 2016): bone metastasis (ischium)

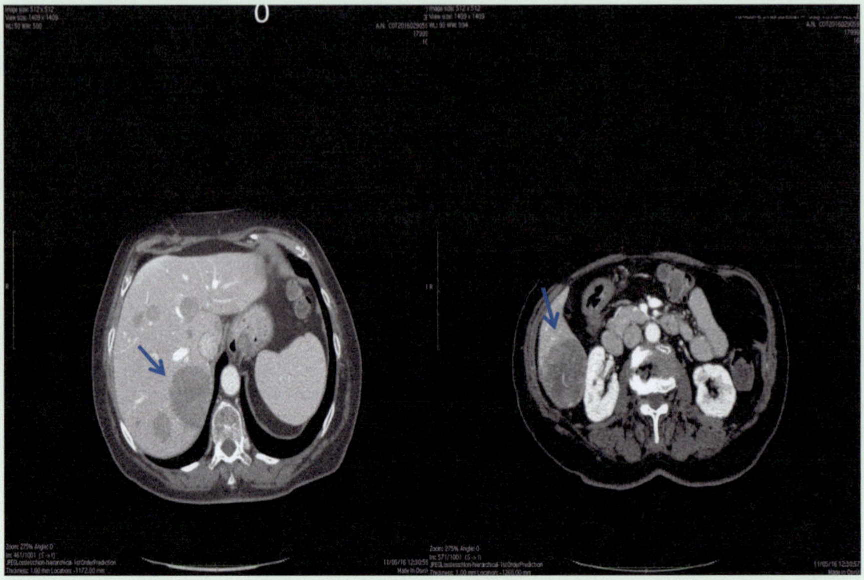

Fig. 20.10 CT scan (May 2016): liver progression (*blue arrows*)

20.3 Comments to the Case

For G1-G2 lesions <10 mm and no involvement of the muscularis propria, endoscopic mucosal resection (EMR) is adequate. EMR band-assisted ligation may improve the percentage of complete resections. If an incomplete resection was performed, endoscopic submucosal dissection (ESD) or transanal endoscopic microsurgery (TEMS) may be indicated as salvage treatment. TEMS leads to more complications [1, 3]. EMR or other techniques should be discussed on a case-per-case. Recently, the cutoff size has also been challenged. Local resection was considered safe in tumors between 10 and 16 mm, and no metastases were observed for tumors <9 mm. No recurrence was seen in about 250 cases after transanal resection and endoscopic polypectomy. It is not clear whether radical resection is better than local resection for 10–20 mm with and without lymph nodes involvement, but radical resection reduces quality of life. New evidence is needed to conclude that local resection is safe for the intermediate tumors. Anterior resection/TME was indicated for tumors >2 cm without metastases, if N1 G2/G3 T4 adjuvant systemic therapy should be considered. In patients with metastases and obstruction, palliative resection/stent/ chemotherapy was indicated, whereas chemotherapy/radiotherapy was indicated in the absence of obstruction.

In non-resectable disease, systemic therapeutic choices should be considered for tumor growth control, quality of life, and/or carcinoid syndrome when present. SSAs are an established therapy for antiproliferative control in both intestinal and pancreatic NET, based on two placebo-controlled trials (the PROMID and the CLARINET studies). Octreotide-LAR and lanreotide autogel are indicated as first-line systemic therapy in midgut NET to control tumor growth. Based on the CLARINET study, the use of SSA in GEP-NET is recommended up to a Ki-67 of 10%; however, there was no consensus among experts on a clear Ki-67 cutoff value for the recommendations of SSA for tumor growth control in the whole group of neuroendocrine neoplasm (NEN). Preferably, in intestinal/pancreatic NET, SSA should be used if Ki-67 is <10%. Prospective data are required to evaluate the appropriate Ki-67 cutoff for treatment stratification to SSA or more aggressive therapies. In liver metastatic disease with over 25% of the liver tumor burden, the recommendations for the applications of SSAs are extended (according to CLARINET study). On this basis, SSA may be used in patients with rectal NET when the SSTR status is positive (on somatostatin imaging or histology) if the tumor is slowly growing, preferably G1/G2 with Ki-67 < 10%. However, in a CLARINET study, only 14 cases of colorectal NET were included, so it is impossible to predict real benefit in this subgroup of patients also with overexpression of somatostatin receptors. Data on combination of everolimus and octreotide has been reported for treatment of advanced NET associated with carcinoid syndrome (RADIANT-2). In a post hoc analysis, there was an improved progression-free survival compared to placebo in the RADIANT-2 study using this combination in well-differentiated G1/G2 colorectal NET; however, this remains to be verified. Most studies recommended that increase in the dose/frequency of SSAs should be considered in patients with radiological progression where disease was previously stabilized at a standard dose also without carcinoid syndrome.

Systemic chemotherapy is indicated in progressive/bulky pancreatic NET and in G3 NEN. Compared to targeted drugs, chemotherapy is also indicated in a symptomatic patients, in case of rapid tumor progression (<6–12 months) and in patients with a possible chance of achieving a response to allow for surgery (neoadjuvant approach). Streptozotocin with 5-fluorouracil (STZ/5-FU) represents the cytotoxic therapies applied and doxorubicin with STZ as an alternative therapy; however, the use of doxorubicin is limited (by a cumulative dose of 500 mg/m^2 due to the risk of cardiotoxicity).

Chemotherapy is not recommended in non-pancreatic NET unless G2 NET with Ki-67 > 15% and RECIST progression in 3–6 months, in patients which are SSTR-negative and/or after failure of other therapies. On this basis, chemotherapy may be considered in NET of other sites (stomach, colon, rectum, lung, and thymus). In G2 NET or in SSTR-negative NET, metronomic chemotherapy may be an option using temozolomide and/or capecitabine +/− SSA or capecitabine + bevacizumab after failure of other treatments (such as locoregional treatments or everolimus).

Phase III NETTER-1 trial compared 177 Lu-DOTATATE to high dose of octreotide-LAR (60 mg/4 weekly) in progressive midgut NET and showed significantly prolonged PFS in PRRT-treated patients. Based on this registrational trial, PRRT may be indicated in midgut NET as a second-line therapy after failure of SSA if all inclusion criteria are fulfilled. In pancreatic NET, PRRT is indicated in progressive G1/G2 with SSTR positive expression in all metastatic lesions after failure of SSA, novel targeted drugs, and chemotherapy. 90Y and/or 177 Lu-labeled SSA are the most frequently used in NET, but 177 Lu-labeled SSA is characterized by a lower toxicity. However, potential increasing toxicity after previous treatments needs to be considered, requires close surveillance, and might justify an earlier use of PRRT in selected patients.

Management of colorectal NET represents a diagnostic and therapeutic challenge, and multidisciplinary approach in specialized centers for NET is highly recommended. Presented patient was offered treatment options in accordance to ENETS guidelines for the management of distant metastatic disease of intestinal (colorectal) tumors.

Questions

1. Which predictors of outcome in rectal NET?
2. There was no consensus on a clear Ki-67 cutoff value for the recommendation of SSA for antiproliferative purposes. General trend supports the use of high dose of octreotide-LAR for control of carcinoid syndrome. Poor data supports the use of high-dose octreotide-LAR for control of tumor progression in patients with GEP-NET. What about Ki-67 cutoff and high-dose schedule in treatment with SSA?

Answers

1. Tumor size and depth predict lymph node metastasis. Intramucosal tumors <1 cm have a 4% risk of lymph node metastasis. Patients with tumors >2 cm metastasize in 60%. The majority of patients appear cured once full resections of small (<10 mm) rectal NET with favorable biology are performed. Predictors of survival continue to be examined and the strongest predictor of survival is the stage.
2. SSA can be recommended for the inhibition of tumor growth in intestinal NET. Some experts feel that 5% might be a more appropriate Ki-67 cutoff threshold, preferably SSA should be used if Ki-67 < 10%. SSA may also be used in rectal NET when the SSTR status is positive (on somatostatin imaging or histology), when tumor is slowly growing, G1 or G2 and preferably with Ki-67 < 10%. Most experts suggest that higher doses of octreotide-LAR should be used in cases of radiological tumor progression. No evidence of increased toxicity was reported.

Up to Date of the Topic

GEP-NET, traditionally considered as rare diseases, has become the topic of great interest in the last few years. The new evidence in the field of histological classification, the identification of nosographic criteria-related clinical aggressiveness, and the new knowledge of molecular biology have made NET the object of great ferment both for basic research and for clinical studies. Currently, the landscape of therapeutic drugs available has greatly expanded, thanks to several phase III studies which led to the registration of new drugs that have proven effective for the treatment of NET. Somatostatin analogues (SSA) are analogues of the native somatostatin. Over 80% of GEP-NET expresses on the surface of its membrane cell, the «SSTR receptors,» in particular the low-grade forms. The SSA-approved and used in our country are the octreotide and lanreotide. They are able to produce an improvement of the clinical symptoms in more than 60% of the cases, a stabilization of tumor growth in the 30–50% of cases. The antiproliferative activity of the SSA has been assessed recently with two clinical studies of equal importance: the study PROMID [1] and the study CLARINET [2]. Both are randomized; prospective studies have demonstrated the antiproliferative activity of these molecules in vivo. Today we can say that thanks to these studies, which definitely showed critical issues and limitations, we have seen a change in terms of perception of the two drugs, which by pure drug palliation care should be understood now as drugs to antiproliferative activity and able to impact positively on PFS of patients with GEP-NET. The therapeutic approach to the GEP-NET has certainly revolutionized by the use of molecular targeted drugs such as everolimus, an inhibitor of mTOR, and sunitinib, an inhibitor of tyrosine kinase. Everolimus is a selective inhibitor of mTOR (mammalian target of rapamycin), a serine-threonine kinase whose activity is known to be involved in a several human cancers, and is a potent inhibitor of the growth and proliferation of tumor cells. Everolimus is indicated for the treatment of NET of pancreatic origin, well or moderately differentiated, inoperable or in metastatic stage, at a dose of 10 mg daily. Recently we published the results of the study RADIANT 4 [4] (RAD001 in advanced NET), a prospective multicenter phase III, double-blind, randomized trial which examined the efficacy and safety of everolimus plus the best therapy support (BSC, best supportive care) versus placebo plus BSC in 302 patients with well-differentiated, nonfunctional, and advanced NET of gastrointestinal or pulmonary origin. The patients treated with everolimus showed a prolonged median progression-free survival compared to those treated with placebo (11.0 vs 3.9 months, HR 00:48; 95% CI 0.35–0, 67; $p < 0.00001$). At the time of the interim analysis of OS, a trend toward improved survival [HR = 0.64; 95% CI, 0.40–1.05; $p = 0.037$] was observed, with a total of 70 deaths recorded at the time of data cutoff (42 [20.5%] in the everolimus arm and 28 [28.6%] in the placebo arm). The result was not statistically significant, as the significance threshold interim analysis was $p = 0.000213$. Even sunitinib [5] is a biologic inhibitor of tyrosine kinase associated with the receptor, it is indicated for the treatment of pancreatic NET (pNET) well-differentiated, inoperable, or metastatic disease (median PFS was 11.4 months with sunitinib arm compared to 5.5 months in the placebo arm [hazard ratio, 0.418 (95% CI 0.263, 0.662), p-value = 0.0001]). The pivotal study with sunitinib in pancreatic NET was terminated prematurely, and the primary endpoint of the Drug Evaluation was based on investigator assessment: both conditions may have affected the estimate of the treatment. Chemotherapy has been, for years, the only therapeutic option for the treatment of metastatic pNET and GEP-NET, with very various results. Therefore, the regimen with cisplatin and etoposide is usually the preferred treatment schedule for the treatment of poorly differentiated NET. Even if such platinum-based treatment scheme has historically shown interesting results in terms of response rate on undifferentiated forms [6], the impact on overall survival is minimal, so these results remain controversial, and the question of what is the best treatment scheme to use for these forms is still debated. The traditional use of this scheme comes from old studies, with little statistical evidence because of the small number of patients enrolled in clinical trials. Also other drugs such as gemcitabine, oxaliplatin, or temozolomide streptozotocin can be evaluated in the treatment of NEC. The activity of temozolomide in patients with metastatic NET has been evaluated in several studies [7–9] that showed interesting activity by the ORR point of view, ranging from 25% to 70%. TMZ has shown good activity in patients with NET and was taken alone or in combination with other anticancer drugs such as capecitabine, bevacizumab, or thalidomide. The first randomized phase III study that included the use of chemotherapy in pancreatic

NET (pNET) was performed by Moertel in 1980 that compared the combination of streptozocin (STZ) and 5-fluorouracil (5-FU) versus STZ as a single agent. The combination arm showed results superior to those of the treatment arm monotherapy in terms of overall response rate (ORR) (63% vs 36%, respectively) and median overall survival (MOS) (26 vs 16.5 months), even if the difference of OS was not statistically significant. The disparity of these results may be related to several factors: the lack of standardization in order to assess the response in previous studies, the heterogeneity of these tumors in terms of biological behavior, and the consequent different response to chemotherapy. In order to clarify the most appropriate place in the therapeutic planning of the streptozotocin associated with five fluorouracil in the treatment of pNET advanced stage, an international multicenter randomized phase III trial (study SEQTOR) is ongoing. This trial, which is currently active at the our Institute, comparing the efficacy and safety of everolimus followed by chemotherapy with streptozotocin and 5-fluorouracil until progression in reverse order (chemotherapy with streptozotocin and 5-fluorouracil until progression or unacceptable toxicity, followed by everolimus progression). Immunotherapy has recently found a new field of application. Antibodies directed against the checkpoints PD-1/PD-L1 showed tumor regressions and lasting dynamics, suggesting a rebalancing of host-tumor interaction. Pembrolizumab showed a promising antitumor activity (objective response rate of 56%) also in the treatment of Merkel cell carcinoma (MCC), which is an aggressive neuroendocrine carcinoma of the skin (which can be distinguished from other malignant tumors for the expression of cytokeratin 20). These preliminary results leave assume a hypothetical and future role of immunotherapy in the treatment of other NET.

Bibliography

1. Rinke A, Müller HH, Schade-Brittinger C et al (2009) Placebo-controlled, double-blind, prospective, randomized study on the effect of octreotide LAR in the control of tumor growth in patients with metastatic neuroendocrine midgut tumors: a report from the PROMID Study Group. J Clin Oncol 27(28):4656–4663
2. Caplin ME, Pavel DM, Ćwikła JB et al (2014) Lanreotide in metastatic enteropancreatic neuroendocrine tumors. N Engl J Med 371(3):224–233
3. Yao JC, Tsuchihashi Z, Panneerselvam A et al (2011) Effect of everolimus treatment on markers angiogenesis in patients with advanced pancreatic neuroendocrine tumours (pNET) results from the phase III RADIANT-3 study. Eur J Cancer 47(Suppl. 1)
4. Yao JC, Fazio N, Singh S et al (2016) Everolimus for the treatment of advanced, non-functional neuroendocrine tumours of the lung or gastrointestinal tract (RADIANT-4): a randomised, placebo-controlled, phase 3 study. Fourth Trial (RADIANT-4) Study Group. Lancet 387(10022):968–977. doi:10.1016/S0140-6736(15)00817-X. Epub 2015 Dec 17
5. Lahner H, Rinke A, Unger N et al (2016) Sunitinib efficacy in patients with advanced pNET in clinical practice. Horm Met Res 48(9):575–580
6. Moertel CG, Kvols LK, O'Connell MJ et al (1991) Treatment of neuro-endocrine carcinomas with combined etoposide and cisplatin. Evidence of major therapeutic activity in the anaplastic variants of these neoplasms. Abstr US Endocr Soc 68:227–232

7. Kulke MH, Stuart K, Enzinger PC, Ryan DP, Clark JW, Muzikansky A et al (2006) Phase II study of temozolomide and thalidomide in patients with metastatic neuroendocrine tumors. J Clin Oncol 24:401–406
8. Ekeblad S, Sundin A, Janson ET et al (2007) Temozolomide as monotherapy is effective in treatment of advanced malignant neuroendocrine tumors. Clin Cancer Res 15:2986–2991
9. Kulke M, Blaszkowsky LS, Zhu AX et al (2010) Phase I/ II study of everolimus (RAD001) in combination with temozolomide (TMZ) in patients (pts) with advanced pancreatic neuroendocrine tumors (NET). 2010 ASCO gastrointestinal cancers symposium. Abstract No. 223
10. Strosberg JR, Fine RL, Choi J et al (2011) First-line chemotherapy with capecitabine and temozolomide in patients with metastatic pancreatic endocrine carcinomas. Cancer 117(2):268–275
11. Fjallskog ML, Janson ET, Falkmer UG et al (2008) Treatment with combined streptozotocin and liposomal doxorubicin in metastatic endocrine pancreatic tumors. Neuroendocrinology 88:53–58
12. Moertel CG, Lefkopoulo M, Lipsitz S et al (1992) Streptozocin-doxorubicin, streptozocin-fluorouracil or chlorozotocin in the treatment of advanced islet-cell carcinoma. N Engl J Med 326:519–523
13. Pembrolizumab (MK-3475) in patients (pts) with extensive-stage small cell lung cancer (SCLC): preliminary safety and efficacy results from KEYNOTE-02. Abstract Number:7502, 2015 ASCO Annual Meeting
14. Nghiem PT, Bhatia S, Lipson EJ et al (2016) PD-1 blockade with pembrolizumab in advanced Merkel-cell carcinoma. N Eng J Med 374(26):2542– 2552
15. Delle Fave G et al (2012) ENETS consensus guidelines for the management of patients with gastroduodenal neoplasms. Neuroendocrinology 95:74–87

Therapy for Metastatic Disease: Pancreas

Beata Kos-Kudła, Karolina Poczkaj, and Anna Malczewska

A. Colao et al. (eds.), *Neuroendocrine Tumors in Real Life*,
https://doi.org/10.1007/978-3-319-59024-0_21

21

Overview

We present a clinical course of a female diagnosed at the age of 52 with a well-differentiated neuroendocrine tumour of the pancreas. The patient underwent pancreaticoduodenectomy and liver resection for the metastasized neuroendocrine tumour. Post-operatively, long-acting somatostatin analogues and peptide receptor radionuclide therapy were administered for progressive and advanced metastatic disease. Due to further disease progression, other treatment options, such as molecular targeted therapy, and eventually chemotherapy, were introduced. In the presented case, treatment decisions were based on the patient's clinical presentation, NET markers, biochemical parameters and imaging results (including functional and conventional imaging – ^{68}Ga-DOTA-TATE PET/CT, ^{18}F–FDG PET/CT, CT, MRI scans) and were made by a multidisciplinary team in accordance with the national and European guidelines for pancreatic neuroendocrine neoplasms management. Management of the patients with neuroendocrine neoplasms, especially those with progressive disease, is recommended to be discussed by a multidisciplinary team, and the patients should be offered diagnostic investigations and treatment at highly specialized centres for neuroendocrine neoplasms.

Clinical Case

The patient initially presented in 2005 at the age of 52 with symptoms of recurrent abdominal pain and diarrhoea. Ultrasound of the abdomen visualized a 52 × 20 mm hypoechoic mass in the pancreatic neck. CT scan confirmed a 25 mm lesion. Blood levels of CA19–9, chromogranin A, glucagon, pancreatic polypeptide, gastrin, insulin and 24 h urine 5-HIAA level were normal. Fine-needle aspiration biopsy of the pancreatic lesion was performed twice, in 2005 and 2006. Neither of the cytology tests identified atypical or neoplastic cells. At that time, the patient did not agree to any surgical procedure. The patient stayed under a close follow-up. Imaging such as ultrasound or CT scans of the abdomen were performed every 3–6 months. Throughout this period, the patient was asymptomatic, in a good general condition.

In June 2008 the patient presented with a 10% weight loss in a 3-month time and symptoms of recurrent abdominal pain and diarrhoea (4–5 bowel movements per day). Abdominal ultrasound visualized enlargement of the previously described lesion in the pancreas, up to dimensions of 75 x 32 mm and a new 32 mm lesion in the pancreatic body. CT scan of the abdomen showed another new finding, solitary 14 mm lesion in the right liver lobe, suspected of a metastasis. CgA level was slightly raised while 24 hour urine 5-HIAA level was normal. The patient underwent somatostatin receptor scintigraphy SPECT/CT with ^{99m}Tc-Tektrotyd which showed foci of increased tracer uptake corresponding to the CT scan findings and suggesting neuroendocrine nature of the lesions. Hormonal and biochemical testing towards MEN-1 syndrome were performed with no evidence of its manifestation. The patient agreed to Whipple procedure and liver resection. In November 2008 the patient underwent pancreaticoduodenectomy with resection of the pancreatic head and body, duodenum, spleen, appendix and liver resection of the metastatic lesion. Histology confirmed metastasized to the liver well-differentiated neuroendocrine tumour of the pancreas, on staining the lesions were positive for chromogranin A, synaptophysin and negative for insulin, gastrin or glucagon (NEN G2, Ki-67 10%, p mT3 N1 M1). The patient recovered well from the surgery. Post-operatively, clinical symptoms resolved and CgA level normalized.

In March 2009 regular follow-up blood tests showed raised CgA level (59.9 IU/L, N: 2–18). Other gut hormones and 24-hour urine 5-HIAA levels were normal. ^{68}Ga-DOTA-TATE PET/CT scan revealed multiple foci of increased tracer uptake in the liver and in the pancreatic bed, while ^{18}F–FDG PET/CT showed focally slightly increased glucose metabolism in the liver. Disease progression with new multiple lesions in the liver and in the pancreatic bed was confirmed by a CT scan based on RECIST criteria. The patient commenced long-acting somatostatin analogues administered every 28 days. After 3 months on treatment with SSA, the patient developed symptoms of flushing and diarrhoea (up to 5–7 bowel movements per day). Gut hormone tests showed increased CgA level (80 IU/L). Cross-sectional imaging confirmed further disease progression. Based on high expression of SSTR in the metastatic lesions confirmed by ^{68}Ga-DOTA-TATE PET/CT scan, advanced disease and its progressive course, the patient was qualified for peptide receptor radioisotope therapy (PRRT). Between August 2009 and December 2009, the patient received three cycles of ^{90}Y/^{177}Lu-DOTA-TATE treatment (cumulative activity of 12.95 GBq). Due to anaemia developed secondarily to PRRT, the treatment was discontinued. Nevertheless, three cycles of PRRT resulted in satisfactory resolution of the clinical symptoms, normalization of CgA level and partial response on imaging. The patient continued on 4-weekly SSA injections and a regular follow-up.

In May 2012 the patient presented again with a diarrhoea up to 4–5 bowel movements per day. CgA level was raised and ^{68}Ga-DOTA-TATE PET/CT scan showed two new foci of increased tracer uptake in the pancreatic bed confirmed by a CT scan as metastatic lymph nodes. Following good response to previously administered three cycles of PRRT, post-treatment normalization of haematology parameters and high SSTR expression in the described metastatic lesions, the patient received two further cycles of PRRT for progressive disease. Between August 2012 and October 2012, two cycles of ^{90}Y/^{177}Lu-DOTA-TATE treatment were administered (cumulative activity of 12.95 GBq). Response to the treatment was satisfactory with resolution of clinical symptoms, normalization of CgA level and partial response on imaging (Fig. 21.1). The patient continued on 4-weekly SSA injections and a regular follow-up.

In January 2014 a follow-up CT scan of the abdomen revealed a new metastatic liver lesion and further lymph node metastases in the pancreatic bed. ^{68}Ga-DOTA-TATE PET/CT scan was consistent with the CT scan findings and in addition revealed new foci of increased tracer uptake in the bones – right femur, ischium, right rib 4 and left rib 10 (Fig. 21.2). Due to progressive disease, the patient commenced molecular targeted treatment with mTOR inhibitor (everolimus) combined with long-acting SSA.

Four months later, CT scan showed partial response of the metastatic lesions in the liver, while other metastatic lesions were stable in appearances. In May 2015, liver MRI scan confirmed further response to the treatment of the liver lesions.

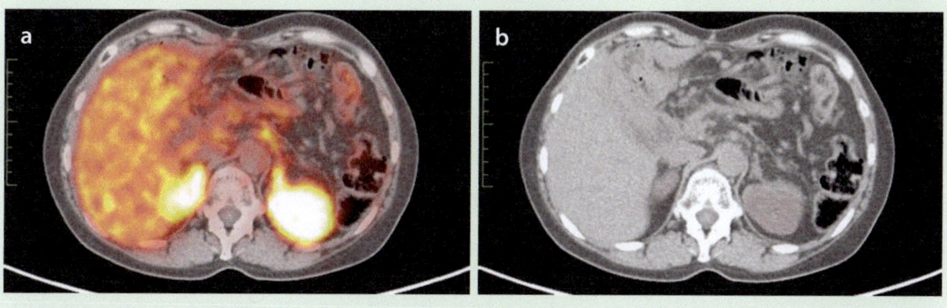

Fig. 21.1 **a** and **b** (August 2013) Stable disease – status post-surgery and 5 cycles of PRRT

In October 2015 new metastatic mesenteric lymph nodes and liver lesions were diagnosed. Everolimus was discontinued (▣ Fig. 21.3).

The patient commenced chemotherapy with capecitabine and temozolomide (CAPTEM) and continued on 4-weekly SSA (▣ Fig. 21.4). Since then, the treatment has been well tolerated, clinical symptoms resolved and the disease maintained stable. The patient stays under a regular follow-up.

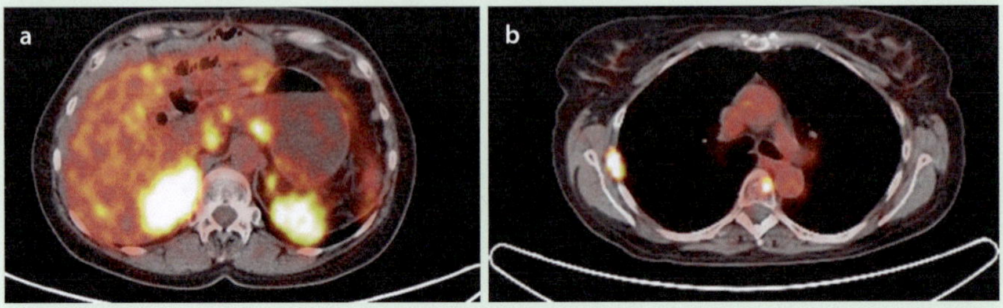

▣ **Fig. 21.2** **a** and **b** (January 2014) Progressive disease – 14 months after 5 cycles of PRRT (new metastatic lesions in the pancreatic bed, liver and bones)

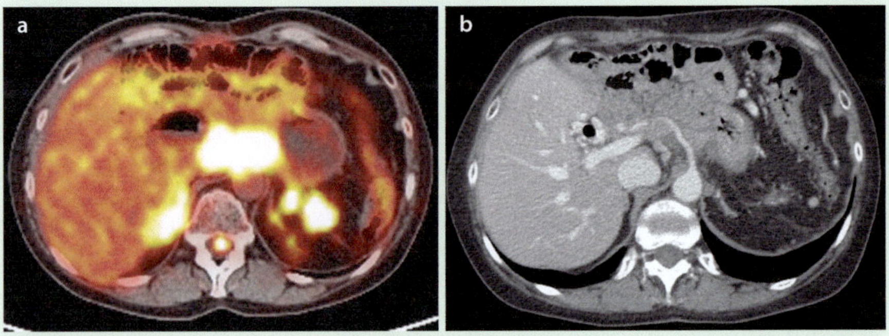

▣ **Fig. 21.3** **a** and **b** (October 2015) Progressive disease – after 15 months on treatment with everolimus

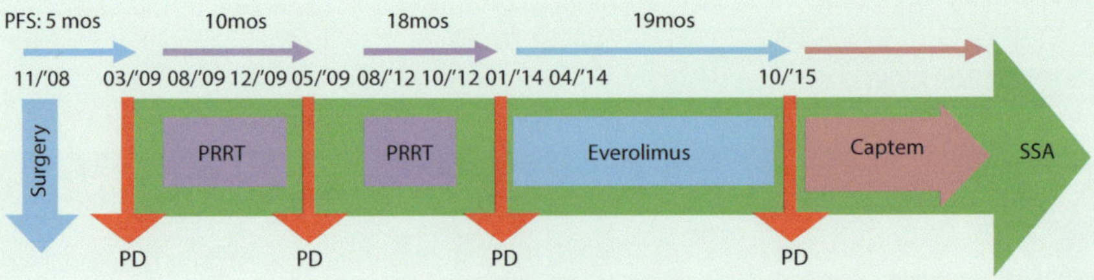

▣ **Fig. 21.4** Treatment response and progression-free survival (PFS). *PD* progressive disease

21.1 Comments to the Case

Management of p-NET patients represents diagnostic and therapeutic challenges.

Presented patient was offered treatment options in accordance with the national and European guidelines for p-NET management.

Management of the patients with neuroendocrine neoplasms, especially those with progressive disease, is recommended to be discussed by a multidisciplinary team, and the patients should be offered diagnostic investigations and treatment at highly specialized centres for neuroendocrine neoplasms.

Questions

1. Is resection of the primary p-NET the treatment of choice?
2. Does treatment with somatostatin analogues show antiproliferative activity?

Answers

1. Surgical resection of p-NET > 2 cm in resectable cases is recommended. In patients with advanced metastatic disease, surgical resection of the primary tumour has been shown to have a positive prognostic role.
2. Placebo-controlled randomized trials have clearly demonstrated that SSA improve progression-free survival of patients with pancreatic NET.

Up to Date of the Topic

Surgery

Surgical resection of p-NET > 2 cm in resectable cases has been reported to be associated with significant improvement in survival [1–3]. For the tumours located in the head of the pancreas, pancreaticoduodenectomy is the procedure of choice while for the tumours located in the body or tail of the pancreas, distal pancreatectomy with or without splenectomy [3, 4]. Recent reports have suggested the value of extended surgical resection in advanced metastatic p-NET. Synchronous resection of primary in the pancreas and focal liver metastases may be performed when it is associated with low morbidity and mortality rates. Pancreaticoduodenectomy with extensive hepatectomy should be avoided due to high morbidity and mortality rates [3, 5, 6].

Somatostatin Analogues

SSA is the treatment of choice for symptoms control in carcinoid syndrome or hormonally active p-NET such as glucagonoma or vipoma. PROMID phase III study showed prolonged PFS in midgut neuroendocrine tumours, both hormonally active or inactive, treated with octreotide LAR (vs. placebo) [7]. CLARINET study showed significantly prolonged PFS in midgut/hormonally inactive p-NET and proliferative index Ki-67 < 10% treated with lanreotide autogel (vs. placebo) [8]. Based on the results of PROMID and CLARINET studies, SSA (octreotide LAR/lanreotide autogel) is an established antiproliferative treatment in patients with intestinal NET [7, 8]. Antiproliferative effect of SSA seems to be a drug-class effect; however, data from a prospective study on octreotide LAR in p-NET are lacking. In terms of lack of toxicity and antiproliferative activity showed by the CLARINET study, lanreotide autogel should be preferably chosen as the therapy for p-NET (Ki-67 < 10%) [8, 9]. SSA can be recommended to prevent or inhibit tumour growth, both in intestinal NET and p-NET [7, 8]. Based on CLARINET study results, SSAs are used as treatment for GEP NET when Ki-67 does not exceed 10%. However, the recommendations do not include cut-offs for the antiproliferative application in the whole group of NEN. For SSA as a first-line treatment in intestinal or p-NET, some experts suggest Ki-67 5% as the most suitable cut-off. In disease metastasized to the liver with liver involvement of over 25%, the recommendations for the application of SSAs are extended (in accordance with the CLARINET study results) [8]. Although the CLARINET study did not demonstrate the positive effect of SSAs on overall survival, it is believed that SSAs positively affect the course of the disease [10].

Peptide Receptor Radionuclide Therapy (PRRT)
^{90}Y–DOTA-TOC or ^{177}Lu-DOTA-TATE have evolved as promising treatment for distant metastatic NET, including p-NET. PRRT could be considered in hormonally active or inactive p-NET, with high and homogenous SSTR expression. Phase III NETTER-1 trial compared ^{177}Lu-DOTATATE with high dose of octreotide LAR (60 mg/4 weekly) in progressive midgut NET and showed significantly prolonged PFS in PRRT-treated group [11]. As part of the phase II study conducted in Europe, over 1000 patients were treated with PRRT; the results showed complete or partial response in 30–40% and 17–40 months of PFS [3, 12, 13]. In general PRRT is recommended in NET G1/G2 following failure of medical treatment (such as SSA, chemotherapy or targeted therapy) [3]. However, introducing PRRT following such treatment lines could potentially increase toxicity of the therapy. Therefore, earlier introduction of PRRT in well-selected patients should be considered [2, 14]. Sequencing of different treatment lines in p-NET, including PRRT, molecular targeted therapy or chemotherapy needs to be defined.

Molecular Targeted Therapy
Based on results of two placebo-controlled randomized phase III trials and in accordance with the ENETS guidelines, molecular targeted therapies (everolimus and sunitinib) are recommended for progressive p-NET G1 or G2. In these studies mean PFS with either of the drugs was around 11 months, while remission occurred in 5% of patients treated with everolimus and in <10% patients treated with sunitinib. The standard dose of everolimus was 10 mg/day or 37.5 mg/day of sunitinib [15, 16]. Comparison between everolimus and sunitinib efficacy in p-NET treatment has not been presented satisfactorily yet. Therefore, up till now selection between everolimus and sunitinib is made mostly on the basis of side effects profiles and general patient's condition/co-morbidities along with regimens availability [14].

Molecular targeted therapy, such as everolimus or sunitinib, is an established treatment for p-NET and can be first- or second-line treatment with respect to chemotherapy or subsequent to SSA. However, these drugs should not be widely used as a first-line treatment due to relatively high potential for toxicity. Sequencing of different treatment lines in p-NET has not been defined yet. Panzuto F. et al. reported results of the retrospective multicentre study of increased everolimus toxicity when the patients were previously treated with PRRT and/or chemotherapy [17]. Contrary to these results, Kamp K. et al. on the basis of a smaller retrospective study did not report increased risk of everolimus toxicity when PRRT was the preceding treatment [18]. Ongoing SEQTOR trial is investigating the best sequencing of everolimus and chemotherapy (STZ/5-FU) in advanced p-NET upon progression [14, 19], while phase II trial, OCCLURANDOM, aims to compare antitumour efficacy of PRRT (^{177}Lu + octreotide) vs. sunitinib in non-resectable progressive p-NET [20].

Locoregional Therapy

In a distant metastatic disease limited to the liver, locoregional therapies may constitute an alternative option to systemic therapies in patients with hormonally inactive tumours. Locoregional therapies may be introduced repetitively during the course of the disease [14, 21–23].

Large randomized studies comparing the efficacy of locoregional therapies for metastatic liver lesions, such as embolization, chemoembolization, radioembolization, selective internal radiation therapy (SIRT), radiofrequency ablation or microwave ablation or systemic treatment are lacking. Selection of the locoregional treatment is based on the extent of liver tumour involvement, number of liver lesions, their localization, vascularization and proliferation index, as well as experience of the NET specialists [14, 21].

Chemotherapy

Systemic chemotherapy is one of the treatment options in well-differentiated p-NET (G1/G2). Commonly applied therapies include streptozotocin with 5-fluorouracil (STZ/5-FU) and doxorubicin with streptozotocin as an alternative therapy; however, the application of doxorubicin is limited due to the risk of cardiotoxicity [14]. Systemic chemotherapy can be a treatment option in patients without preceding disease progression but with high tumour burden. There is no Ki-67 cut-off established for this type of treatment, although most often it is introduced in patients with p-NET and Ki-67 5–20%. Factors favouring chemotherapy over targeted therapy include rapid disease progression within ≤6–12 months, bulky disease, symptomatic presentation and neoadjuvant approach which may potentially enable surgery [14].

Approach to replace STZ/5-FU by temozolomide/capecitabine is gaining popularity, however, it cannot be highly recommended as still the data on temozolomide are lacking, although temozolomide +/− capecitabine could be considered if availability of STZ/5-FU is limited. Small prospective and retrospective studies reported objective response rates between 15% and 70% for temozolomide combined with antiangiogenic drugs or capecitabine [14, 24–26]. Therapeutic value of temozolomide or its combination with capecitabine or antiangiogenic drugs is under investigation in prospective clinical trials (► www.clinicaltrials.gov). After failure of chemotherapy based on STZ, there are other alternative chemotherapy options, including temozolomide +/− capecitabine, oxaliplatin +5-FU or capecitabine. It has not been defined yet which treatment option is superior; however, in p-NET there is data favouring preferential use of temozolomide +/− capecitabine due to promising response rates and low toxicity [14, 25, 27, 28].

21

21.2 Conclusions

Management of p-NET patients is based on clinical presentation, disease stage, course of the disease, SSTR expression in the NET lesions (evaluated by functional imaging) and histological features of the tumour [29]. Best sequencing of different treatment lines in p-NET still needs to be established. Therefore, treatment decisions in p-NET patients should be discussed and made by multidisciplinary team, and the patients should be offered diagnostic investigations and treatment at highly specialized centres for neuroendocrine neoplasms.

Bibliography

1. Ito T, Igarashi H, Jensen RT (2012) Pancreatic neuroendocrine tumors: clinical features, diagnosis and medical treatment: advances. Best Pract Res Clin Gastroenterol 26:737–753
2. Kos-Kudła B, Hubalewska-Dydejczyk A, Kuśnierz K et al (2013) Pancreatic neuroendocrine neoplasms – management guidelines (recommended by the Polish Network of Neuroendocrine Tumours). Endokrynol Pol 64:459–479
3. Falconi M, Eriksson B, Kaltsas G et al (2016) ENETS consensus guidelines update for the management of patients with functional pancreatic neuroendocrine tumors and non-functional pancreatic neuroendocrine tumors. Neuroendocrinology 103:153–171
4. Watzka FM, Laumen C, Fottner C et al (2013) Resection strategies for neuroendocrine pancreatic neoplasms. Langenbeck's Arch Surg 398:431–440
5. Birnbaum DJ, Turrini O, Vigano L et al (2015) Surgical management of advanced pancreatic neuroendocrine tumors: short-term and long-term results from an international multi-institutional study. Ann Surg Oncol 22:1000–1007
6. Gaujoux S, Gonen M, Tang L et al (2012) Synchronous resection of primary and liver metastases for neuroendocrine tumors. Ann Surg Oncol 19:4270–4277
7. Rinke A, Muller HH, Schade-Brittinger C et al (2009) Placebo-controlled, double-blind, prospective, randomized study on the effect of Octreotide LAR in the control of tumor growth in patients with metastatic neuroendocrine midgut tumors: a report from the PROMID Study Group. J Clin Oncol 27:4656–4663
8. Caplin ME, Pavel M, Ćwikła JB et al (2014) Lanreotide in metastatic enteropancreatic neuroendocrine tumors. N Engl J Med 371(3):224–233
9. Martín-Richard M, Massutí B, Pineda E et al (2013) Antiproliferative effects of lanreotide autogel in patients with progressive, well-differentiated neuroendocrine tumours: a Spanish, multicentre, open-label, single arm phase II study. BMC Cancer 13:427
10. Shen C, Shih YC, Xu Y et al (2014) Octreotide long-acting repeatable use among elderly patients with carcinoid syndrome and survival outcomes: a population-based analysis. Cancer 120: 2039–2049
11. Strosberg J, El-Haddad G, Wolin E et al (2017) Phase 3 trial of (177) Lu-dotatate for midgut neuroendocrine tumors. N Engl J Med 376(2):125–135
12. Imhof A, Brunner P, Marincek N et al (2011) Response, survival, and long-term toxicity after therapy with the radiolabeled somatostatin analogue [90Y-DOTA]-TOC in metastasized neuroendocrine cancers. J Clin Oncol 29:2416–2423
13. Kwekkeboom DJ, de Herder WW, Kam BL et al (2008) Treatment with the radiolabeled somatostatin analog [177 Lu-DOTA 0, Tyr3] octreotate: toxicity, efficacy, and survival. J Clin Oncol 26:2124–2130
14. Pavel M, O'Toole D, Costa F et al (2016) ENETS consensus guidelines update for the management of distant metastatic disease of intestinal, pancreatic, bronchial neuroendocrine neoplasms (NEN) and NEN of unknown primary site. Neuroendocrinology 103:172–185
15. Raymond E, Dahan L, Raoul JL et al (2011) Sunitinib malate for the treatment of pancreatic neuroendocrine tumors. N Engl J Med 364:501–513

16. Yao JC, Shah MH, Ito T et al (2011) RAD001 in advanced neuroendocrine tumors, third trial (RADIANT-3) study group. Everolimus for advanced pancreatic neuroendocrine tumors. N Engl J Med 364:514–523
17. Panzuto F, Rinzivillo M, Fazio N et al (2014) Real world study of everolimus in advanced progressive neuroendocrine tumors. Oncologist 19:966–974
18. Kamp K, Gumz B, Feelders RA et al (2013) Safety and efficacy of everolimus in gastrointestinal and pancreatic neuroendocrine tumors after (177)Lu-octreotate. Endocr Relat Cancer 20:825–831
19. Salazar R et al Randomized open label study to compare the efficacy and safety of everolimus followed by chemotherapy with streptozotocin-fluorouracilo (STZ-5FU) upon progression or the reverse sequence, in advanced progressive pancreatic NETs (pNETs). ClinicalTrials.gov identifier: NCT02246127
20. Baudin E et al Antitumor efficacy of peptide receptor radionuclide therapy with 177Lutetium octreotate randomized vs sunitinib in unresectable progressive well-differentiated neuroendocrine pancreatic tumor: first randomized phase II. ClinicalTrials.gov identifier: NCT02230176
21. de Baere T, Deschamps F, Tselikas L et al (2015) GEP-NETS update: interventional radiology: role in the treatment of liver metastases from GEP-NETs. Eur J Endocrinol 172:R151–R166
22. Fiore F, Del Prete M, Franco R et al (2014) Transarterial embolization (TAE) is equally effective and slightly safer than transarterial chemoembolization (TACE) to manage liver metastases in neuroendocrine tumors. Endocrine 47:177–182
23. Benson AB 3rd, Geschwind JF, Mulcahy MF et al (2013) Radioembolisation for liver metastases: results from a prospective 151 patient multi-institutional phase II study. Eur J Cancer 49:3122–3130
24. Chan JA, Stuart K, Earle CC et al (2012) Prospective study of bevacizumab plus temozolomide in patients with advanced neuroendocrine tumors. J Clin Oncol 30:2963–2968
25. Strosberg JR, Fine RL, Choi J et al (2011) First line chemotherapy with capecitabine and temozolomide in patients with metastatic pancreatic endocrine carcinomas. Cancer 117:268–275
26. Kulke MH, Stuart K, Enzinger PC et al (2006) Phase II study of temozolomide and thalidomide in patients with metastatic neuroendocrine tumors. J Clin Oncol 24:401–406
27. Welin S, Sorbye H, Sebjornsen S et al (2011) Clinical effect of temozolomide based chemotherapy in poorly differentiated endocrine carcinoma after progression on first line chemotherapy. Cancer 117:4617–4622
28. Fine RL, Gulati AP, Krantz BA et al (2013) Capecitabine and temozolomide (CAPTEM) for metastatic, well-differentiated neuroendocrine cancers: the pancreas Center at Columbia University experience. Cancer Chemother Pharmacol 71:663–670
29. Rosiek V, Kunikowska J, Kos-Kudła B (2012) A non-functioning pancreatic neuroendocrine tumour: a case report. Endokrynol Pol 63:59–64

Therapy for Metastatic Disease: Ileum

David L. Chan, Eva Segelov, and Simron Singh

A. Colao et al. (eds.), *Neuroendocrine Tumors in Real Life*,
https://doi.org/10.1007/978-3-319-59024-0_22

22

Overview

The ileum is one of the most common primary sites for neuroendocrine tumours and the most common site of GI NETs. Approximately half will present as locoregionally advanced or metastatic disease. Patients with ileal NETs can vary widely in terms of their clinical course, based on underlying histopathological factors and patient characteristics. Recently, large international randomised trials have reported significant progress in the treatment of ileal NETs for the following therapies: somatostatin analogues, the mTOR inhibitor everolimus and peptide receptor radionuclide therapy (PRRT). Other treatments such as debulking surgery, liver-directed therapy chemotherapy and interferon are commonly used albeit with less evidence base. There are few randomised trials in Grade 3 NETs or neuroendocrine carcinoma (NEC), but chemotherapy is the mainstay of systemic treatment for this patient group. Issues remain in defining the optimal sequencing of therapies and detecting of changes in disease that should trigger changes in therapy. The increasing use of functional imaging gives clinicians a greater understanding of individual tumour biology and disease burden. Further research is needed to probe the molecular characteristics across the spectrum of NETs, to allow optimisation of current systemic therapies and develop even more effective approaches.

Clinical Case

A 67-year-old male presented to the emergency room with a 5-year history of abdominal discomfort, bloating and increasingly frequent episodes of constipation. On further questioning, he also reported incidental bouts of diarrhoea and flushing, which were attributed to irritable bowel syndrome by his primary care physician.

Computed tomography (CT) of the abdomen revealed the presence of a 4 cm mesenteric mass and extensive bilobar liver lesions. Core biopsy of the liver revealed the presence of a Grade 1 neuroendocrine tumour (Ki-67 index, 1%), with immunohistochemistry suggestive of a gastrointestinal origin. He was referred to a multidisciplinary NET clinic at this point for further evaluation and management.

CT of the thorax demonstrated no other lesions of concern, but CT enterography revealed the presence of multifocal ileal lesions. His chromogranin A (CgA) level was 167, and the urinary 5-hydroxyindoleacetic acid (5-HIAA) level was 306. After discussion in a multidisciplinary context, the patient underwent partial debulking of hepatic metastases and resection of the ileal primary, with perioperative octreotide. He was commenced on octreotide LAR 30 mg/28 days after recovery from surgery.

After 3 years of stable disease on the above treatment, there was radiological evidence of disease progression in the liver as well as biochemical progression (CgA 389, 5-HIAA 673). He was referred for consideration of PRRT in the context of a clinical trial. At the same time, asymptomatic tricuspid regurgitation was noted on echocardiogram. He remains well on follow-up in the clinic.

22.1 Comments to the Case

- Delayed diagnosis is the norm for neuroendocrine tumours, particularly those in the small bowel. A recent survey [1] of 1928 patients showed that the mean time from first symptom onset to diagnosis was 52 months. CT enterography should be considered for patients without an obvious primary and also for patients scheduled for small bowel surgery, as the presence of multifocal disease may alter the surgical plan.
- Initial systemic treatment of metastatic NET consists of somatostatin analogues. The use of either octreotide or lanreotide is supported by phase III trial evidence. On progression, systemic options include everolimus, PRRT and clinical trials.
- Screening for carcinoid heart disease should be considered for all patients with carcinoid syndrome.

Questions

1. Should small bowel primaries be resected in the presence of unresectable metastatic disease?
2. What is the optimal treatment strategy for a patient with refractory carcinoid syndrome?

Answers

1. Removal of the small bowel primary may be performed in the presence of metastatic disease to prevent future complications from local fibrosis and disease progression, resulting in mesenteric ischemia and bowel obstruction. Although several studies suggest a potential survival benefit [2], there is currently no high-quality trial evidence for this approach. We consider resection of the primary in a multidisciplinary setting if mesenteric ischaemia or bowel obstruction is thought to be likely complications from fibrosis or if the patient is symptomatic from the primary.
2. The management of refractory carcinoid syndrome is challenging in clinical practice because of the paucity of effective treatment options. Dose escalation of somatostatin analogue is often employed. However, increasing doses past octreotide LAR 120 mg/28 day or lanreotide 120 mg/14 days may not produce further symptom improvement, and QT prolongation as noted in patients with acromegaly [3] is a clinical concern. Telotristat, a novel oral serotonin synthesis inhibitor, decreased the frequency of bowel movements in a phase III trial [4], but this drug is not widely available at present. Liver-directed therapies (such as chemoembolisation, bland embolisation or selective internal radiotherapy) or surgical debulking may be considered in difficult cases.

22

Up to Date of the Topic

Introduction

Ileal tumours comprise 20% of all NETs [5], and the ileum is one of the most common primary sites for neuroendocrine tumours and is the most common site of GI NETs. Approximately half will present as locoregionally advanced or metastatic disease. Patients with ileal NETs can vary widely in terms of their clinical course, based on underlying histopathological factors and patient characteristics. Whilst surgery is the standard of cure for resectable disease, approximately 50% of patients present with either locoregionally advanced or metastatic disease [6].

There has been an increasing recognition of the heterogeneity in behaviour of metastatic NETs, and those of ileal origin also demonstrate considerable variation in biological aggressiveness and clinical course. The World Health Organization (WHO) 2010 histological classification of NETs [7] has successfully explained much of this clinical heterogeneity. This schema classifies tumours into Grades 1–3 based on the mitotic count and Ki-67 index (◘ Table 22.1). Grade 1–2 tumours (those with a Ki-67 index of <20% and mitotic count of <=20 mitoses per ten high power fields) tend to progress more slowly and are amenable to multiple treatment regimens. In contrast, Grade 3 tumours may progress rapidly, and chemotherapy is often the only effective systemic treatment.

However, the presence of intra-tumoural heterogeneity and change in tumour behaviour over time mean that optimal selection of therapy and accurate identification of the patient with aggressive disease remain challenging. A deeper understanding of the molecular phenotype and correlation with functional imaging (particularly somatostatin receptor-based nuclear medicine scans) may define groups of patients with poor prognosis who require more aggressive therapy. Treatment of ileal NETs is further complicated by symptoms of hormones produced by some NETs such as serotonin, prostaglandins and substance P. Some of these patients present with symptoms of diarrhoea, flushing and/or bronchospasm and are classified as having functional NETs. Urinary levels of 5-hydroxyindoleacetic acid, a serotonin metabolite, are elevated in 68% of patients [8], but the frequency of the other vasoactive substances is less well defined.

◘ Table 22.1 2010 World Health Organization (WHO) classification of neuroendocrine tumours

Grade	Mitotic count (mitoses per ten high power fields)	Ki-67 index	WHO/ENETS nomenclature
Grade 1	<2 mit/10 HPF	<3%	Neuroendocrine tumour (Grade 1)
Grade 2	2–20 mit/10 HPF	3–20%	Neuroendocrine tumour (Grade 2)
Grade 3	>20 mit/10 HPF	>20%	Neuroendocrine carcinoma (large cell or small cell type)
Mixed adenoneuroendocrine carcinoma (MANEC)			
Hyperplastic and preneoplastic lesions			

Treatment of this heterogeneous and relatively uncommon disease requires multidisciplinary care from specialties including surgery, diagnostic and interventional imaging, nuclear medicine, gastroenterology, endocrinology and medical oncology. Presentation of patients at multidisciplinary clinics within recognised NET specialist centres may increase the use of efficacious therapies and potentially improve outcome [9]. Whilst the use of surgery and liver-directed therapies is important in many patients, this chapter will focus on current systemic therapies for metastatic Grade 1–2 ileal NETs. Multiple trials published in the last decade have established the effectiveness of various modalities of treatment in this setting (◘ Table 22.2). The challenge remains to avoid overtreatment of relatively indolent disease whilst exposing patients to all effective therapies during their disease course.

◘ Table 22.2 Randomised trials in metastatic ileal NET

Trial (phase)	Intervention	Population	Progression-free survival (PFS), HR, *p*-value, median	Overall survival, HR, *p*-value	Objective response rate
PROMID (III)	Octreotide vs placebo	Midgut NET	Time to progression 14.3 vs 6 months, HR 0.34, $p = 0.000072$	HR 0.81 P = 0.77	2.4% vs 2.3%
CLARINET (III)	Lanreotide vs placebo	Mixed gastrointestinal NET	Not reached vs 18 months, HR 0.47, $p = 0.0002$	No difference, $P = 0.88$	Not reported
Yao 2008 (II)	Octreotide + bevacizumab vs Octreotide + interferone-alpha-2b	Mixed gastrointestinal NET	16.5 vs 14 months, $p = 0.34$	No difference observed. Exact figure not reported	50% vs 45%
Kolby 2003	Interferon + octreotide vs octreotide	Midgut NET	Not reported	HR 0.62, $p = 0.132$	Not reported
Faiss 1999	Interferon alpha + lanreotide vs lanreotide vs interferon alpha	Mixed gastrointestinal NET	Not reported	Not reported	Lanreotide 4%; IFN-a 3.7%; combination 7.1%
Arnold 2005 (II)	Interferon + octreotide vs octreotide	Mixed gastrointestinal NET	Not reported	HR 0.82, $p = 0.38$	50% vs 45%

(continued)

Table 22.2 (continued)

RADIANT-2 (III)	Everolimus + octreotide LAR vs octreotide LAR	Mixed gastrointestinal NET	11 vs 4.6 months, HR 0.35, $p < 0.001$	HR 1.05, $p = 0.59$	5% vs 2%
RADIANT-4 (III)	Everolimus vs placebo	Gastrointestinal and lung NET	11.0 vs 3.9 months, HR 0.48, $p < 0.00001$	Median not reached	2% vs 1%
NETTER-1 (III)	PRRT vs octreotide LAR 60 mg	Midgut NET, progressing on octreotide LAR 30 mg	Not reached vs 8.4 months, HR 0.21, $p < 0.0001$	Not reported yet	18% vs 3%

Somatostatin Analogues

Somatostatin analogues (SSAs: octreotide, lanreotide, pasireotide) act on the somatostatin receptors and inhibit release of various pro-growth hormones such as growth hormone, glucagon and insulin. They have been used to control symptoms of carcinoid syndrome related to excess hormonal secretion since the 1980s. Following observations of tumour stabilisation and even regression, clinical trials were undertaken to investigate the anti-proliferative effect of SSAs in metastatic NETs, initially of pancreatic origin and later of gastrointestinal origin.

Two pivotal trials conducted in the last decade have led to the demonstration that SSAs can achieve tumour control. PROMID was a single-centre, phase III trial which randomised patients with advanced midgut NETs (95% Grade 1) to octreotide LAR 30 mg every 28 days or best supportive care. The primary endpoint, time to progression, was prolonged from 6 to 14.3 months (HR 0.34, 95% CI 0.20–0.59, $p = 0.00072$) [10]. The later larger phase III trial, CLARINET, randomised patients with gastrointestinal NETs (36% midgut, 45% pancreatic origin) with Ki-67 < 10% to lanreotide ATG 120 mg every 28 days or placebo [11]. This similarly demonstrated prolongation of progression-free survival (PFS), the primary endpoint, the median of which was not reached in the lanreotide group versus 18 months in the placebo group (HR 0.47, 95% CI 0.30–0.73, $p < 0.001$). There are subtle but important differences between these two trials (Table 22.3). A trial of pasireotide versus escalated dose octreotide (60 mg every 28 days) in 110 patients with metastatic NET and carcinoid symptoms (75% of small bowel origin) resulted in median progression-free survival of 11.8 months for pasireotide and 6.8 months for octreotide (HR 0.46, 95% CI 0.20–0.98, $p = 0.045$), although this was not the primary endpoint [12]. Nevertheless, this robust evidence supports a class effect of somatostatin analogues in preventing tumour proliferation.

Table 22.3 Differences between CLARINET and PROMID

Trial characteristic	CLARINET	PROMID
SSA used	Lanreotide 120 mg/28 days	Octreotide 30 mg/28 days
Patient population	Gastroenteropancreatic	Midgut/unknown primary
Functionality	Non-functioning	Both functioning and non-functioning
Response assessment	RECIST	WHO
Primary endpoint	Progression-free survival	Time to progression
Disease status	Stable disease (95%)	Unknown
Proliferation index (Ki-67)	<2% in 68% of patients; 2–10% in 32% of patients	<2% in 95% of patients; ≥2% in 5% of patients
Liver involvement	<10% in 49% of patients; >25% in 39% of patients	<10% in 77% of patients; >25% in 19% of patients

SSAs have become the cornerstone of medical therapy for G1–G2 metastatic ileal NETs due to their efficacy, favourable side effect profile and the availability of long-acting formulations. SSAs are currently recommended as first-line treatment by multiple guidelines: ENETS [13], ESMO [14] and NANETS [15].

Treatment of Functional NETs/Hormonal Syndromes: Dose Escalation of SSAs
Vasoactive substances such as serotonin are secreted by some NETs, resulting in the classic symptoms of episodic flushing, diarrhoea and bronchospasm known as carcinoid syndrome. Whilst serotonin is usually metabolised by the liver, high levels of hormone production (from large tumour burden) may overwhelm this metabolic pathway; additionally, bulky liver metastases can result in bypass of the pathway altogether. Functional NETs comprise a minority of tumours, but the exact proportion in ileal NETs is difficult to determine, measuring from 5% to 20% depending on the exact population investigated [16–18].

It is important to screen patients with carcinoid syndrome or elevated 5-HIAA level for valvular heart disease, particularly right-sided (tricuspid) valve abnormalities which can present precipitously with advanced right heart failure. Long-term administration of serotonin induced cardiac valve fibrosis in rats [19], implicating it in the pathogenesis of valve disease. Early detection of abnormality on echocardiogram may allow timely surgical intervention. Patients with refractory carcinoid symptoms despite administration of SSA, high-dose conventional antidiarrhoeals and appropriate antitumour therapy remain a challenging clinical problem. Dose escalation of SSAs (e.g. octreotide up to 60 mg every 2 weeks or lanreotide 120 mg up to every 2 weeks) has been trialled in small series, with response rates ranging from 20% to 79% for diarrhoea and 79% to 91% for flushing [20–22]. Dose escalation may have some effects on tumour control as well with disease control rates from 30% to 100% [12, 23, 24], but response rates are modest at 0–31% [24–26].

Telotristat etiprate is an oral inhibitor of tryptophan hydroxylase, an enzyme in the serotonin production pathway. A recent phase III trial, TELESTAR, demonstrated reduction in the number of bowel movements and urinary 5-hydroxyindoleacetic acid (5-HIAA) levels in 135 patients with functional NET who had at least four bowel movements per day [27]. However, the frequency of flushing and abdominal pain was not significantly reduced. TELECAST is a similar study in 85 patients with less than four bowel movements per day and the presence of carcinoid symptoms, but full results have not yet been reported.

Everolimus: An mTOR Inhibitor
The mammalian target of rapamycin (mTOR) pathway plays a critical path in cell cycle control [28] and cell growth [29]. It is a serine/threonine kinase from the phosphoinositide-3 kinase (PI3K) family and forms the complexes mTORC1 and mTORC2. Several key observations led to the investigation of mTOR inhibitors in NET. Patients with tuberous sclerosis (TSC1/TSC2) and neurofibromatosis (NF1) – mediated by the TSC1/TSC2 pathway – have an increased risk of NET. TSC1/TSC2 is intimately related to mTOR regulation, and mTOR is constitutively activated in NF1-deficient cells [30]. A series of 99 GEPNETs reported a 70% rate of mutation in foregut NET and 53% in midgut NETs [31]. It is therefore biologically plausible that inhibition of the mTOR pathway would result in downregulation of NET growth.

The RADIANT trials are a series of studies which have firmly established everolimus in the management of patients with metastatic NETs. After promising results in single-arm studies of everolimus, an oral mTOR inhibitor [32], several randomised trials [33–35] were conducted investigating its efficacy in gastrointestinal NETs.

The RADIANT-2 trial randomised 427 patients with metastatic low-to-intermediate grade functional and non-functional GI NET to everolimus plus octreotide or octreotide alone. Included sites of origin were the small intestine (52%), lung (10%) and other GI primary sites (colon 6%, pancreas 6%, liver 4%, others 21%) [33]. Median progression-free survival, the primary endpoint, was 11.3 months for the octreotide alone arm and 16.4 months in the everolimus arm, with HR 0.77 (95% CI 0.59–1.00, $p = 0.026$). As the significance boundary for the p-value had been set at 0.0246 due to adjustment for two interim analyses, this result did not reach the prespecified significance level. Subsequent retrospective analyses demonstrated imbalance in the arms based on known prognostic indicators (high proportion of patients with lung primary, ECOG 1–2 and moderately differentiated disease in the everolimus arm) as well as discrepancy between central and local radiological reviews, reflecting a common issue of response assessment in NETs. Reanalysis with adjustment for the imbalance yielded a significant result in favour of everolimus [36]. Common side effects of everolimus were stomatitis, diarrhoea and fatigue. Grade 3–4 hyperglycaemia was noted in 5% and all-grade pneumonitis in 12%.

RADIANT-4 [35] followed from the somewhat difficult to interpret RADIANT-2 results. This trial restricted enrolment to 302 patients with well-differentiated NETs from GI tract or lung without evidence of carcinoid syndrome, randomised to everolimus or placebo. The most common primary tumour sites were the lung (30%), ileum (24%) and rectum (13%). The primary endpoint – centrally assessed progression-free survival (PFS) – was met with median of 11 months in the everolimus arm versus 3.9 months for placebo and HR of 0.48 (0.35–0.67, $p < 0.00001$). Preliminary OS analyses indicated a trend to improved overall survival (HR 0.64, $p = 0.037$), but formal conclusions for this endpoint require further maturation of the trial cohort. Objective RR was 2% in the everolimus arm and 1% in placebo arm; disease stabilisation was achieved in 81% of the everolimus arm compared to 64% with placebo. The adverse event profile was similar to RADIANT-2 with treatment discontinuation rate 12% in the everolimus arm and a 16% incidence of pneumonitis (1% Grade 3; no Grade 4). Preplanned subgroup analysis by primary tumour origin suggested consistent PFS benefit in patients with gastrointestinal primaries (HR 0.56, 95% CI 0.37–0.84) [37]. Based on this data, everolimus recently received FDA approval for the treatment of progressive, well-differentiated, non-functional, advanced NET of GI origin.

Anti-angiogenic Agents

Neuroendocrine tumours are known to be vascular, with microvessel density increased in higher grade NETs [38, 39]. As a result, there has been interest in the use of anti-angiogenic agents (monoclonal antibodies and small-molecule tyrosine kinase inhibitors (TKIs)). A phase II trial investigated the combination of temozolomide and bevacizumab in 34 patients (19 with ileal NET) and demonstrated a response rate of 33% in the pancreatic NET population [40]. Unfortunately, the responses were less marked in the ileal NET population with response rate of 0% and median progression-free survival of 7.3 months. A trial reported at ASCO 2015 [41] randomised 427 patients to the combination of octreotide and bevacizumab against a «standard» arm of octreotide and interferon. The primary endpoint of median PFS was not significantly different (16.6 mo in bevacizumab arm vs 15.4 mo in interferon arm; HR 0.93, $p = 0.55$).

Several tyrosine kinase inhibitors (TKIs) have been investigated for treatment of metastatic ileal NETs, but none have entered routine clinical practice as yet, unlike the situation with pancreatic NET. Sunitinib, a TKI with multiple targets including vascular endothelial growth factor receptor (VEGFR) and platelet-derived growth factor receptor (PDGFR), was investigated in a single-arm phase II study [42]. Forty-one of the 107 patients receiving treatment had an ileal NET. The objective response rate was 2.4%, but 83% of patients had stable disease. Commonly observed Grade 3 or greater toxicities included fatigue (24%), hypertension (10%), neutropenia (29%), nausea and vomiting (5% each); there was one fatal GI haemorrhage. Treatment was associated with increase in serum VEGF and decrease in VEGFR2/VEGFR3 levels, with non-significantly greater decreases in sVEGFR3 in patients with partial response [43]. A randomised phase III trial [44] established that sunitinib improved PFS in pancreatic NETs, but no further trials have been undertaken to date in the ileal NET population.

Pazopanib, another TKI targeting VEGFR1–VEGFR3, has been studied in two phase II trials involving patients with ileal NETs. Treatment with the combination of pazopanib and octreotide resulted in no responses from the 20 patients with ileal NET [45]. A trial of pazopanib monotherapy [46] enrolled 15 patients with GI NET from a total of 44; the overall response rate was 4/44 (9%), but subgroup results were not reported. The toxicity profile of pazopanib is similar to that of sunitinib with the most frequent adverse events being fatigue, nausea, diarrhoea and hypertension.

In summary, unlike pNET, there is no data to support anti-angiogenic agents in the treatment pathway of GI NET. No further trials with currently existing agents in the class are likely to be undertaken.

Chemotherapy
Chemotherapy has been used for many years in NET treatment, despite a paucity of data. Original regimens used the combination of streptozotocin and 5-fluorouracil (more recently capecitabine), cisplatin and/or doxorubicin, with response rates ranging from 5% to 15% [47]. Oxaliplatin-based regimens (such as FOLFOX with bevacizumab or CAPOX with bevacizumab) have shown response rates of 20–25% [48, 49] but need larger trials to confirm the degree of clinical benefit for patients with ileal NETs. More recently, temozolomide, an alkylating agent analogue of dacarbazine, has been investigated for NET treatment. The combination of the oral agents temozolomide and capecitabine achieved a response rate of 41% in 12 patients with well-moderately differentiated ileal NET [50]. Due to a lack of alternatives and a desire to avoid the toxicity of older regimens, this has been widely adopted with a level of evidence lower than that usually accepted for chemotherapy. Even though MGMT methylation status is receiving increasing acceptance in neuro-oncology [51], it has not been definitively shown to predict for temozolomide efficacy in neuroendocrine tumours, with mixed results from trials [52, 53]. With the now robust body of evidence for the targeted therapies, chemotherapy particularly for low and even intermediate grade disease is being used less often and reserved for refractory patients.

Interferon
Interferon-alpha is another stalwart of NET treatment dating from the 1980s when it was observed that classic midgut carcinoids had low levels of natural killer cells. Whilst interferon monotherapy improves symptoms in around 60% of patients with functional tumours with biochemical responses in up to 45%, objective response rates remain modest at 5–10%, with an objective response rate of 5–10% and biochemical response in around 45% [23, 54, 55]. Two RCTs published in the 2000s failed to show benefit of adding octreotide to interferon, although case series reported some benefit [23, 56, 57]. The chronic toxicities of fever, flu-like symptoms, significant fatigue and mood depression are significant such that in the context of well-established new therapies, IFN is now not commonly used outside of Europe. It is still recommended as a potential disease-modifying agent in the ENETS 2016 guidelines.

Surgery and Locoregional Therapies
Surgery for metastatic ileal NET includes removal of the small bowel primary, debulking of metastatic disease and even liver transplantation aiming to cure in carefully selected cases. Perioperative somatostatin analogues should be considered in patients with functional NETs who are planned to undergo surgery, due to the potential to develop carcinoid crisis although the benefit has never actually been proven.

Removal of the primary may be performed to improve quality of life when there are symptoms from local disease such as pain from venous ischemia or recurrent bowel obstruction [58] or prophylactically. Resection of the primary in metastatic midgut NET was addressed in a recent systematic review [2] which identified six retrospective studies, three showing significantly improved overall survival in resected patients. However, the potential for selection bias towards fitter patients in the surgical cohort needs to be acknowledged. Whilst prospective trials of this approach would be ideal, adequate accrual may prove difficult in practice. Debulking of liver metastases may be performed to reduce hormone production or with aggressive intent in patients with small-volume liver disease and stability of disease on systemic treatment.

Locoregional therapies such as radiofrequency ablation, trans-arterial embolisation, chemotherapy or a combination of them and selective internal radiation therapy with ^{90}Yttrium microspheres are all important techniques in treatment of liver-predominant metastatic NET with liver-predominant disease (see ► Chap. 21).

Peptide Receptor Radionuclide Therapy (PRRT)

PRRT has been used in specialist international centres over the past 15 years and is increasingly gaining traction as a viable treatment for metastatic NETs. PRRT utilises a peptide which attaches to the somatostatin receptor expressed on NETs, linked to a radionuclide (most commonly ^{177}Lutetium or ^{90}Yttrium). After intravenous administration, the radionuclide is internalised by the somatostatin receptor-expressing cell and emits beta radiation causing cellular damage.

The landmark randomised phase III NETTER-1 trial enrolled 230 patients with metastatic GI NET whose disease had progressed on octreotide 30 mg every 4 weeks [59]. Patients were randomised to increased dose of octreotide (60 mg every 4 weeks) or the combination of PRRT with ^{177}Lu-DOTATATE plus standard-dose octreotide. Seventy-four percent of the patients had an ileal primary; 69% of the patients had Grade 1 disease and 31% had Grade 2 disease. PRRT improved progression-free survival compared to increased-dose octreotide; median PFS was not reached for the PRRT group compared to 8.4 months for the higher dose octreotide group (HR 0.21, 95% CI 0.13–0.34, $p < 0.00001$). Whilst the response rate was only 19% for the PRRT group (3% for the octreotide group), 96% of patients had at least stable disease (76% for octreotide group). Grade 3 side effects occurred in 26% of the PRRT group leading to 5% withdrawing from treatment. Potential short-term adverse events from PRRT include nausea, vomiting, cytopenias, acute kidney injury and flare of symptoms; long-term adverse events include renal impairment and bone marrow toxicity although these are only significant in <1% of treated patients.

PRRT is usually administered as an intravenous injection every 6–8 weeks, with four cycles of treatment. «Maintenance» treatment (giving further cycles at a reduced frequency after completion of four cycles) is used in some centres but has not been investigated in large numbers of patients to date. Cumulative radiation dose to the kidneys and bone marrow limits the long-term use of PRRT, but the use of prophylactic amino acid infusions on the day of treatment is thought to lessen the risk of renal injury. The optimal dose and frequency of PRRT, the impact of lesions with low somatostatin receptor uptake, the efficacy of concomitant radiosensitising chemotherapy (such as capecitabine alone or in combination with temozolomide) and the optimal sequencing of PRRT with other agents are all unresolved questions of clinical importance.

Nuclear Imaging in Guiding Treatment Choice

The concept of theranostics in NET was a natural evolution from the ability to selectively target the somatostatin receptor for imaging. Nuclear imaging has been used in NET imaging due to its unique ability to correlate tumour biology (i.e. the expression of somatostatin receptors) with anatomical location and thus potentially predict the efficacy of somatostatin-targeting treatment for a particular patient. Whilst multiple modalities are now available, the 111In-pentetreotide scan (OctreoScan) was in use for decades and remains the only modality available in many centres worldwide. OctreoScan has been limited by the lack of spatial resolution and the difficulty inherent in obtaining quantitative measurements for particular lesions. The development of somatostatin receptor-based positron emission tomography (PET) (such as ^{68}Ga-DOTATATE/DOTATOC/DOTANOC PET – Fig. 22.1) has provided a much-needed breakthrough. This allows for correlation with co-localising CT, as well as quantitative measurements of uptake, resulting in a deeper understanding of

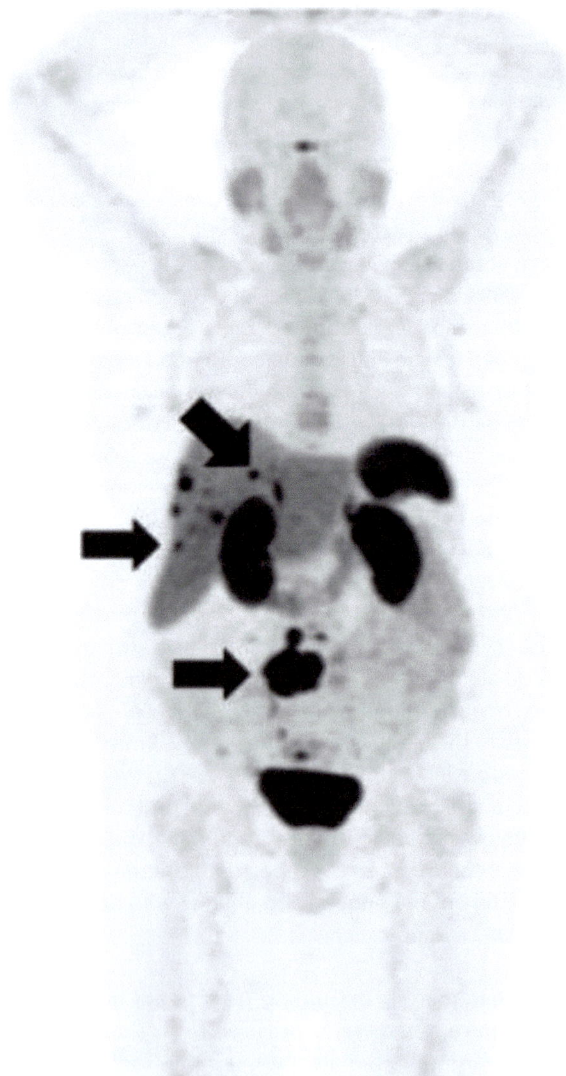

Fig. 22.1 An example of a ^{68}Ga-DOTATATE PET scan in a patient with metastatic Grade 1 neuroendocrine tumour of the small bowel. The *arrows* indicate areas of avidity in hepatic lesions as well as the small bowel primary

intra-patient tumour heterogeneity and potentially directing the choice of medical treatment. The improvement in resolution with Ga-labelled DOTATATE/TOC/NOC PET has also allowed for more accurate imaging of somatostatin receptor density, thus identifying suitable patients for PRRT.

Two of the trials providing seminal treatment evidence (CLARINET and NETTER-1) required uptake on somatostatin receptor scintigraphy (either OctreoScan or 68Ga-based PET) for eligibility. More importantly, PRRT is thought to require sufficient somatostatin receptor density (evidenced by uptake on OctreoScan or ^{68}Ga-based PET) to have clinical effect. In practice, the cutoff for OctreoScan is uptake more than the baseline intensity of the liver (Krenning score > =2) and an unresolved issue for ^{68}Gallium PET. Although analysis of a small series suggests correlation between ^{68}Ga SUV_{max} and likelihood of response on a lesional basis [60], there have been few prospective trials in this area. The use of ^{68}Ga-based PET as a potential quantitative predictive biomarker in PRRT is an important clinical question.

Frequency and Mode of Follow-Up

The optimal frequency of follow-up and disease reassessment in metastatic NETs is unknown. Whilst frequent follow-up may detect early tumour progression, the benefit of early switch (or initiation) of therapy is unknown. A large proportion of patients will have relatively indolent, Grade 1 disease which may be well controlled with SSA therapy alone over a period of years. Frequent follow-up for this cohort of patients may be less appropriate. Factors to consider in formulation of a follow-up plan include the anxiety caused to patients and family as well as travel and other costs to the patient and the healthcare system.

Current guidelines vary widely in terms of suggested follow-up regimens even for the same grade and stage of disease. For instance, ENETS guidelines suggest yearly (or longer) follow-up with ultrasound, computed tomography (CT) or magnetic resonance imaging (MRI) for metastatic Grade 1 ileal NETs after the first year [56], but ESMO guidelines suggest 3–6 monthly CT/MRI [14]; NANETS does not state any particular frequency. Nuclear imaging may play an increasing role in following disease and assessment of treatment response with the introduction of ^{68}Ga-based PET. There are no studies comparing different follow-up regimens in the metastatic setting. Whilst awaiting such evidence, follow-up should be individualised to both patient and tumour factors, taking into account grade, burden of disease, symptom load (both functional and related to tumour burden) and comorbidities/quality of life.

Management Strategy: Integrating Available Modalities in G1–G2 NET

Recent progress in developing new therapeutic modalities for metastatic Grade 1–2 ileal NETs has led to the dilemma of sequencing these agents. Upfront observation for the patient with small-volume, non-functioning nonprogressive Grade 1 NET is a reasonable option which may reduce the number of investigations and preserve quality of life. If upfront treatment is needed, or progression occurs on observation, SSAs represent the most common first-line management [13], given the relative low toxicity and the accumulated clinical trial evidence. However, the optimal choice of agents after progression on SSAs is not defined, with randomised evidence for both PRRT and everolimus. The choice may depend on the anticipated side effect profile (the choice of everolimus in a patient with renal impairment or PRRT in a patient with poorly controlled diabetes mellitus), access to therapy (cost and regional availability) and tumour characteristics (uptake on nuclear imaging). Dose escalation of SSAs is also a reasonable strategy for patients with significant functional symptoms or slowly progressive disease.

Chemotherapy and interferon are all potential options which are largely reserved now for refractory disease, sequenced with debulking surgery, liver directed therapy and even retreatment with PRRT where appropriate. Re-biopsy or additional nuclear imaging (such as FDG-PET to define more aggressive disease) should be considered over the course of disease, particularly if the clinical course observed does not correspond to the initial histological grade. Clinical trial participation should be encouraged so that further progress can be made in this uncommon tumour building on the achievements of the past decade.

Grade 3 NETs and NECs

Grade 3 NETs are rare but present with more aggressive behaviour. There is a wide spectrum of clinical behaviours observed in traditionally classified Grade 3 NETs, which can be divided into well-differentiated NETs and poorly differentiated neuroendocrine carcinomas (NECs), the latter being associated with a higher Ki-67 and poorer prognosis [61]. The most recent histopathological classification may separate these two categories, reserving NEC for high-grade cancers akin to small cell cancers of the lung.

In contrast to Grade 1–2 NETs, chemotherapy is the preferred treatment in Grade 3 disease. Poorly differentiated NECs with Ki-67 index above 55% may show a superior response rate to platinum-based doublet chemotherapy (such as cisplatin/etoposide) compared to those with Ki-67 index below 55% [62]. Current trials exist comparing different regimens for Grade 3 NEC such as cisplatin/etoposide or carboplatin/etoposide, capecitabine/temozolomide (CAPTEM) (NCT02595424) and nab-paclitaxel (NCT02215447). Evidence for second-line therapies is sparse. Retreatment with regimens which provided a good period of disease control is reasonable; alternate chemotherapy agents including CAV (cyclophosphamide, doxorubicin and vincristine) and those used in other gastrointestinal tumours (e.g. combinations of 5-fluorouracil, oxaliplatin and irinotecan) have been used but have relatively little data to support any particular approach.

Quality of Life and Patient Experience in Metastatic Ileal NETs

NETs are characterised by their vast heterogeneity on the background of relatively low incidence. This means that the patient journey for a patient with indolent Grade 1 NET may differ vastly to another patient with a NEC. A recent global survey of 1928 patients with NETs showed that a diagnosis of NET had negative impacts on personal and work lives, with the problem compounded by delayed diagnosis and limited availability to NET experts or specialist centres [1]. Further research into patient experiences with NET can help direct research and scarce resources, so as to minimise the impact of living with NET.

Future Research

Although significant progress in diagnosis and treatment of metastatic ileal NETs has been made, a number of important clinical questions remain (▶ Box 22.1). Large clinical trials are needed to study NET according to site of origin and account for the large variation in disease behaviour. New agents including immunotherapy are being explored. Sequencing and combination of existing therapies are also important.

Box 22.1 Future Directions in NETs

- *Future directions in NETs*
- *Pathology*
  - Reaching consensus regarding classification of Grade 3 NETs and NECs
- *Management*
  - Sequencing of currently available treatments
  - Optimisation of SSA dosages; understanding SSA pharmacokinetics
  - New systemic options for Grade 3 NETs/NECs
  - Treatment of refractory carcinoid syndrome
- *Follow-up*
  - Follow-up intervals for patients being observed only
  - Follow-up intervals for patients on systemic treatment

22.2 Conclusion

Metastatic ileal NETs are a heterogeneous entity, best classified by the WHO 2010 histological grade. Multiple options in Grade 1–2 NETs have been proven in randomised controlled trials over the last decade. After observation or SSAs in the first-line setting, everolimus, PRRT, interferon, chemotherapy, surgery and liver-directed treatment all play a part in management. As a result, a multidisciplinary approach to the patient is essential, taking into account patient and tumour factors as well as local availability and expertise.

Grade 3 NETs are rare, and chemotherapy is the mainstay of treatment. More trials are needed in this setting to provide further treatment options.

The development of nuclear medicine – both diagnostic (somatostatin receptor-based PET scans) and therapeutic (PRRT) – represents a new and impressive modality with recent randomised evidence supporting its efficacy. Further developments have the potential both to change our understanding of NET heterogeneity and to redefine the treatment landscape. There is an ongoing need for clinical trials and translational research to continue improving outcomes from this uncommon and complex disease.

Acknowledgements We acknowledge the help of Professor Dale Bailey in providing ◘ Fig. 22.1.

References

1. Singh S, Granberg D, Wolin E, Warner R, Sissons M, Kolarova T et al (2016) Patient-reported burden of a neuroendocrine tumor (NET) diagnosis: results from the first global survey of patients with NETs. J Glob Oncol [Internet] [Cited 2016 Sep 5]. Available from: http://jgo.ascopubs.org/cgi/doi/10.1200/JGO.2015.002980
2. Capurso G, Rinzivillo M, Bettini R, Boninsegna L, Delle Fave G, Falconi M (2012) Systematic review of resection of primary midgut carcinoid tumour in patients with unresectable liver metastases. Br J Surg 99(11):1480–1486
3. Fatti LM, Scacchi M, Lavezzi E, Pecori Giraldi F, De Martin M, Toja P et al (2006) Effects of treatment with somatostatin analogues on QT interval duration in acromegalic patients. Clin Endocrinol 65(5):626–630
4. Kulke MH, Hörsch D, Caplin ME, Anthony LB, Bergsland E, Öberg K et al (2017) Telotristat ethyl, a tryptophan hydroxylase inhibitor for the treatment of carcinoid syndrome. J Clin Oncol Off J Am Soc Clin Oncol 35(1):14–23
5. Hallet J, Law CHL, Cukier M, Saskin R, Liu N, Singh S (2015) Exploring the rising incidence of neuroendocrine tumors: a population-based analysis of epidemiology, metastatic presentation, and outcomes. Cancer 121(4):589–597
6. Yao JC, Hassan M, Phan A, Dagohoy C, Leary C, Mares JE et al (2008) One hundred years after "carcinoid": epidemiology of and prognostic factors for neuroendocrine tumors in 35,825 cases in the United States. J Clin Oncol 26(18):3063–3072
7. Bosman FT, World Health Organization, International Agency for Research on Cancer (eds) (2010) WHO classification of tumours of the digestive system. 4th edn. International Agency for Research on Cancer, Lyon, 417 p (World Health Organization classification of tumours)
8. Meijer WG, Kema IP, Volmer M, Willemse PH, de Vries EG (2000) Discriminating capacity of indole markers in the diagnosis of carcinoid tumors. Clin Chem 46(10):1588–1596
9. Townsend A, Price T, Yeend S, Pittman K, Patterson K, Luke C (2010) Metastatic carcinoid tumor: changing patterns of care over two decades. J Clin Gastroenterol 44:195–199
10. Rinke A, Müller H-H, Schade-Brittinger C, Klose K-J, Barth P, Wied M et al (2009) Placebo-controlled, double-blind, prospective, randomized study on the effect of octreotide LAR in the control of tumor growth in patients with metastatic neuroendocrine midgut tumors: a report from the PROMID Study Group. J Clin Oncol Off J Am Soc Clin Oncol 27(28):4656–4663
11. Caplin ME, Pavel M, Ćwikła JB, Phan AT, Raderer M, Sedláčková E et al (2014) Lanreotide in metastatic enteropancreatic neuroendocrine tumors. N Engl J Med 371(3):224–233
12. Wolin E, Jarzab B, Eriksson B, Walter T, Toumpanakis C, Morse MA et al (2015) Phase III study of pasireotide long-acting release in patients with metastatic neuroendocrine tumors and carcinoid symptoms refractory to available somatostatin analogues. Drug Des Devel Ther 9:5075–5086
13. Pavel M, O'Toole D, Costa F, Capdevila J, Gross D, Kianmanesh R et al (2016) ENETS consensus guidelines update for the Management of Distant Metastatic Disease of intestinal, pancreatic, bronchial neuroendocrine neoplasms (NEN) and NEN of unknown primary site. Neuroendocrinology 103(2):172–185
14. Oberg K, Akerstrom G, Rindi G, Jelic S (2010) Neuroendocrine gastroenteropancreatic tumours: ESMO clinical practice guidelines for diagnosis, treatment and follow-up. Ann Oncol 21(Suppl 5):v223–v227
15. Kunz PL, Reidy-Lagunes D, Anthony LB, Bertino EM, Brendtro K, Chan JA et al (2013) Consensus guidelines for the management and treatment of neuroendocrine tumors. Pancreas 42:557–577
16. Ito T, Tanaka M, Sasano H, Osamura YR, Sasaki I, Kimura W et al (2007) Preliminary results of a Japanese nationwide survey of neuroendocrine gastrointestinal tumors. J Gastroenterol 42(6):497–500
17. Marshall JB, Bodnarchuk G (1993) Carcinoid tumors of the gut. Our experience over three decades and review of the literature. J Clin Gastroenterol 16(2):123–129
18. Shen C, Dasari A, Zhou S, Chu Y, Xu Y, Shih Y-CT et al (2016) Functional status of neuroendocrine tumors among elderly patients: a large population-based study using SEER-Medicare data. ASCO Meet Abstr 34(15_suppl):4097
19. Gustafsson BI, Tømmerås K, Nordrum I, Loennechen JP, Brunsvik A, Solligård E et al (2005) Long-term serotonin administration induces heart valve disease in rats. Circulation 111(12):1517–1522

20. di Bartolomeo M, Bajetta E, Buzzoni R, Mariani L, Carnaghi C, Somma L et al (1996) Clinical efficacy of octreotide in the treatment of metastatic neuroendocrine tumors. A study by the Italian trials in medical oncology group. Cancer 77(2):402–408
21. Strosberg JR, Benson AB, Huynh L, Duh MS, Goldman J, Sahai V et al (2014) Clinical benefits of above-standard dose of octreotide LAR in patients with neuroendocrine tumors for control of carcinoid syndrome symptoms: a multicenter retrospective chart review study. Oncologist 19(9):930–936
22. Al-Efraij K, Aljama MA, Kennecke HF (2015) Association of dose escalation of octreotide long-acting release on clinical symptoms and tumor markers and response among patients with neuroendocrine tumors. Cancer Med 4(6):864–870
23. Faiss S, Pape U-F, Böhmig M, Dörffel Y, Mansmann U, Golder W et al (2003) Prospective, randomized, multicenter trial on the antiproliferative effect of lanreotide, interferon alfa, and their combination for therapy of metastatic neuroendocrine gastroenteropancreatic tumors – the International Lanreotide and Interferon Alfa Study Group. J Clin Oncol Off J Am Soc Clin Oncol 21(14):2689–2696
24. Ferolla P, Faggiano A, Grimaldi F, Ferone D, Scarpelli G, Ramundo V et al (2012) Shortened interval of long-acting octreotide administration is effective in patients with well-differentiated neuroendocrine carcinomas in progression on standard doses. J Endocrinol Investig 35(3):326–331
25. Anthony L, Johnson D, Hande K, Shaff M, Winn S, Krozely M et al (1993) Somatostatin analogue phase I trials in neuroendocrine neoplasms. Acta Oncol Stockh Swed 32(2):217–223
26. Faggiano A, Carratù AC, Guadagno E, Tafuto S, Tatangelo F, Riccardi F et al (2016) Somatostatin analogues according to Ki67 index in neuroendocrine tumours: an observational retrospective-prospective analysis from real life. Oncotarget 7(5):5538–5547
27. Kulke MH, Horsch D, Caplin M, Anthony L, Bergsland E, Oberg K et al (2015) 37LBA Telotristat etiprate is effective in treating patients with carcinoid syndrome that is inadequately controlled by somatostatin analog therapy (the phase 3 TELESTAR clinical trial). Eur J Cancer 51:S728
28. Hashemolhosseini S, Nagamine Y, Morley SJ, Desrivières S, Mercep L, Ferrari S (1998) Rapamycin inhibition of the G1 to S transition is mediated by effects on cyclin D1 mRNA and protein stability. J Biol Chem 273(23):14424–14429
29. Dufner A, Thomas G (1999) Ribosomal S6 kinase signaling and the control of translation. Exp Cell Res 253(1):100–109
30. Johannessen CM, Reczek EE, James MF, Brems H, Legius E, Cichowski K (2005) The NF1 tumor suppressor critically regulates TSC2 and mTOR. Proc Natl Acad Sci U S A 102(24):8573–8578
31. Kasajima A, Pavel M, Darb-Esfahani S, Noske A, Stenzinger A, Sasano H et al (2011) mTOR expression and activity patterns in gastroenteropancreatic neuroendocrine tumours. Endocr Relat Cancer 18(1):181–192
32. Yao JC, Lombard-Bohas C, Baudin E, Kvols LK, Rougier P, Ruszniewski P et al (2010) Daily oral everolimus activity in patients with metastatic pancreatic neuroendocrine tumors after failure of cytotoxic chemotherapy: a phase II trial. J Clin Oncol 28(1):69–76
33. Pavel ME, Hainsworth JD, Baudin E, Peeters M, Hörsch D, Winkler RE et al (2011) Everolimus plus octreotide long-acting repeatable for the treatment of advanced neuroendocrine tumours associated with carcinoid syndrome (RADIANT-2): a randomised, placebo-controlled, phase 3 study. Lancet 378(9808):2005–2012
34. Yao JC, Shah MH, Ito T, Bohas CL, Wolin EM, Van Cutsem E et al (2011) Everolimus for advanced pancreatic neuroendocrine tumors. N Engl J Med 364:514–523
35. Yao JC, Fazio N, Singh S, Buzzoni R, Carnaghi C, Wolin E et al (2016) Everolimus for the treatment of advanced, non-functional neuroendocrine tumours of the lung or gastrointestinal tract (RADIANT-4): a randomised, placebo-controlled, phase 3 study. Lancet Lond Engl 387(10022):968–977
36. Yao JC, Hainsworth JD, Wolin EM, Pavel ME, Baudin E, Gross D et al (2012) Multivariate analysis including biomarkers in the phase III RADIANT-2 study of octreotide LAR plus everolimus (E+O) or placebo (P+O) among patients with advanced neuroendocrine tumors (NET). J Clin Oncol 30(suppl):Abstr 4014
37. Singh S, Carnaghi C, Buzzoni R, Raderer M, Lahner H, Valle JW et al (2016) Everolimus for advanced, progressive, nonfunctional neuroendocrine tumors (NET) of the gastrointestinal (GI) tract: efficacy and safety from a RADIANT-4 subgroup analysis. ENETS 2016. P. Abstr L20
38. Yazdani S, Kasajima A, Tamaki K, Nakamura Y, Fujishima F, Ohtsuka H et al (2014) Angiogenesis and vascular maturation in neuroendocrine tumors. Hum Pathol 45(4):866–874

39. Kuiper P (2011) Angiogenic markers endoglin and vascular endothelial growth factor in gastroenteropancreatic neuroendocrine tumors. World J Gastroenterol 17(2):219
40. Chan JA, Blaszkowsky L, Stuart K, Zhu AX, Allen J, Wadlow R et al (2013) A prospective, phase 1/2 study of everolimus and temozolomide in patients with advanced pancreatic neuroendocrine tumor. Cancer 119:3212–3218
41. Yao J, Guthrie K, Moran C, Strosberg JR, Kulke MH, Chan JA et al (2015) SWOG S0518: Phase III prospective randomized comparison of depot octreotide plus interferon alpha-2b versus depot octreotide plus bevacizumab (NSC #704865) in advanced, poor prognosis carcinoid patients (NCT00569127). J Clin Oncol 33(Suppl):Abstr 4004
42. Kulke MH, Lenz HJ, Meropol NJ, Posey J, Ryan DP, Picus J et al (2008) Activity of sunitinib in patients with advanced neuroendocrine tumors. J Clin Oncol 26:3403–3410
43. Bello C, Deprimo SE, Friece C, Smeraglia J, Sherman L, Tye L et al (2006) Analysis of circulating biomarkers of sunitinib malate in patients with unresectable neuroendocrine tumors (NET): VEGF, IL-8, and soluble VEGF receptors 2 and 3. ASCO Meet Abstr 24(18_suppl):4045
44. Raymond E, Dahan L, Raoul JL, Bang YJ, Borbath I, Lombard-Bohas C et al (2011) Sunitinib malate for the treatment of pancreatic neuroendocrine tumors. N Engl J Med 364:501–513
45. Phan AT, Halperin DM, Chan JA, Fogelman DR, Hess KR, Malinowski P et al (2015) Pazopanib and depot octreotide in advanced, well-differentiated neuroendocrine tumours: a multicentre, single-group, phase 2 study. Lancet Oncol 16:695–703
46. Grande E, Capdevila J, Castellano D, Teulé A, Durán I, Fuster J et al (2015) Pazopanib in pretreated advanced neuroendocrine tumors: a phase II, open-label trial of the Spanish Task Force Group for Neuroendocrine Tumors (GETNE). Ann Oncol 26(9):1987–1993
47. Wong MH, Chan DL, Lee A, Li BT, Lumba S, Clarke SJ et al (2016) Systematic review and meta-analysis on the role of chemotherapy in advanced and metastatic neuroendocrine tumor (NET). Stemmer SM, editor. PLoS One 11(6):e0158140
48. Venook AP, Ko AH, Tempero MA, Uy J, Weber T, Korn M et al (2008) Phase II trial of FOLFOX plus bevacizumab in advanced, progressive neuroendocrine tumors. ASCO Meet Abstr 26(15_suppl):15545
49. Kunz PL, Kuo T, Zahn JM, Kaiser HL, Norton JA, Visser BC et al (2010) A phase II study of capecitabine, oxaliplatin, and bevacizumab for metastatic or unresectable neuroendocrine tumors. ASCO Meet Abstr 28(15_suppl):4104
50. Fine RL, Gulati AP, Tsushima D, Mowatt KB, Oprescu A, Bruce JN et al (2014) Prospective phase II study of capecitabine and temozolomide (CAPTEM) for progressive, moderately, and well-differentiated metastatic neuroendocrine tumors. ASCO Meet Abstr 32(3_suppl):179
51. Wick W, Weller M, van den Bent M, Sanson M, Weiler M, von Deimling A et al (2014) MGMT testing—the challenges for biomarker-based glioma treatment. Nat Rev Neurol 10(7):372–385
52. Kulke MH, Hornick JL, Frauenhoffer C, Hooshmand S, Ryan DP, Enzinger PC et al (2009) O6-methylguanine DNA methyltransferase deficiency and response to temozolomide-based therapy in patients with neuroendocrine tumors. Clin Cancer Res 15(1):338–345
53. Cives M, Ghayouri M, Morse B, Brelsford M, Black M, Rizzo A et al (2016). Analysis of potential response predictors to capecitabine/temozolomide in metastatic pancreatic neuroendocrine tumors. Endocr Relat Cancer 23(9):759–767
54. Granberg D, Eriksson B, Wilander E, Grimfjärd P, Fjällskog ML, Oberg K et al (2001) Experience in treatment of metastatic pulmonary carcinoid tumors. Ann Oncol Off J Eur Soc Med Oncol ESMO 12(10):1383–1391
55. Mirvis E, Mandair D, Garcia-Hernandez J, Mohmaduvesh M, Toumpanakis C, Caplin M (2014) Role of interferon-alpha in patients with neuroendocrine tumors: a retrospective study. Anticancer Res 34(11):6601–6607
56. Arnold R, Chen Y-J, Costa F, Falconi M, Gross D, Grossman AB et al (2009) ENETS consensus guidelines for the standards of care in neuroendocrine tumors: follow-up and documentation. Neuroendocrinology 90(2):227–233
57. Kolby L, Persson G, Franzen S, Ahren B (2003) Randomized clinical trial of the effect of interferon alpha on survival in patients with disseminated midgut carcinoid tumours. Br J Surg 90:687–693
58. Gulec SA, Mountcastle TS, Frey D, Cundiff JD, Mathews E, Anthony L et al (2002) Cytoreductive surgery in patients with advanced-stage carcinoid tumors. Am Surg 68(8):667. -671-672

59. Strosberg JR, Wolin EM, Chasen B, Kulke MH, Bushnell DL, Caplin ME et al (2016) NETTER-1 phase III: Progression-free survival, radiographic response, and preliminary overall survival results in patients with midgut neuroendocrine tumors treated with 177-Lu-Dotatate. J Clin Oncol 34(Suppl 4S): Abstr 194
60. Kratochwil C, Stefanova M, Mavriopoulou E, Holland-Letz T, Dimitrakopoulou-Strauss A, Afshar-Oromieh A et al (2015) SUV of [68Ga]DOTATOC-PET/CT predicts response probability of PRRT in neuroendocrine tumors. Mol Imaging Biol 17(3):313–318
61. Basturk O, Yang Z, Tang LH, Hruban RH, Adsay V, McCall CM et al (2015) The high-grade (WHO G3) pancreatic neuroendocrine tumor category is morphologically and biologically heterogeneous and includes both well differentiated and poorly differentiated neoplasms. Am J Surg Pathol 39(5):683–690
62. Sorbye H, Welin S, Langer SW, Vestermark LW, Holt N, Osterlund P et al (2013) Predictive and prognostic factors for treatment and survival in 305 patients with advanced gastrointestinal neuroendocrine carcinoma (WHO G3): the NORDIC NEC study. Ann Oncol Off J Eur Soc Med Oncol ESMO 24(1):152–160

Therapy for Metastatic Disease: Bronchi

Kjell Öberg

A. Colao et al. (eds.), *Neuroendocrine Tumors in Real Life*,
https://doi.org/10.1007/978-3-319-59024-0_23

23

Overview

The clinical management for advanced metastatic lung-NETs requires a multidisciplinary approach involving surgeons, medical and radiation oncologist, as well as endocrinologist. The main aims of the management of lung-NETs are to control the tumor growths as well as endocrine secretory activity. Surgical removal is the treatment of choice for lung-NETs with the aim to remove as much tumor tissue as possible, preserving the lung tissue. Pulmonary surgery is considered in patients with typical and atypical lung-NETs with low proliferation and slow growths, with the aim to remove as much as 90% of metastatic disease. For symptomatic control somatostatin analogs are still the major treatment modality but can sometimes be complimented by interferon and PRRT. To control tumor growth, somatostatin analogs are still a valid alternative for low-proliferating, well-differentiated lung-NETs, supplemented sometimes by local regional therapies such as radiofrequency ablation, embolization, and radioembolization. Systemic cytotoxic treatments include temozolomide alone or in combination with capecitabine. Significant antitumor activity has not been seen in low-grade lung-NETs. Carboplatin plus etoposide is applied in high-grade tumors. Everolimus has now demonstrated in at least two big trials and significant antitumor activity for lung-NETs and is registered for the treatment of low- and intermediate-grade lung-NETs. PRRT is an important adjunct to the treatment arsenal, but there are still limited results published. Combinations of several treatment modalities concomitantly or sequentially are most often applied.

Clinical Case

The case is as follows: The patient is a 42-year-old male from outside Sweden that came in 2006 for second opinion and treatment of an atypical lung-NET with Ki-67 of 95%. Cis-platinum and etoposide had failed. He was started on the triple combination with capecitabine, temozolomide, and bevacizumab (◘ Fig. 23.1). After 4 months of therapy, he was almost free of disease and at 6 moths he was tumor-free. Regular checkups twice a year showed no recurrence, and in June 2016 he is still free of disease, after 10 years.

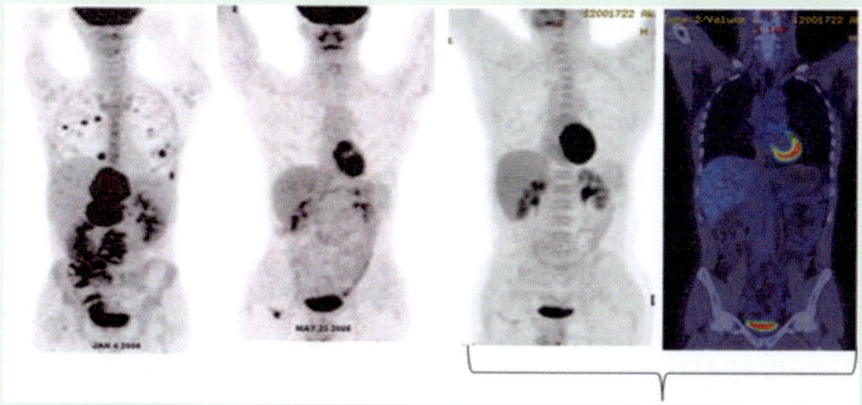

Fig. 23.1 FDG-PET/CT – Patient with atypical lung carcinoid with Ki-67 of 95% responding to the triple combination of capecitabine, temozolomide, and bevacizumab

Questions

1. Which type of chemotherapy is to take into consideration as possible therapeutic option in high-proliferating well-differentiated NETs of the lung (atypical carcinoid)?
2. Is FDG-PET to prefer to Octreoscan/gallium PET in high-proliferating well-differentiated NETs of the lung (atypical carcinoid)?

Answers

1. Platinum/etoposide chemotherapy is to be used in the lung as in gastroentero-pancreatic NET in the poorly differentiated subgroup. Temozolomide ± capecitabine is a potentially effective and safe option in this setting.
2. Even well-differentiated NET could be highly proliferating and of consequence be characterized by intense glucose metabolism. In addition, metabolic changes could be rapid and predict volume changes. For this reason, FDG-PET could be one of the main imaging procedures to detect tumor lesions in these patients as well as to evaluate changes after therapy.

Up-to-Date of the Topic

The clinical management of advanced metastatic lung-NETs, typical (TC) and atypical (AC), requires a multidisciplinary approach involving surgeons, medical and radiation oncologists, as well as endocrinologists. The main aims of the management of lung-NETs are to control the tumor growths and/or endocrine secretory activity, at times also paraneoplastic syndromes. In the absence of curative options in case of metastatic disease, it is to make the quality of life a predominant objective [1–3].

Surgical removal is the treatment of choice for lung-NETs; the aim is to remove the tumor and to preserve as much lung tissue as possible. The surgical approach is dependent on the size, location, and the tissue type [4–6]. Surgery for metastatic disease as part of a multimodality management of the patients is not fully explored.

If pulmonary surgery is considered, the consensus would be to reserve surgery for patients with limited sites of disease with curative intent where radical treatment is possible for all sites [7]. Such surgery usually applies to TC and perhaps sometimes AC carcinoid with low mitotic counts. Surgical resection of liver metastases can be considered with curative intent to aid symptom control or for debulking where more than 90% of tumor can be removed [7]. Complete resection of liver metastases has increased 5-year overall survival rate. The minimal requirements for curative intent are [8]:

1. Resectable G1–G2 liver disease with acceptable morbidity and <5% mortality
2. Absence of right heart insufficiency
3. Absence of unresectable lymph node and extra abdominal metastases
4. Absence of diffuse or unresectable peritoneal carcinomatosis

Symptomatic Control

Lung-NETs (the percentage compared to gastroenteropancreatic ones (10–12% vs 30%) [1]. Somatostatin analog constitutes the gold standard for symptomatic control. Flushing and diarrhea improved in >50% of cases [9]. When Cushing's syndrome is present, it can be treated with the commonly available drugs such as ketoconazole, metyrapone, etomidate, or mifepristone [2]. In the absence of hormonal control, many patients may benefit from somatostatin analogs or interferon associated with local regional therapy (liver palliative surgery, radiofrequency ablation, and transarterial chemoembolization) [8, 10, 11]. Some patients with ectopic ACTH syndrome might respond to somatostatin analogs but usually in combination with alpha interferon and PRRT in selected patients [2, 8, 12, 13]. Prophylaxis against carcinoid crisis should be carried out before surgical or local regional intervention using an adequate dosage of somatostatin analog. For major procedures, a preoperative intravenous bolus of 100–200 μg followed by a continued infusion of 50–100 μg/h during the procedure is recommended, and the dose can be increased if required. Infusion should continue for 24 h postoperatively before being slowly tapered out over the next 48 h. In such cases it is likely that patients will require long-acting somatostatin analog [8, 14].

Tumor Control

There are very few prospective trials dedicated to lung-NETs that may guide treatment; most literatures consist of case series or studies that deal with a mixed population of primary NET patients. In asymptomatic patients, mainly with advanced TC or AC with low proliferative index as well as low tumor burden, a watch-and-wait policy might be considered and explained to the patient on the basis of regular cross-sectional imaging, initially every 3–6 months [2].

Somatostatin analogs can induce stabilization in 30–70% of patients with well-differentiated NETs, as demonstrated in multiple prospective and retrospective studies that include lung-NETs [15, 16]. There are no dedicated trials available for lung primary NETs except for the so-called LUNA trial where pasireotide is included in one of the arms or in combination with the mTOR inhibitor everolimus in a second arm. The third arm contains everolimus alone; the data from this trial are not available yet but will be presented at ESMO 2016. The randomized placebo-controlled PROMID study with octreotide LAR 30 mg vs placebo in midgut NETs demonstrates antitumor control with median time to progression significantly longer in the octreotide LAR group than placebo, 14.3 months vs 6 months, respectively [17]. The phase III randomized placebo-controlled CLARINET study in 204 patients with nonfunctioning enteropancreatic NETs, allocated either lanreotide autogel 120 mg every 28 days or placebo, shows significantly prolonged progression-free survival over placebo ($p = 0.0002$) [18]. The most commonly used long-acting somatostatin analogs are octreotide LAR by deep intramuscular injection and lanreotide autogel given deep subcutaneously, both administrated every 28 days. Due to their excellent safety profile, somatostatin analogs should be considered as first-line systemic treatment of patients with advanced lung-NETs with low proliferation index (TC and AC) and positive somatostatin receptor scintigraphy [2]. In patients with slowly progressive tumors, multiple local regional therapies aiming at reducing burden and targeting the bronchial primary and liver, bone, or lung metastases should be considered [14, 18].

Local Regional Therapies

Radiofrequency ablation or cryoablation of the primary tumor is occasionally considered as an adjuvant to surgery or whenever resection is not possible. Liver but also bone or lung metastases constitute potential targets of RF ablation. Embolization of liver metastases is another option for local regional therapy, either using bland particles or cytotoxics combined with particles or radioactive beads. Radiological responses rate between 30% and 70%. There is no evidence of beneficial response of chemoembolization over particle embolization alone. There is emerging evidence of using radioactive microspheres as yttrium-90 beads in liver metastases (SIRT) [8, 10, 19, 20].

Peptide Radio-Receptor Therapy (PRRT)

Well-differentiated lung-NETs frequently express subtype 2 of the somatostatin receptor family; PRRT may be used to treat metastases of TCs and ACs with yttrium^{90}-DOTADOC-octreotide or ^{177}lutetium-DOTA-octreotide [12, 13, 21]. This treatment has proven to be particularly promising in selected patients with high uptake of SRS [13]. So far no randomized controlled trials have been performed, but small numbers of patients from various European centers have reported interesting response rates, up to 50% partial remission. Although most studies are limited to single centers, a large retrospective study looks at 1100 metastatic NETs including 84 lung-NETs of which 28% showed a morphological response as estimated by RECIST criteria and 38% showed a clinical response with a median survival of 40 months. Grade 3–4 toxicity was reported in 10–33% of the patients, mainly renal or hematological toxicity [12].

Systemic Chemotherapy

Systemic chemotherapy should be considered in patients with advanced unresectable, progressive lung-NETs. In general, results with chemotherapy have been largely disappointing, and survival data have to be interpreted with caution due to the small number of patients and the mixed population of primary tumors. Overall response rates above <30% have been described with 5-FU-dacarbacin and temozolomide alone or in combination, but also a combination of 5-FU with streptozotocin or oxaliplatin [22–28]. The value in the management of advanced lung-NETs remains unclear, but grade 3–4 toxicity is expected in about 10%. Temozolomide could be considered in cases with brain metastases, and analysis of methylguanine-DNA-methyltransferase expression in NETs may help to select responders [29]. A triple combination of temozolomide plus capecitabine plus bevacizumab has sometimes been effective in patients with AC with very high proliferation, above 50% Ki-67 (personal experience) (▪ Fig. 23.1). Cisplatin plus etoposide or carboplatin plus etoposide should be reserved for patients with high-grade tumors due to its significant rate of toxicity [28].

mTOR Inhibitors

The main target of rapamycin (mTOR) has been identified as a kinase activated in the PI3-kinase signaling pathway of lung-NETs. Recently, activation of PI3-kinase pathway was reported in both TC and AC lung-NETs [30]. In the randomized phase III trial, RADIANT-2 assessed everolimus 10 mg plus octreotide LAR vs placebo plus octreotide LAR in 429 patients in non-pancreatic tumors, where 44 primaries were of bronchial origin. The study demonstrated a clinically significant 5.1-month increasing median progression-free survival [31]. The RAMSETE study analyzed the antitumor benefit of everolimus in 119 foregut-derived NETs with progression-free survival of 189 days reported [32]. As previously mentioned, the LUNA study, a three-arm phase II trial, assesses everolimus alone vs pasireotide alone vs the combination of both. The study is closed and the result will be presented in the next few months. The randomized phase III study, RADIANT-4 which assessed everolimus 10 mg vs placebo in 279 patients with nonfunctioning NETs including lung-NETs, has recently been finished. The median PFS in the treatment arm was 11 months vs 3.9 months in the placebo arm [33]. The hazard ratio was 0.48, 50 patients with lung-NETs that had a HR ratio of 0.50 presenting a clear efficacy of everolimus in this group of both typical and atypical lung carcinoids.

Anti-angiogenic Therapy

The place of anti-angiogenic therapy in lung-NETs remains uncertain. Sunitinib is an orally administered kinase inhibitor (small molecule) with activity against a number of tyrosine kinase receptors including VGFR-1, VGFR-2, and VGFR-3 and PDGFR-α and PDGFR-β. A phase II study evaluated the activity of sunitinib in 109 NET patients including 41 with carcinoids of which 14 were foregut tumors including lung-NETs. In the carcinoid patients, overall response rate was 2.4%, stable disease in 83%, and time to tumor progression of 10.2 months. The PAZONET study with pazopanib as a sequencing in treatment in progressive metastatic NET showed clinical benefit in 85% of patients treated with pazopanib including patients with lung carcinoids [34].

Bevacizumab is an anti-vascular endothelial growth factor (VEGF) monoclonal antibody. In a phase II study, patients were randomized to bevacizumab or pegylated interferon; 21 out of 22 patients demonstrated partial response in the bevacizumab group where 4 patients have lung-NETs [35]. One phase II study evaluated the antitumor efficacy of sorafenib plus bevacizumab combination in 44 NETs including 19 foreguts. A 10% overall response rate was reported in digestive NETs [36]. Promising results have been published with a combination with bevacizumab and chemotherapy [37].

23.1 Conclusions

Somatostatin analogs may be considered as first-line systemic antiproliferative treatment of patients with advanced and non-resectable lung-NETs with low proliferative index and slowly progressive. Local regional options including surgery for primary metastases will always be considered for slow progressive lung-NETs. Cytotoxic treatment has been the standard for aggressive metastatic lung-NETs and demonstrates activity in TC and AC lung-NETs with high proliferation. Temozolomide alone or in combination with capecitabine plus/minus bevacizumab demonstrates a clinical benefit. The combination has been particularly useful in patients with high-proliferating tumors. The PRRT is an option in patients with tumors that demonstrate high expression of somatostatin receptors. Publication of data from the RADIANT-4 study is reporting on activity of everolimus in typical and atypical lung-NETs. Everolimus should be considered as a treatment of choice for many patients with low- to intermediate-grade lung-NETs. Data from the LUNA study is still pending but might further support the role of everolimus in the treatment of lung-NETs.

Bibliography

1. Ferolla P (2014) Medical treatment of advanced thoracic neuroendocrine tumors. Thorac Surg Clin 24(3):351–355
2. Caplin ME et al (2015) Pulmonary neuroendocrine (carcinoid) tumors: European Neuroendocrine Tumor Society expert consensus and recommendations for best practice for typical and atypical pulmonary carcinoids. Ann Oncol 26(8):1604–1620
3. Filosso PL et al (2015) Multidisciplinary management of advanced lung neuroendocrine tumors. J Thorac Dis 7(Suppl 2):S163–S171
4. Daddi N et al (2004) Surgical treatment of neuroendocrine tumors of the lung. Eur J Cardiothorac Surg 26(4):813–817
5. Detterbeck FC (2010) Management of carcinoid tumors. Ann Thorac Surg 89(3):998–1005
6. Lim E et al (2005) The impact of stage and cell type on the prognosis of pulmonary neuroendocrine tumors. J Thorac Cardiovasc Surg 130(4):969–972
7. Glazer ES et al (2010) Long-term survival after surgical management of neuroendocrine hepatic metastases. HPB (Oxford) 12(6):427–433
8. Pavel M et al (2012) ENETS consensus guidelines for the management of patients with liver and other distant metastases from neuroendocrine neoplasms of foregut, midgut, hindgut, and unknown primary. Neuroendocrinology 95(2):157–176
9. Filosso PL et al (2002) Long-term survival of atypical bronchial carcinoids with liver metastases, treated with octreotide. Eur J Cardiothorac Surg 21(5):913–917

10. Steinmuller T et al (2008) Consensus guidelines for the management of patients with liver metastases from digestive (neuro)endocrine tumors: foregut, midgut, hindgut, and unknown primary. Neuroendocrinology 87(1):47–62
11. Kos-Kudla B et al (2010) ENETS consensus guidelines for the management of bone and lung metastases from neuroendocrine tumors. Neuroendocrinology 91(4):341–350
12. Imhof A et al (2011) Response, survival, and long-term toxicity after therapy with the radiolabeled somatostatin analogue [90Y-DOTA]-TOC in metastasized neuroendocrine cancers. J Clin Oncol 29(17):2416–2423
13. van Essen M et al (2007) Peptide receptor radionuclide therapy with 177Lu-octreotate in patients with foregut carcinoid tumours of bronchial, gastric and thymic origin. Eur J Nucl Med Mol Imaging 34(8):1219–1227
14. Phan AT et al (2010) NANETS consensus guideline for the diagnosis and management of neuroendocrine tumors: well-differentiated neuroendocrine tumors of the thorax (includes lung and thymus). Pancreas 39(6):784–798
15. Aparicio T et al (2001) Antitumour activity of somatostatin analogues in progressive metastatic neuroendocrine tumours. Eur J Cancer 37(8):1014–1019
16. Ducreux M et al (2000) The antitumoral effect of the long-acting somatostatin analog lanreotide in neuroendocrine tumors. Am J Gastroenterol 95(11):3276–3281
17. Rinke A et al (2009) Placebo-controlled, double-blind, prospective, randomized study on the effect of octreotide LAR in the control of tumor growth in patients with metastatic neuroendocrine midgut tumors: a report from the PROMID Study Group. J Clin Oncol 27(28):4656–4663
18. Öberg K et al (2012) Neuroendocrine bronchial and thymic tumors : ESMO Clinical Practice Guidelines for diagnosis, treatment and follow-up. Ann Oncol **23**(Suppl 7):vii120–vii123
19. Kennedy AS et al (2008) Radioembolization for unresectable neuroendocrine hepatic metastases using resin 90Y-microspheres: early results in 148 patients. Am J Clin Oncol 31(3):271–279
20. Cao CQ et al (2010) Radioembolization with yttrium microspheres for neuroendocrine tumour liver metastases. Br J Surg 97(4):537–543
21. Kwekkeboom DJ et al (2008) Treatment with the radiolabeled somatostatin analog [177 Lu-DOTA 0,Tyr3]octreotate: toxicity, efficacy, and survival. J Clin Oncol 26(13):2124–2130
22. Ekeblad S et al (2007) Temozolomide as monotherapy is effective in treatment of advanced malignant neuroendocrine tumors. Clin Cancer Res 13(10):2986–2991
23. Crona J et al (2013) Effect of temozolomide in patients with metastatic bronchial carcinoids. Neuroendocrinology 98(2):151–155
24. Sun W et al (2005) Phase II/III study of doxorubicin with fluorouracil compared with streptozocin with fluorouracil or dacarbazine in the treatment of advanced carcinoid tumors: Eastern Cooperative Oncology Group Study E1281. J Clin Oncol 23(22):4897–4904
25. Bajetta E et al (2007) Are capecitabine and oxaliplatin (XELOX) suitable treatments for progressing low-grade and high-grade neuroendocrine tumours? Cancer Chemother Pharmacol 59(5):637–642
26. Pavel M et al (2010) ENETS consensus guidelines for the management of brain, cardiac and ovarian metastases from neuroendocrine tumors. Neuroendocrinology 91(4):326–332
27. Turner NC et al (2010) Chemotherapy with 5-fluorouracil, cisplatin and streptozocin for neuroendocrine tumours. Br J Cancer 102(7):1106–1112
28. Meyer T et al (2014) Capecitabine and streptozocin +/− cisplatin in advanced gastroenteropancreatic neuroendocrine tumours. Eur J Cancer 50(5):902–911
29. Kulke MH, Scherubl H (2009) Accomplishments in 2008 in the management of gastrointestinal neuroendocrine tumors. Gastrointest Cancer Res 3(5 Suppl 2):S62–S66
30. Hay N (2005) The Akt-mTOR tango and its relevance to cancer. Cancer Cell 8(3):179–183
31. Pavel ME et al (2011) Everolimus plus octreotide long-acting repeatable for the treatment of advanced neuroendocrine tumours associated with carcinoid syndrome (RADIANT-2): a randomised, placebo-controlled, phase 3 study. Lancet 378(9808):2005–2012
32. Pavel M et al (2012) Ramsete: a single-arm, multicenter, single-stage phase ii trial of rad001 (everolimus) in advanced and metastatic silent neuro-endocrine tumours in Europe: analysis by tumor origin. 37th congress of the European-Society-for-Medical-Oncology (ESMO), Sept 28–Oct 02, 2012, Vienna. 23(S9):377–377

33. Yao JC et al (2016) Everolimus for the treatment of advanced, non-functional neuroendocrine tumours of the lung or gastrointestinal tract (RADIANT-4): a randomised, placebo-controlled, phase 3 study. Lancet 387(10022):968–977
34. Pulido EG, Castellano DE, Garcia-Carbonero R et al (2012) PAZONET: results of a phase II trial of pazopanib as a sequencing treatment in progressive metastatic neuroendocrine tumors (NETs) patients (pts), on behalf of the Spanish task force for NETs (GETNE)—NCT01280201
35. Yao JC et al (2008) Targeting vascular endothelial growth factor in advanced carcinoid tumor: a random assignment phase II study of depot octreotide with bevacizumab and pegylated interferon alpha-2b. J Clin Oncol 26(8):1316–1323
36. Castellano D et al (2013) Sorafenib and bevacizumab combination targeted therapy in advanced neuroendocrine tumour: a phase II study of Spanish Neuroendocrine Tumour Group (GETNE0801). Eur J Cancer 49(18):3780–3787
37. Chan JA et al (2012) Prospective study of bevacizumab plus temozolomide in patients with advanced neuroendocrine tumors. J Clin Oncol 30(24):2963–2968

Therapy for Metastatic Disease with Unknown Primary Tumor

Nicola Fazio and Manila Rubino

A. Colao et al. (eds.), *Neuroendocrine Tumors in Real Life*,
https://doi.org/10.1007/978-3-319-59024-0_24

24

Overview

Metastatic neuroendocrine neoplasms (NENs) with an unknown primary (UP) represent a specific subset that can concern both well-differentiated neuroendocrine tumors (NETs) and poorly differentiated neuroendocrine carcinomas (NECs). An appropriate diagnostic work-up is necessary to conclude for UP NEN, including complete pathological report and morphological and functional imaging. Therapeutical approach to UP NEN is controversial and nonevidence based, as only few clinical trials include UP NEN as a specific entity. While in UP NETs the identification of the primary site can have relevant therapeutic implications, it is not the case for UP NECs, where the high grade of the neoplasm usually indicates starting chemotherapy soon. In patients with a metastatic UP NENs, ENETS guidelines suggest to base treatment decisions on grading, functionality, somatostatin receptor status, tumor extent, and hepatic tumor burden.

Metastatic UP NECs are usually approached with chemotherapy, mainly platinum-based; by contrast metastatic UP NETs are managed in a multimodal manner, and they should be discussed within a multidisciplinary NEN-dedicated team given that several different therapies can be proposed and integrated.

Clinical Case

A 39-year-old man undergoes abdominal ultrasound (US) due to persistent dyspepsia. A 3 cm hypoechoic lesion is detected at the epi-mesogastric region. A subsequent esophagogastroduodenoscopy (EGDS) does not show alterations. Then a pancreatic endoscopic US (EUS) is performed, showing a 35 × 25 mm solid lesion that does not look as originating from pancreas, and it is more similar to a lymphadenopathy. Further adenopathies are visible close to pancreatic isthmus and hepatic hilus. A cholangio-magnetic resonance imaging (MRI) does not show dilation of biliary tract, confirming a probable adenopathy with a maximal diameter of 25 mm between pancreas and duodenum, next to the median wall of the second part of duodenum. There is a narrow cleavage with the head of the pancreas. A further 25 mm adenopathy is visible under the uncinate process, and two more adenopathies, 17 and 20 mm, are next to the tail. A Chest X-ray is negative.

On the basis of a suspected lymphoma, no fine needle aspiration (FNA) is performed during EUS, while an explorative laparotomy is performed to obtain histological material. Laparotomy shows the peripancreatic nodes previously detected at MRI. Inspection and manual exploration of the liver and abdominal cavity is negative. In the uncinate process, one lymph node is removed, and intraoperative histological exam indicates a clear cell carcinoma. The definitive histological exam concludes for a well-differentiated NET, Ki-67 = 3%, chromogranin A (CgA), and synaptophysin (SYN) positive.

Based on this diagnosis a total-body somatostatin receptor scintigraphy (SRS) is performed, without any evidence of uptake areas. Then an entero-computed tomography (CT) is performed without any evidence of possible primary site. Blood CgA is normal.

No antitumor therapy is prescribed, and a chest-abdomen CT scan is performed after 3 months, showing stability of the peripancreatic adenopathies.

At this time the patient presents at a NET referral center for a second opinion. He is still asymptomatic, with a good performance status.

A pathology second opinion is requested confirming the initial diagnosis of well-differentiated NET, with 4% Ki-67, CgA positive, and SYN positive. No further immunohistochemical (IHC) analysis has been performed due to the poorness of material. Then a total-body ^{68}gallium-positron emission tomography (PET)-CT-DOTA-TOC ++showed an area of high uptake next to the pancreatic head, probably corresponding to a lymph node, and another area on the wall of jejunum. An entero-CT is performed, showing two adenopathies close to the second portion of the duodenum, corresponding to the uptake areas at PET; no small bowel intrinsic lesion is visible; a contrast-enhancement area in the wall of the first portion of duodenum is detected. Inter-porto-caval and retro-pancreatic adenopathies are showed (maximum diameter 2 cm). Thereafter an EUS is performed showing periduodenal adenopathies infiltrating the duodenal wall.

A multidisciplinary discussion of the case is performed within the NET-dedicated tumor board, and the decision is starting octreotide LAR 30 mg/4 weeks, as the surgical approach is judged at high risk. After around 3 years of therapy the patient is asymptomatic, with a good performance status and good tolerance of octreotide LAR. The adenopathies are morphologically stable at CT scan and functionally stable at ^{68}Ga-PET-CT. Therapy is ongoing.

24.1 Comments to the Case

In this clinical case, the patient has a diagnosis of nodal localizations from a well-differentiated NET with an UP. The stage of the disease is advanced due to the distant nodal spread. A morphological and functional imaging was performed without no evidence of primary site. However a colonoscopy with terminal ileum exploration was not performed; this is a tool often considered to study the distal part of the ileum, possible site of primary NET. Uptake on the jejunum wall at ^{68}gallium-PET-CT-DOTA-TOC suggested a possible primary site in small intestine, but no evidence of morphological lesion at the same site was detected with the entero-CT. Entero-MRI is a possible alternative to the entero-CT to study the small bowel, and video capsule is a further option.

IHC analysis of the metastatic tumor sample can help to suppose the possible primary site even though no IHC test can be considered pathognomonic. In this case the pathologist who reported the second opinion did not receive enough tumor tissue material to perform specific IHC indicating a possible primary site. However it was not considered mandatory given that an explorative laparotomy was performed.

Surgical exploration to identify the primary site of a NET in metastatic NET patients is debated. In this case it was not successful, but it should be considered that no intraoperative further diagnostic tools were performed. For instance intraoperative US, if performed, could have been shown the presence of pancreatic lesions, not visible with CT and MRI.

Questions

1. What is the correct staging work-up to define an unknown primary NET?
2. Should the unknown primary NET be included in clinical trials?
3. What is the utility of searching for the primary site in a patient with metastatic high-grade neuroendocrine carcinoma?

24

Answers

1. In patients who have a histological diagnosis of NET on a metastatic site, a Chest-abdomen CT scan with contrast medium is usually performed to stage the disease; therefore, this is a tool routinely included often as a first exam in patients with a UP NET. An MRI is indicated when abdomen CT scan cannot be performed or is not conclusive [1]. Then, an appropriate work-up of patients with metastatic UP NET should include a total-body ^{68}gallium-DOTA-TOC/–NOC/–TATE-PET-TC. Gallium-PET is superior to SRS for detecting a NET primary site; therefore, SRS should not be used to this scope [2, 3].

   Nevertheless, not all NETs have a high expression of somatostatin type 2 receptors (SSTR2), in particular high-grade NECs; consequently 18-fluorodeoxyglucose (18FDG) PET-CT is recommended in high-grade NECs [4]. Scanning with specific tracers such as 11 carbon-5-hydroxytryptophan (^{11}C-5HTP) or 18 fluorodihydroxyphenylalanine (^{18}F-DOPA) can be used in low-intermediate-grade NETs when gallium-PET is negative, but they are not of routine use (5–6). After a negative work-up for detecting a NET primary site with morphological (chest CT scan + abdomen CT scan or MRI) and functional (^{68}gallium-DOTA-TOC/–NOC/–TATE-PET-TC) total-body staging, then endoscopic exams (EGDS and ileocolonoscopy) +/– entero-CT or entero-MRI may be considered [7, 8]. Colonoscopy should always study the terminal part of the ileum, which sometimes represents the site of the primary tumor. Video capsule is indicated instead of entero-CT or entero-MRI to detect a primary NET in the small bowel [9]. Endoscopic ultrasound (EUS) can be helpful when a pancreatic primary NET is suspected. The pathology report can represent a help to define the instrumental work-up. Although no IHC parameter can be considered conclusive for a NET primary site, some staining can make highly suspected a primary site, such as caudal-type homeobox transcription factor 2 (CDX-2) for the GI tract, thyroid transcription factor 1 (TTF-1) for lung and thyroid, paired box gene 8 (PAX-8) or insulin gene enhancer binding protein Isl-1 (ISLET-1) for pancreas, and serotonin for small bowel [10, 11].

   Some reports suggest abdomen surgical exploration to detect a UP NET. However all these reports are based on retrospective series, where the decision to perform or not a laparotomy or laparoscopy was arbitrary and prior imaging to detect the primary site was different among the various studies.

   Begum et al. showed a survival advantage of a complete surgical tumor resection, in patients who had NETs of UP; therefore, they suggest that all patients with well-differentiated NETs and suspected intestinal neoplasia should be explored to look for a primary tumor [12, 13].

2. The UP NETs should be included in clinical trials, to avoid that patients with this condition lose the opportunity to receive novel therapies. However the characteristics of the UP NET should be well defined in the inclusion criteria of the study to homogenize the population and make the results more reliable.

   In this way also regulatory authorities could have more data to approve new drugs also in this category of NET patients, and clinicians could be more confident to prescribe some drugs to patients with UP NET. Several regulatory trials with new drugs (CLARINET, RADIANT-4, PROMID) included patient with UP NETs [14–16].

3. Neuroendocrine carcinomas are very aggressive malignancies, with 5-year survival rates of 5% and 13 to 57% for small cell neuroendocrine carcinomas (SCNECs) and large cell neuroendocrine carcinomas (LCNECs), respectively [17, 18]. NECs are rare in the gastrointestinal tract, whereas they are frequent in the lung as SCLCs. Survival is poor in NECs, ranging from 38 months for patients with localized disease to 5 months in the metastatic setting [19]. In patients with a metastatic NEC, the morphological staging with CT scan and/or MRI detects a primary site in most cases. When this is not the case, a ^{18}FDG-PET-CT may be helpful as well as IHC. However therapy of a real poorly differentiated metastatic NEC is always a chemotherapy, in the vast majority of cases represented by cisplatin or carboplatin and etoposide [20, 21]. Therefore the primary site usually does not condition the therapeutic choice in these cases. Unlike NETs in NECs, the primary site surgical removal is not considered useful to improve prognosis. Furthermore debulking or cytoreductive surgery and surgical resection of metastasis are not recommended [22].

Up to Date of the Topic

Cancer of unknown primary (CUP) has been traditionally considered as metastatic cancer in the absence of a clinically detectable anatomically defined primary tumor site after an "adequate" diagnostic evaluation [23]. Most CUP are adenocarcinoma. The UP condition can concern also NENs, both well differentiated, as the NETs, and poorly differentiated, as the NECs. Unknown primary incidence in NENs was reported as slightly over 10% [24]. Of course this frequency is related to the diagnostic/staging work-up performed that is different in several series. So far no conventional validated work-up exists to define an UP NEN.

Once a metastatic UP NEN has been defined, the therapeutic approach depends on the biological characteristics of the tumor and clinical picture of the patient. Well-differentiated NETs with SSTR2 functional expression are usually treated as G1-G2 GEP NETs or typical/atypical lung carcinoids. Advanced poorly differentiated NECs are usually approached with platinum-based chemotherapy [25].

Surgical exploration is quite debated. In a series of patients with metastatic disease and occult primary tumors examined surgically, primary tumors were found in the small bowel, appendix, colon, or rectum in 74.6%, and only 3.2% were found in the pancreas [23].

A retrospective study that analyzed 38 trials showed that patients with UP NEN were older (65 years vs 56 years; $p \leq 0.01$) and had a shorter median survival (66 months vs median not reached, respectively) than patients with gastrointestinal or lung NETs. Among patients with NENs UP, 63% had grade 1 G1-G2, 26% G3 tumors, and 11% unknown [26]. In this study survival was significantly influenced by patient's age, chemotherapy, WHO performance status, WHO grade, number of metastatic sites, and surgery, and WHO performance status and surgery were independent predictors of survival. In a subgroup analysis, restricted to patients who have undergone explorative surgery, only a complete tumor resection was associated with good overall survival; on the contrary the overall survival of operated patients with macroscopic tumor remnant was comparable with patients who were not treated with an operative procedure. Authors conclude that a complete tumor resection should be performed when possible, also if primary tumor could not be detected [13]. Other studies also indicated a role for explorative surgery in identification and treatment of primary tumor, in patients with well-differentiated UP NETs and liver metastasis [12, 27]. In a recent published report, 138/800 patients (17%) with a UP NET who have undergone surgical cytoreduction had the primary site discovered intraoperatively in 124 cases (124/138, 90%). The primary tumor could not be identified intraoperatively in 14 patients (14/138, 11%) who underwent 15 surgical cytoreductions (15/1001, 1%) [28]. Stoyianni et al. reviewed 38 articles about UP NENs patients; among a total of 500 patients diagnosed with UP NEN, specific treatment data were available for 336 patients. Forty-eight percent of patients received platinum-based chemotherapy incorporating bleomycin, etoposide, 5-fluorouracil, or taxanes, while 37% patients were administered non-platinum-based regimens. They found, moreover, that in the course of time, there was a shift from platinum salts toward biological targeted therapies. Stoyianni et al. identified three groups of patients with UP NENs: patients with low-grade NETs who do not take advantage of aggressive therapy and experience a protracted disease course, patients with high-grade NECs who respond to systemic chemotherapy, and patients with high-grade NECs who either do not respond to therapy or initially respond to systemic chemotherapy but derive modest survival benefit [29]. Extensive disease, high mitotic index, and immunohistochemically positive markers have been reported as negative prognostic parameters [30].

In patients with UP NENs, ENETS guidelines suggest to base therapeutic decision on grading, functional status, somatostatin receptor status, tumor extent, and hepatic tumor burden [31].

Somatostatin analogs (SSA), octreotide and lanreotide, are recommended as first-line therapy in low-grade functioning NETs, for syndrome controls and also in nonfunctioning NETs, for their antiproliferative effects; PROMID and CLARINET studies also included patients with UP, so SSA may be considered also in this category [14, 15]. Moreover chemotherapy with capecitabine and temozolomide could also be considered in UP NEC G3 [32]. In NEC G3 platinum-based chemotherapy is recommended as first-line therapy [22]. Peptide receptor radionuclide therapy (PRRT) could also be considered in patients with a strong SSTR expression at somatostatin receptor imaging, while extensive hepatic or bone disease may limit its use [33]. Everolimus is recommended in progressing advanced nonfunctional NET of gastrointestinal, lung, or even UP on the basis of the results from the RADIANT-4 trial [16].

Bibliography

1. Kaltsas G, Rockall A, Papadogias D, Reznek R, Grossman AB (2004) Recent advances in radiological and radionuclide imaging and therapy of neuroendocrine tumours. Eur J Endocrinol 151:15–27
2. Schreiter NF, Bartels AM, Froeling V, Steffen I, Pape UF, Beck A, Hamm B, Brenner W, Röttgen R (2014) Searching for primaries in patients with neuroendocrine tumors (NET) of unknown primary and clinically suspected NET: evaluation of Ga-68 DOTATOC PET/CT and in-111 DTPA octreotide SPECT/CT. Radiol Oncol 48(4):339–347
3. Santhanam P, Chandramahanti S, Kroiss A, Yu R, Ruszniewski P, Kumar R, Taïeb D (2015) Nuclear imaging of neuroendocrine tumors with unknown primary: why, when and how? Eur J Nucl Med Mol Imaging 42(7):1144–1155

4. Deroose CM, Hindié E, Kebebew E, Goichot B, Pacak K, Taïeb D, Imperiale A (2016) Molecular imaging of gastroenteropancreatic neuroendocrine tumors: current status and future directions. J Nucl Med 57(12):1949–1956
5. Orlefors H, Sundin A, Garske U, Juhlin C, Oberg K, Skogseid B, Langstrom B, Bergstrom M, Eriksson B (2005) Whole-body (11)C-5-hydroxytryptophan positron emission tomography as a universal imaging technique for neuroendocrine tumors: comparison with somatostatin receptor scintigraphy and computed tomography. J Clin Endocrinol Metab 90:3392–3400
6. Koopmans KP, de Vries EG, Kema IP, Elsinga PH, Neels OC, Sluiter WJ, van der Horst-Schrivers AN, Jager PL (2006) Staging of carcinoid tumours with 18F-DOPA PET: a prospective, diagnostic accuracy study. Lancet Oncol 7:728–734
7. Kamaoui I, De-Luca V, Ficarelli S, Mennesson N, Lombard-Bohas C, Pilleul F (2010) Value of CT enteroclysis in suspected small-bowel carcinoid tumors. AJR Am J Roentgenol 194:629–633
8. Masselli G, Polettini E, Casciani E, Bertini L, Vecchioli A, Gualdi G (2009) Small-bowel neoplasms: prospective evaluation of MR enteroclysis. Radiology 251:743–750
9. Frilling A, Smith G, Clift AK, Martin J (2014) Capsule endoscopy to detect primary tumour site in metastatic neuroendocrine tumours. Dig Liver Dis 46(11):1038–1042
10. Lin X, Saad RS, Luckasevic TM, Silverman JF, Liu Y (2007) Diagnostic value of CDX-2 and TTF-1 expressions in separating metastatic neuroendocrine neoplasms of unknown origin. Appl Immunohistochem Mol Morphol 15(4):407
11. Bellizzi AM (2013) Assigning site of origin in metastatic neuroendocrine neoplasms: a clinically significant application of diagnostic immunohistochemistry. Adv Anat Pathol 20(5):285–314
12. Wang SC, Parekh JR, Zuraek MB, Venook AP, Bergsland EK, Warren RS, Nakakura EK (2010) Identification of unknown primary tumors in patients with neuroendocrine liver metastases. Arch Surg 145(3):276–280
13. Begum N, Wellner U, Thorns C, Brabant G, Hoffmann M, Bürk CG, Lehnert H, Keck T (2015) CUP syndrome in neuroendocrine neoplasia: analysis of risk factors and impact of surgical intervention. World J Surg 39(6):1443–1451
14. Caplin ME, Pavel M, Ćwikła JB, Phan AT, Raderer M, Sedláčková E, Cadiot G, Wolin EM, Capdevila J, Wall L, Rindi G, Langley A, Martinez S, Blumberg J, Ruszniewski P, CLARINET Investigators (2014) Lanreotide in metastatic enteropancreatic neuroendocrine tumors. N Engl J Med 371(3):224
15. Yao JC, Fazio N, Singh S et al (2016) Everolimus for the treatment of advanced, non-functional neuroendocrine tumours of the lung or gastrointestinal tract (RADIANT-4): a randomised, placebo-controlled, phase 3 study. Lancet 387:968–977
16. Rinke A, Müller HH, Schade-Brittinger C, Klose KJ, Barth P, Wied M, Mayer C, Aminossadati B, Pape UF, Bläker M, Harder J, Arnold C, Gress T, Arnold R, PROMID Study Group (2009) Placebo controlled, double-blind, prospective, randomized study on the effect of octreotide LAR in the control of tumor growth in patients with metastatic neuroendocrine midgut tumors: a report from the PROMID Study Group. J Clin Oncol 27(28):4656
17. Gridelli C, Rossi A, Airoma G et al (2013) Treatment of pulmonary neuroendocrine tumours: state of the art and future developments. Cancer Treat Rev 39:466–472. 43
18. Sgambato A, Casaluce F, Maione P et al (2013) Medical treatment of small cell lung cancer: state of the art and new development. Expert Opin Pharmacother 14:2019–2031
19. Nicholson SA, Beasley MB, Brambilla E et al (2002) Small cell carcinoma (SCLC). A clinicopathological study of 100 cases with surgical specimens. Am J Surg Pathol 26:1184–1197
20. Yamaguchi T et al (2014) Multicenter retrospective analysis of systemic chemotherapy for advanced neuroendocrine carcinoma of the digestive system. Cancer Sci 105:1176–1181
21. Mitry E et al (1999) Treatment of poorly differentiated neuroendocrine tumours with etoposide and cisplatin. Br J Cancer 81:1351
22. Sørbye H et al (2013) Predictive and prognostic factors for treatment and survival in 305 patients with advanced gastrointestinal neuroendocrine carcinoma (WHO G3): the NORDIC NEC study. Ann Oncol 24:152–160
23. Greco FA, Hainsworth JD (2008) Cancer of unknown primary site. In: DeVita VT Jr, Hellman S, Rosenberg S (eds) Cancer: principles and practice of oncology, 8th edn. Lippincott, Philadelphia, pp 2363–2387

24. Yao JC, Hassan M, Phan A, Dagohoy C, Leary C, Mares JE, Abdalla EK, Fleming JB, Vauthey JN, Rashid A et al (2008) One hundred years after "carcinoid": epidemiology of and prognostic factors for neuroendocrine tumors in 35,825 cases in the United States. J Clin Oncol 26:3063–3072
25. Spigel DR, Hainsworth JD, Greco FA (2009) Neuroendocrine carcinoma of unknown primary site. Semin Oncol 36(1):52–59
26. Klimstra DS, Arnold R, Capella C et al (2010) WHO classification of tumours of the digestive system. Lyon, IACR
27. Massimino KP, Han E, Pommier SJ et al (2012) Laparoscopic surgical exploration is an effective strategy for locating occult primary neuroendocrine tumors. Am J Surg 203:628–631
28. Woltering EA, Voros BA, Beyer DT, Wang YZ, Thiagarajan R, Ryan P, Wright A, Ramirez RA, Ricks MJ, Boudreaux JP (2017) Aggressive surgical approach to the management of neuroendocrine tumors: a report of 1,000 surgical cytoreductions by a single institution. J Am Coll Surg 224(4):434–447
29. Stoyianni A, Pentheroudakis G, Pavlidis N (2011) Neuroendocrine carcinoma of unknown primary: a systematic review of the literature and a comparative study with other neuroendocrine tumors. Cancer Treat Rev 37(5):358–365
30. Faggiano A, Sabourin JC, Ducreux M, Lumbroso J et al (2007) Pulmonary and extrapulmonary poorly differentiated large cell neuroendocrine carcinomas: diagnostic and prognostic features. Cancer 110(2):265–274
31. Pavel M, O'Toole D, Costa F, Capdevila J, Gross D, Kianmanesh R, Krenning E, Knigge U, Salazar R, Pape UF, Öberg K, Vienna Consensus Conference participants (2016) ENETS consensus guidelines update for the management of distant metastatic disease of intestinal, pancreatic, bronchial neuroendocrine neoplasms (NEN) and NEN of unknown primary site. Neuroendocrinology 103(2):172–185
32. Fine RL, Gulati AP, Krantz BA, Moss RA, Schreibman S, Tsushima DA, Mowatt KB, Dinnen RD, Mao Y, Stevens PD, Schrope B, Allendorf J, Lee JA, Sherman WH, Chabot JA (2013) Capecitabine and temozolomide (CAPTEM) for metastatic, well-differentiated neuroendocrine cancers: the Pancreas Center at Columbia University experience. Cancer Chemother Pharmacol 71(3):663–670
33. Kwekkeboom DJ, Krenning EP, Lebtahi R, Komminoth P, Kos-Kudła B, de Herder WW et al (2009) ENETS consensus guidelines for the standards of care in neuroendocrine tumors: peptide receptor radionuclide therapy with radiolabeled somatostatin analogs. Neuroendocrinology 90:220–226

Supplementary Information

A. Colao et al. (eds.), *Neuroendocrine Tumors in Real Life*,
https://doi.org/10.1007/978-3-319-59024-0

Index

H

I

J

K

L

O

P

R

S

T

U

V

W

Z

MIX
Papier aus verantwortungsvollen Quellen
Paper from responsible sources
FSC® C105338

If you have any concerns about our products,
you can contact us on
ProductSafety@springernature.com

In case Publisher is established outside the EU,
the EU authorized representative is:
Springer Nature Customer Service Center GmbH
Europaplatz 3, 69115 Heidelberg, Germany

Printed by Libri Plureos GmbH
in Hamburg, Germany